The Electrodiagnosis of Neuromuscular Disorders

Editor

MICHAEL D. WEISS

PHYSICAL MEDICINE AND REHABILITATION CLINICS OF NORTH AMERICA

www.pmr.theclinics.com

Consulting Editor
GREGORY T. CARTER

February 2013 • Volume 24 • Number 1

ELSEVIER

1600 John F. Kennedy Boulevard • Suite 1800 • Philadelphia, Pennsylvania 19103

http://www.theclinics.com

PHYSICAL MEDICINE AND REHABILITATION CLINICS OF NORTH AMERICA Volume 24, Number 1
February 2013 ISSN 1047-9651, ISBN-13: 978-1-4557-4958-4

Editor: Jessica McCool

Reprints. For copies of 100 or more of articles in this publication, please contact the Commercial Reprints Department, Elsevier Inc., 360 Park Avenue South, New York, NY 10010-1710. Tel.: 212-633-3812; Fax: 212-462-1935; E-mail: reprints@elsevier.com.

Physical Medicine and Rehabilitation Clinics of North America (ISSN 1047-9651) is published quarterly by Elsevier Inc., 360 Park Avenue South, New York, NY 10010-1710. Months of issue are February, May, August, and November. Business and Editorial Offices: 1600 John F. Kennedy Blvd., Suite 1800, Philadelphia, PA 19103-2899. Customer Service Office: 3251 Riverport Lane, Maryland Heights, MO 63043. Periodicals postage paid at New York, NY and additional mailing offices. Subscription price per year is $263.00 (US individuals), $459.00 (US institutions), $140.00 (US students), $320.00 (Canadian individuals), $598.00 (Canadian institutions), $200.00 (Canadian students), $395.00 (foreign individuals), $598.00 (foreign institutions), and $200.00 (foreign students). Foreign air speed delivery is included in all *Clinics* subscription prices. All prices are subject to change without notice. **POSTMASTER:** Send address changes to *Physical Medicine and Rehabilitation Clinics of North America*, Customer Service Office: Elsevier Health Sciences Division, Subscription Customer Service, 3251 Riverport Lane, Maryland Heights, MO 63043. **Customer Service: 1-800-654-2452 (US). From outside of the United States, call 314-447-8871. Fax: 314-447-8029. E-mail: JournalsCustomer Service-usa@elsevier.com (for print support); JournalsOnlineSupport-usa@elsevier.com (for online support).**

Physical Medicine and Rehabilitation Clinics of North America is indexed in *Excerpta Medica, MEDLINE/ PubMed (Index Medicus), Cinahl,* and *Cumulative Index to Nursing and Allied Health Literature.*

Printed and bound by CPI Group (UK) Ltd, Croydon, CR0 4YY

Transferred to digital print 2012

Contributors

CONSULTING EDITOR

GREGORY T. CARTER, MD, MS
Medical Director, Muscular Dystrophy Association Regional Neuromuscular Center, Providence Medical Group, Department of Clinical Neurosciences; Physical Medicine and Rehabilitation Division, Olympia, Washington

GUEST EDITOR

MICHAEL D. WEISS, MD
Director, EMG Laboratory, Director, MDA/ALS Center, Associate Professor, Division of Neuromuscular Diseases, Department of Neurology, University of Washington Medical Center, Seattle, Washington

AUTHORS

ANTHONY AMATO, MD
Professor of Neurology, Department of Neurology, Brigham and Women's Hospital, Harvard Medical School, Boston, Massachusetts

KAREN BARR, MD
Associate Professor, Rehabilitation Medicine, University of Washington, Seattle, Washington

MARK B. BROMBERG, MD, PhD
Department of Neurology, University of Utah, Salt Lake City, Utah

WILLIAM W. CAMPBELL, MD, MSHA
Department of Neurology, Uniformed Services University of the Health Sciences, Bethesda, Maryland

B. JANE DISTAD, MD
Associate Professor, Division of Neuromuscular Diseases, Department of Neurology, University of Washington Medical Center, Seattle, Washington

ANURADHA DULEEP, MD
Assistant Professor, Department of Neurology, SUNY Upstate Medical University, Syracuse, New York

P. JAMES B. DYCK, MD
Professor of Neurology, Department of Neurology; Peripheral Neuropathy Research Laboratory, Mayo Clinic Rochester, Rochester, Minnesota

KEVIN HAKIMI, MD
Assistant Professor, Director, Rehabilitation Care Services, Department of Rehabilitation Medicine, VA Puget Sound, University of Washington School of Medicine, Seattle, Washington

MICHAEL K. HEHIR, MD
Assistant Professor, Department of Neurology, University of Vermont, Burlington, Vermont

JAMES F. HOWARD Jr, MD
Distinguished Professor of Neuromuscular Disease, Chief, Neuromuscular Disorders Section, Department of Neurology, The University of North Carolina at Chapel Hill, Chapel Hill, North Carolina

MARK E. LANDAU, MD
Department of Neurology, Walter Reed National Military Medical Center, Bethesda, Maryland

RUPLE S. LAUGHLIN, MD
Assistant Professor of Neurology, Department of Neurology, Mayo Clinic Rochester, Rochester, Minnesota

ERIC L. LOGIGIAN, MD
Professor, Department of Neurology, University of Rochester, Rochester, New York

CHRISTINA MARCINIAK, MD
Associate Professor, Northwestern University, Feinberg School of Medicine, The Rehabilitation Institute of Chicago, Chicago, Illinois

SABRINA PAGANONI, MD, PhD
Instructor in Physical Medicine and Rehabilitation, Department of Physical Medicine and Rehabilitation, Spaulding Rehabilitation Hospital, Harvard Medical School, Boston, Massachusetts

JEREMY SHEFNER, MD, PhD
Chair and Professor, Department of Neurology, SUNY Upstate Medical University, Syracuse, New York

ZACHARY SIMMONS, MD
Director, Neuromuscular Program and ALS Center, Penn State Hershey Medical Center, Professor of Neurology, Penn State College of Medicine, Hershey, Pennsylvania

DAVID SPANIER, MD
Clinical Assistant Professor, Rehabilitation Care Services, Department of Rehabilitation Medicine, VA Puget Sound, University of Washington School of Medicine, Seattle, Washington

LEILEI WANG, MD, PhD
Clinical Assistant Professor, Department of Rehabilitation Medicine, University of Washington, Seattle, Washington

LEO H. WANG, MD, PhD
Assistant Professor, Department of Neurology, University of Washington Medical Center, University of Washington, Seattle, Washington

MICHAEL D. WEISS, MD
Director, EMG Laboratory, Director, MDA/ALS Center, Associate Professor, Division of Neuromuscular Diseases, Department of Neurology, University of Washington Medical Center, Seattle, Washington

Contents

Cervical radiculopathy is a common diagnosis with a peak onset in the fifth decade. The most commonly affected nerve root is C7, C6, and C8. The etiology is often compressive, but may arise from noncompressive sources. Patients commonly complain of pain, weakness, numbness, and/or tingling. Examination may reveal sensory or motor disturbance in a dermatomal/myotomal distribution. Neural compression and tension signs may be positive. Diagnostic tests include imaging and electrodiagnostic study. Electrodiagnostic study serves as an extension of the neurologic examination. Electrodiagnostic findings can be useful for patients with atypical symptoms, potential pain-mediated weakness, and nonfocal imaging findings.

This article describes the normal anatomy of the brachial plexus and its major terminal branches, as well as the major causes and clinical presentations of lesions of these structures. An approach to electrodiagnosis of brachial plexopathies and proximal upper extremity neuropathies is provided, with an emphasis on those nerve conduction studies and portions of the needle examination, which permit localization of lesions to specific trunks, cords, and terminal branches. The importance of specific sensory nerve conduction studies for differentiating plexopathies from radiculopathies and mononeuropathies is emphasized.

The radial nerve is the major nerve serving the extensor compartment of the arm. This article describes the anatomic features, clinical features based on lesion location, electrodiagnostic assessment, prognosis, and treatment of radial neuropathies. Numerous traumatic causes have been reported to result in radial neuropathies, including compression or stretch injury, surgical insult, or trauma. Entrapment is a rare cause of radial neuropathy. Electrodiagnostic testing has been used to distinguish radial neuropathy from other disorders presenting with wrist or finger drops. In addition, its use may aid in determining the prognosis for recovery of functional movement.

In this review, we delineate clinical, electrodiagnostic, and radiographic features of ulnar mononeuropathies. Ulnar neuropathy at the elbow (UNE) is most commonly due to lesions at the level of the retroepicondylar groove (RTC), with approximately 25% at the humeroulnar arcade (HUA). The term 'cubital tunnel syndrome' should be reserved for the latter. The diagnostic accuracy of nerve conduction studies is limited by biological (e.g. low elbow temperature) and technical factors. Across-elbow distance measurements greater than 10 cm improve diagnostic specificity at the expense of decreased sensitivity. Short-segment incremental studies can differentiate lesions at the HUA from those at the RTC.

This article discusses the historical aspects related to the understanding of carpal tunnel syndrome (CTS) and its diagnosis, highlighting observations about this disease that have yet to be challenged. This is followed by a discussion regarding the use of electrodiagnostic testing as a diagnostic tool for CTS, as well as the author's approach to making the diagnosis of CTS. Finally, conclusions about future directions in the diagnosis and treatment of this disorder are presented.

The evaluation of patients with suspected lumbar radiculopathy is one of the most common reasons patients are referred for electrodiagnostic testing. The utility of this study depends on the expertise of the physician who plans, performs, and completes the study. This article reviews the strengths and weaknesses of electrodiagnosis to make this diagnosis, as well as the clinical reasoning of appropriate study planning. The current use of electrodiagnostic testing to determine prognosis and treatment outcomes is also discussed.

Patients presumed to have lower limb symptoms localizing to the lumbar or lumbosacral plexus require rigorous electrophysiological evaluation. Entities that cause lumbosacral plexopathies may be patchy, asymmetrical and more diffuse than initially suspected. As a result, bilateral nerve conduction studies and needle examination outside those routinely tested and clinically affected may be needed to document the extent of involvement including needle examination of the thoracic paraspinals and consideration of upper limb studies. This article outlines the lumbar and lumbosacral plexus anatomy, and discusses a differential diagnosis and electrophysiological approach in assessing patients with presumed lumbosacral plexopathies.

Sciatic neuropathy is the second most common neuropathy of the lower extremity and a common cause of foot drop. This article reviews the anatomy, clinical features, pathophysiology, and electrodiagnostic assessment of sciatic neuropathies. There are multiple potential sites of pathology, determined in part by the mechanism of insult, including trauma, compression, masses, inflammation, and vascular lesions. Diagnosis is augmented by careful electrodiagnostic studies and imaging to help distinguish sciatic neuropathy from other sources of pathology. Electrodiagnostic studies may also help in assessing for early recovery and in determining prognosis.

Peroneal or fibular neuropathy is the most frequent mononeuropathy encountered in the lower limb. In this article, the causes, clinical features, electrodiagnostic assessment, and the treatment of peroneal neuropathies are described. Numerous causes have been reported to result in peroneal neuropathies, with mechanisms including compression, stretch, surgery, or trauma. Electrodiagnostics have been used to distinguish peroneal neuropathy from other disorders presenting with ankle dorsiflexor weakness. In addition, their use may aid in identifying the potential for recovery of functional movement.

Electrodiagnostic testing has proved useful in helping to establish the diagnosis of amyotrophic lateral sclerosis by eliminating possible disease mimics and by demonstrating abnormalities in body areas that are clinically unaffected. Electrodiagnosis begins with an understanding of the clinical features of the disease, because clinical correlation is essential. To improve the sensitivity of the electrophysiologic evaluation, the Awaji criteria have been proposed as a modification to the revised El Escorial criteria. Although techniques to evaluate corticomotor neuron abnormalities and to quantify lower motor neuron loss have been developed, they remain primarily research techniques and have not yet influenced clinical practice.

Electrodiagnosis, which includes nerve conduction and needle electromyographic studies, is an essential element in the evaluation of peripheral neuropathies. A systematic approach to the electrodiagnostic evaluation aids in clarifying the distribution and extent of involvement, type of nerve damage, and time course. When these data are combined with clinical information, a full characterization of the neuropathy is possible leading to

PHYSICAL MEDICINE & REHABILITATION CLINICS OF NORTH AMERICA

NOW AVAILABLE FOR YOUR iPhone and iPad

Foreword

The Electrodiagnosis of Neuromuscular Disorders

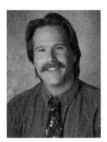

Gregory T. Carter, MD, MS
Consulting Editor

As the consulting editor for the *Physical Medicine and Rehabilitation Clinics of North America*, it is my job to recruit guest editors for our core topics. When it came time to find an editor for this issue of the *Physical Medicine and Rehabilitation Clinics of North America* on "The Electrodiagnosis of Neuromuscular Disorders," I immediately thought of my very close friend and colleague, Dr Michael Weiss. Michael does everything with excellence and attention to detail and this project is no exception. Serving as the Director of the Electrodiagnostics Laboratory at the University of Washington, Michael is one of the best electrodiagnosticians I know.

Here he brings us an issue that should really be a very "hands-on," "user-friendly" text that I suspect will be found lying next to EMG machines in offices and labs of many physiatrists and neurologists as well. I can tell you it will be in my office. This text contains some of the best graphics I have ever seen in this area, making it easy to reference and use right in the lab. The anatomic diagrams really help define the physiology and make it easier to understand some of the more complex pathophysiology. In addition to diagrams, there are highlights of each diagnosis and excellent coverage of some of the more common diagnostic dilemmas one is likely to encounter when doing these studies. This makes the text easy to use quickly to reference. Yet the level of detail provided here also makes it an excellent text to study for board exams, and as an information source to cite in lectures.

All major topics are covered in-depth, including the electrodiagnosis of cervical and lumbar radiculopathy, brachial plexopathies, proximal upper extremity neuropathies and plexopathies, radial, ulnar, and median neuropathies, ulnar neuropathies, lumbosacral plexopathies, sciatic neuropathies, fibular (peroneal) neuropathies, motor neuron diseases, peripheral neuropathies, disorders of neuromuscular transmission, and myopathies, including myotonic disorders.

Phys Med Rehabil Clin N Am 24 (2013) xi–xii
http://dx.doi.org/10.1016/j.pmr.2012.09.004
1047-9651/13/$ – see front matter © 2013 Elsevier Inc. All rights reserved.

Among the authors Michael recruited for this project are some of the true masters in the field, including Zachary Simmons, MD, P. James "Jim" B. Dyck, MD, Jeremy Shefner, MD, Mark B. Bromberg, MD, PhD, James F. "Chip" Howard Jr, MD, Anthony "Tony" Amato, MD, William "Bill" Campbell, MD, MSHA, and Eric L. Logigian, MD. All of these authors are among the world's foremost experts in the electrodiagnosis of neuromuscular diseases. It is an honor to have all of these authors here and I want to express my sincerest thanks to each and every one of these esteemed authors, all of whom dedicated much time and energy to bring us this issue of the *Physical Medicine and Rehabilitation Clinics of North America*. I also, as always, want to thank our Elsevier editor, Jessica McCool, for her patience, dedication, and wisdom, which is crucial to bringing this all together.

Gregory T. Carter, MD, MS
Muscular Dystrophy Association Regional Neuromuscular Center
Providence Medical Group, Department of Clinical Neurosciences
Physical Medicine and Rehabilitation Division
410 Providence Lane, Building 2
Olympia, WA 98506, USA

E-mail address:
gtcarter@uw.edu

Preface

The Electrodiagnosis of Neuromuscular Disorders

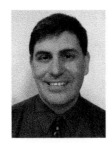

Michael D. Weiss, MD
Guest Editor

When Dr Greg Carter asked me to guest edit an issue of *Physical Medicine and Reha-bilitation Clinics of North America* devoted to the electrodiagnostic evaluation of neuro-muscular disorders, I thought this to be a daunting task. There are many textbooks that cover this topic in full, some quite extensively. After accepting the offer, I chose to select nationally renowned authors with known expertise in the diagnosis and electro-diagnosis of specific disorders with an emphasis on their particular method for ap-proaching such patients. I gathered together a number of such neurologists and physiatrists, who have helped me fashion an outstanding issue.

The goal of this issue is to be of stand-alone value to electrodiagnosticians who diagnosis patients with a wide variety of neuromuscular conditions ranging from carpal tunnel syndrome to cervical radiculopathy to diabetic lumbosacral radiculoplexus neuropathy to motor neuron disease. When appropriate, emphasis is placed in the arti-cles on consensus guidelines for the electrodiagnosis of certain disorders put forth by the American Association of Neuromuscular and Electrodiagnostic Medicine. However, more importantly, each expert has outlined a detailed approach to the elec-trodiagnostic evaluation of these conditions. Each expert was also given latitude to discuss ancillary testing, such as neuroimaging and pathologic evaluation, which broadens the scope and appeal of the articles, in a manner that most textbooks in elec-trodiagnosis do not. The end result is an issue that is both comprehensive and practical.

It is my belief that this issue will be of great value to both neurologists and physiat-rists with an interest in neuromuscular medicine. I also hope that it will sit on the book-shelf of these practitioners as a practical compendium to traditional textbooks in

Phys Med Rehabil Clin N Am 24 (2013) xiii–xiv
http://dx.doi.org/10.1016/j.pmr.2012.08.024
1047-9651/13/$ – see front matter

electrodiagnostic medicine. I thank Dr Carter for giving me the opportunity to participate in such an important issue and all of the authors for their stellar contributions.

Michael D. Weiss, MD
Department of Neurology
University of Washington Medical Center
1959 NE Pacific Street Room NN282A, Box 356115
Seattle, WA 98195, USA

E-mail address:
mdweiss@u.washington.edu

Electrodiagnosis of Cervical Radiculopathy

Kevin Hakimi, MD*, David Spanier, MD

KEYWORDS

- Cervical • Radiculopathy • Electrodiagnosis • Electromyography

KEY POINTS

- To properly diagnose cervical radiculopathy, a combination of clinical signs/symptoms, imaging, and electrodiagnostic studies should be used.
- Differential diagnosis must consider various causes of neuropathic and musculoskeletal pain, which may be affecting the extremity.
- Needle electromyography is the most useful electrodiagnostic technique and provides moderate sensitivity in the diagnosis of radiculopathies.
- Appropriate sampling of muscles must be done including paraspinals, if possible, to ensure a diagnostically accurate study.
- Electrodiagnostic findings can be particularly useful for patients with atypical symptoms, potential pain-mediated weakness, and nonfocal imaging findings.

INTRODUCTION

Cervical radiculopathy is a common disorder effecting people most often in the fourth and fifth decades of life. Symptoms of pain, numbness, and/or tingling may be mild, but in severe cases, cervical radiculopathy will be associated with motor weakness. Efficient diagnosis can minimize pain and disability and also minimize the direct and indirect costs of care. Treatment of cervical radiculopathy is based on a clear understanding of its natural history, clinical evaluation, diagnostic testing, and therapeutic options for this disorder. This article will provide an overview of the pathophysiology, pertinent anatomy, history/examination findings, and imaging options. It will focus on the electrodiagnosis of cervical radiculopathy. Electrodiagnosis is a critical part of the evaluation of patients presenting with signs and symptoms of neuropathic upper extremity dysfunction, especially when coexisting with neck pain. This article will review developing an appropriate differential diagnosis and

Rehabilitation Care Services, Department of Rehabilitation Medicine, VA Puget Sound, Rehabilitation Care Services (RCS-117), 1660 South Columbian Way, Seattle, WA 98108, USA
* Corresponding author.
E-mail address: khakimi@uw.edu

Phys Med Rehabil Clin N Am 24 (2013) 1–12
http://dx.doi.org/10.1016/j.pmr.2012.08.012
1047-9651/13/$ – see front matter Published by Elsevier Inc.

choosing appropriate electrodiagnostic techniques with a focus on needle electro-myography (EMG).

EPIDEMIOLOGY

An epidemiologic study of cervical radiculopathy was performed at the Mayo Clinic between 1976 and 1990.[1] Five hundred sixty-one cases were included in this study. This research revealed the following:

Age ranged from 13 to 91 years (332 males, mean age 47.6 ± 13.1 years; 229 females, mean age 48.2 ± 13.8 years)

History of trauma or exertion was found in only 14.8% of cases

Previous history of lumbar radiculopathy was found in 41% of cases

Median duration of symptoms before diagnosis was 15 days

Monoradiculopathy involving nerve root C7 was most common, followed by nerve roots C6, C8, and then C5 in decreasing frequency

Etiology included confirmed disc protrusion (21.9%) and spondylosis, disc, or both (68.4%)

Recurrence over 4.9 years = 31.7%

Surgery was performed in 26% of patients

Ninety percent of patients were asymptomatic or only mildly incapacitated at last follow-up

A more recent study looked at the incidence of cervical radiculopathy in the US military from 2000 to 2009.[2] They found that age (40 years old and above) was the greatest risk factor for cervical radiculopathy, and that female sex, white race, senior military position, and service in the Army or Air Force were also risk factors.

ANATOMY

The cervical spine is comprised of 7 vertebrae. The first vertebra (C1, also called the atlas) is a ring-shaped bone without a spinous process. It serves as the point of attachment of the skull to the spine via the occipital condyles articulating with the superior aspect of the C1 vertebra. C1 articulates directly with C2 without the presence of an intervertebral disc. C2 has a bony superior process called the dens, which projects into the ring of the atlas and serves as the axis of rotation.

Facet Joints (Zygapophyseal Joints)

Vertebrae C3 through C7 have posteriorly placed facet joints that serve as points of articulation between the vertebrae. These are paired joints that arise at the junction of the pedicle and the lamina. The superior facets project upward to articulate with the inferior facets of the superior adjacent vertebra. The inferior facets project downward to articulate with the superior facets of the inferior adjacent vertebra. These joints are synovial with a surrounding capsule. The joints are innervated by the medial branch of the dorsal primary ramus of the exiting spinal nerve. The joints provide directional stability and prevent relative translation of 1 vertebra upon another. They lie posterior to the exiting spinal nerve root.

Uncovertebral Joints (Joints of Luschka)

Extending off the lateral surface of the cervical vertebral bodies are small bony projections called uncinate processes. The uncinate process makes contact with the disc and vertebral body above. The points of contact are called uncovertebral joints, and they are located anteromedial to the exiting nerve roots.

Intervertebral Disc

Between cervical vertebrae C2 through C7 is a supporting intervertebral disc. The disc is comprised of 2 layers; the outer layer is called the annulus fibrosis, which is made up of approximately 20 concentric lamellae of orthogonally oriented fibers. The inner layer is called the nucleus pulposis, comprised of 90% water, which desiccates with age. The anterior annulus is reinforced by the anterior longitudinal ligament (ALL), and posteriorly by the posterior longitudinal ligament (PLL). The PLL is not very broad, and accordingly there is greater chance of nucleus pulposis herniation laterally as opposed to centrally.

Spinal Canal

The spinal canal is made up of the consecutive vertebral foramen. In the intervertebral spaces, the canal is protected posteriorly by the ligamentum flavum and anteriorly by the PLL. The spinal canal has its greatest Anterior-Posterior (A-P) diameter in the upper cervical spine between C1 and C3. During maximal cervical spine extension, the canal narrows an additional 2 to 3 mm.

Spinal Motion

The specific motions of each cervical segment have been thoroughly described elsewhere. Broadly speaking, most rotational movement of the head occurs in the upper cervical spine, where flexion and extension occur predominantly in the lower cervical spine. Accordingly, spondylotic disease arises most commonly in the lower cervical spine.

Intervertebral Foramina

The foramina are bordered anteriorly by the vertebral body and disc, and posteriorly by the facet joint. The pedicles form the superior and inferior margins of the foramen. Additionally the uncinate processes are located at the anteromedial margin of the foramen.

Neural Elements

The spinal cord is located within the central canal. There is an enlargement of the cord diameter within the cervical spine from C3 through T2, and in the lumbar spine from L1 to S3. The spinal nerve is comprised of sensory fibers traveling through the dorsal root and motor fibers from the ventral root. The dorsal root ganglia (DRG) are located on the dorsal nerve roots, usually in the intervertebral foramen, just outside the spinal dural layer. The DRG of C4 and C5 are located closer to the spinal cord than the lower roots.[3] The dorsal and ventral roots fuse to form the spinal nerve in the intervertebral foramen. The spinal nerve continues for a few millimeters before it separates into the dorsal and ventral rami. The dorsal rami supply the cervical paraspinals (PSPs) and skin of the back of the neck. The ventral rami form the cervical and brachial plexuses.

The cervical nerve roots exit through the intervertebral foramen above the corresponding cervical vertebral body. For example, the C5 nerve root exits through the C4 to C5 intervertebral foramen. The C8 nerve root exits below the C7 vertebral body and above the T1 vertebral body. Subsequent nerve roots exit below the corresponding vertebral body.

Understanding the anatomy of the exiting spinal nerve with regards to both the innervation of the PSP musculature and position of the DRG is critical in understanding the results of the electrodiagnostic evaluation of cervical radiculopathy.

ETIOLOGY

Radiculopathy arises from a process that affects the nerve root. These processes can be divided into compressive and noncompressive causes. The compressive causes include cervical spondylosis and disc herniation.

Compressive Causes

Cervical spondylosis

As the nerve root enters the foramen medially, it lies at the level of the superior articular facet of the inferior vertebrae. Hypertrophy of either the uncovertebral joints or the facets joints may impinge mechanically on an exiting nerve root to cause radiculopathy. The process of degenerative change in these joints is called spondylosis. Degenerative change may also result in bone formation in these areas, producing an osteophyte or hard disc.

Disc herniation The anatomy of the intervertebral disc has been discussed previously. Circumferential tears in the annulus fibrosis begin to be present around the age of 20 and progress to fraying and splitting of collagen fibers. With the progression of degeneration, there is continued loss of the fluid properties of the nucleus pulposis, which undergoes replacement with fibrous tissue. The combination of intervertebral pressure and degenerative change of the disc can lead to tears in the annulus, which allow for disc bulging and/or prolapse of the nucleus pulposis. This often results in deformation of the DRG. The mechanical deformation (either compression or tension) causes release of substance P, phospholipase 2, and vasoactive intestinal peptide from the nucleus pulposis. This produces a chemical inflammation that is an additional insult to the nerve root on top of any mechanical pressure.

Noncompressive causes

Although less common, noncompressive causes should always be considered. These include demyelination, infection, tumor infiltration, root avulsion, and nerve root infarction. The dorsal and ventral roots may be affected (much more so than in compressive etiologies). Deficits of noncompressive radiculopathies may span multiple myotomes and dermatomes, and may be more complete or dense than are commonly seen in compressive etiologies.

KEY HISTORY FINDINGS

The patient's history is critical in evaluating a suspected radiculopathy, because there is an extensive differential diagnosis to be considered. Symptoms may develop acutely with an initial episode of neck pain followed by radiation in a dermatomal pattern or weakness in the affected extremity. A herniated disk more often causes acute radiculopathy, while spondylitic narrowing results in a more indolent course. Patients may complain of neck pain, arm pain, chest or shoulder pain, pain in the interscapular region, or pain in the face.[4]

Dermatomal paresthesia or numbness develops in 80% of patients. Subjective weakness is less common than paresthesia.[1] The patient may describe positions that alleviate symptoms, such as rotating the head away from the affected side, and the abducted shoulder sign, in which the patients describe pain relief with the affected shoulder abducted and the hand resting on top of the head.

Some patients may describe a recent history of physical exertion or trauma preceding symptom onset; however, most cases have no readily identifiable causative event.[4]

More concerning complaints that may suggest not only radiculopathy but also myelopathy or infection must also be sought. Lhermitte sign (shock-like paresthesias occurring with neck flexion), difficulty walking, or bowel and bladder symptoms are suggestive of myelopathy or intramedullary pathology. Any history of fever, chills, weight loss, or cancer should raise suspicion for tumor or infection.[5]

KEY PHYSICAL EXAMINATION FINDINGS

The initial physical examination includes observation of the patient, noting the position of the head and neck contours. Atrophy can be detected with more severe or long-standing lesions. Muscle wasting may suggest particular nerve root involvement:

C5 or C6: supra- or infrascapular fossae or deltoid
C7: triceps
C8: thenar eminence
T1: first dorsal interossei

Manual muscle testing has greater specificity than reflex or sensory abnormalities, and might need to be performed repetitively or with the muscle at a mechanical disadvantage to elicit subtle weakness.[6] Severe weakness (<3/5 on the Medical Research Council grade) is less consistent with a single root lesion and should prompt the examiner to search for multilevel pathology. Sensation to light touch, pinprick, and vibration should be assessed. Upper motor neuron signs should also be assessed including Hoffman sign and Babinski response.

Provocative maneuvers such as Spurling maneuver may be performed. This test is performed by extending and rotating the neck to the painful side followed by the application of downward pressure to the head.[7] The test is positive if it reproduces limb pain and/or paresthesia. Neck pain alone does not signify a positive test. The Spurling maneuver has a high specificity but moderate-to-low sensitivity for cervical radiculopathy.[8] A negative test does not rule out radicular pathology.

DIAGNOSTIC IMAGING
Plain Radiographs

Conventional radiographs are often obtained in the evaluation of neck pain, but their utility in establishing a diagnosis is somewhat limited. Radiographs have relatively low sensitivity in detecting tumor, infection, and disc herniation. Plain radiographs may be completely normal in patients with tumor or infection. Conversely, patients with compressive radiculopathy will likely have multilevel pathology identified on plain radiographs. Furthermore, there is limited value in the finding of cervical intervertebral narrowing in predicting nerve root compression.[9]

Magnetic Resonance Imaging

Magnetic resonance imaging (MRI) is the imaging modality of choice when investigating cervical radiculopathy.[10] MRI generally provides superior evaluation of the soft tissues when compared with computed tomography (CT), although bony abnormalities may be underestimated, while stenosis is often overestimated.[11] T1 weighted images show bone spurs and disc herniations as hypointense, making it difficult to distinguish these structures from bone and ligament. T2 weighted images create a myelographic effect as fluid (both cerebrospinal fluid [CSF] and water within the nucleus pulposis) appears bright. Gadolinium enhanced images should be obtained if there is suspicion of metastatic disease, osteomyelitis, or other inflammatory conditions. Radiographic abnormalities should always be interpreted within a clinical context.

Computed Tomography

CT myelography is considered the gold standard in evaluating foraminal compression. CT myelography is superior to MRI in distinguishing osteophyte from soft tissue material, although there is some evidence that CT myelography may be inadequate to assess developing osteophytes.[12] Due to the exposure to ionizing radiation, CT and CT myelography are usually reserved for patients who are claustrophobic or when MRI is contraindicated or nondiagnostic.

The clinician should always be cognizant of the fact that normal age-related changes may occur in the cervical spine in the absence of symptoms. Matsumoto and colleagues[13] recently reported a study of asymptomatic middle-aged patients (mean age 48 years) in which over 90% of patients had cervical degenerative changes on MRI – including posterior disc protrusion, anterior compression of the thecal sac, and decrease in disc height.

DIFFERENTIAL DIAGNOSIS OF POTENTIAL UPPER EXTREMITY RADICULAR SIGNS/SYMPTOMS

Patients with classical symptoms of neck pain and radicular type pain are often referred to the electrodiagnostic laboratory to be evaluated for cervical radiculopathy. However, often signs or symptoms will be more vague. The electromyographer following a thorough history and directed physical examination should also consider other diseases that may be mimicking a cervical radiculopathy and design an electrodiagnostic study to evaluate for these other possibilities as appropriate. Differential diagnoses are discussed in the following sections.

Peripheral Nerve Lesions

Median and ulnar neuropathies are very common and must always be considered a possibility in patients with neurologic finding in the upper extremity. Even if a patient has evidence of cervical radiculopathy, it is important to realize that peripheral nerve entrapments often occur concomitantly and should be documented. Questioning should include identification of numbness, paresthesias into the hand, repetitive motion history, and other potential risk factors for nerve entrapments.

Brachial Plexopathies

While brachial plexus lesions are less common then peripheral nerve entrapments, they must also be considered in the differential diagnoses. Traumas or mass lesions are common causes of plexopathies. When considering the possibility of a mass lesion, one should inquire about weight loss, fevers, night sweats, and smoking history. Idiopathic brachial neuritis (Parsonage-Turner syndrome) should also be considered, especially with a presentation of acute shoulder pain followed by muscle weakness.

Other Conditions

It is important also to consider other conditions such as myelopathy secondary to central spinal stenosis, which may present with more bilateral weakness, upper motor neuron signs, and possible bowel/bladder involvement. Motor neuron disease should be considered in a patient presenting with upper extremity weakness without radicular-type pain or sensation changes on examination. Neurogenic thoracic outlet syndrome may also be considered but is a rare diagnosis to make in the electrodiagnostic laboratory. Non-neurologic causes of upper extremity pain should also be considered such as facet disease, subacromial bursitis rotator cuff pathology, and lateral/medial epicondylitis. Each of these processes may mimic radicular pain.

ROLE OF ELECTRODIAGNOSIS

Electrodiagnosis plays a critical role in the assessment of patients with symptoms and signs of cervical radiculopathy. Electrodiagnosis is often referred to as an extension of the neurologic examination, as it is able to provide physiologic evidence of nerve dysfunction. The electrodiagnostic study can aid in clarifying the presumed diagnosis of radiculopathy and is critical in identifying other possible nonroot-level causes of neurologic dysfunction. The electrodiagnostic information and history, physical, and imaging findings are combined to confirm the most likely diagnosis and to guide future treatment. Electrodiagnostic findings can be particularly useful for patients with atypical symptoms, potential pain-mediated weakness, and nonfocal imaging findings.

Various types of electrodiagnostic studies may be considered when evaluating a patient for cervical radiculopathy in the electrodiagnostic laboratory. Potential tests include EMG, motor and sensory nerve conduction studies, late responses, and somatosensory evoked potentials. These tests can all be considered based on the clinical scenario and will be discussed individually.

ELECTROMYOGRAPHY

EMG is the most useful test for evaluating for radiculopathy. The EMG portion of the examination can localize lesions to a particular root level and can provide information on acuity of the disease process. The goal of EMG is to find a pattern of spontaneous and/or chronic motor unit changes in a clear myotomal pattern. It is also important to note the limitations of EMG. EMG can only detect change in the motor nervous system; furthermore, it primarily detects damage to the axonal component of the nerve versus myelin. Many early radiculopathies may have a primary sensory and demyelinating component, and these types of radiculopathies would not be detected with needle sampling.

Diagnostic Criteria for Needle EMG

To diagnose radiculopathy electrodiagnostically, needle study of 2 muscles that receive innervation from the same nerve root, preferably via different peripheral nerves, should be abnormal. Adjacent nerve roots should be unaffected unless a multi-level radiculopathy is present. Since muscles receive innervation from multiple levels, the pattern of abnormalities should point to a nerve root level that is primarily affected. Various myotomal maps are available to assist the electromyographer in determining the root level affected (**Fig. 1**).

Sensitivity of Needle EMG

The utility of needle EMG in diagnosing cervical radiculopathy with regards to sensitivity was thoroughly reviewed in 1999 by the American Association for Electrodiagnostic Medicine (AAEM), now known as the American Association for Neuromuscular and Electrodiagnostic Medicine (AANEM), and published as a practice parameter.[14] Establishing the sensitivity of electrodiagnostic testing (as well as many radiological procedures) is difficult, because there is no gold standard by which one can definitively true presence of disease.

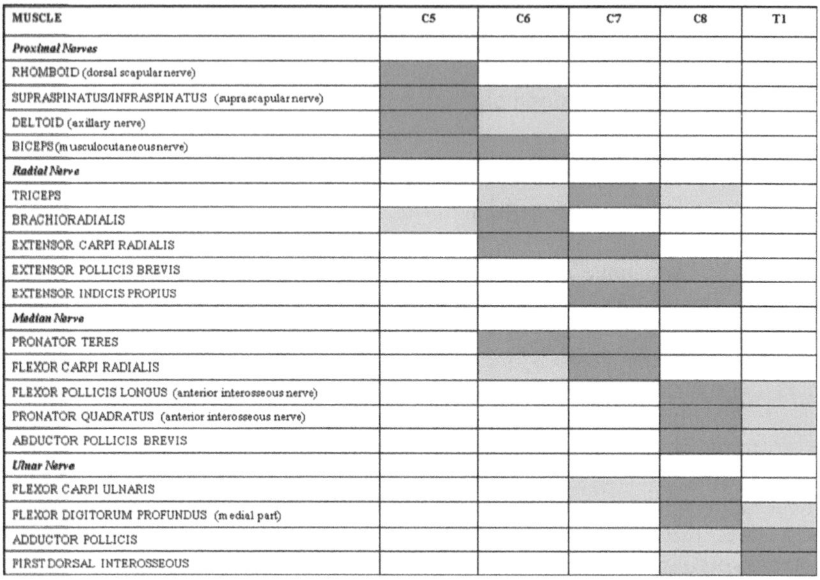

MUSCLE	C5	C6	C7	C8	T1
Proximal Nerves					
RHOMBOID (dorsal scapular nerve)	▓				
SUPRASPINATUS/INFRASPINATUS (suprascapular nerve)	▓				
DELTOID (axillary nerve)	▓				
BICEPS (musculocutaneous nerve)	▓	▓			
Radial Nerve					
TRICEPS			▓		
BRACHIORADIALIS	▓	▓			
EXTENSOR CARPI RADIALIS		▓			
EXTENSOR POLLICIS BREVIS			▓	▓	
EXTENSOR INDICIS PROPIUS			▓	▓	
Median Nerve					
PRONATOR TERES		▓			
FLEXOR CARPI RADIALIS		▓	▓		
FLEXOR POLLICIS LONGUS (anterior interosseous nerve)			▓	▓	
PRONATOR QUADRATUS (anterior interosseous nerve)				▓	
ABDUCTOR POLLICIS BREVIS				▓	
Ulnar Nerve					
FLEXOR CARPI ULNARIS			▓	▓	
FLEXOR DIGITORUM PROFUNDUS (medial part)				▓	
ADDUCTOR POLLICIS				▓	▓
FIRST DORSAL INTEROSSEOUS				▓	▓

Fig. 1. Upper extremity myotomal chart showing major and significant nerve root innervation of upper extremity muscles. Boxes shaded in green represent a dominant contribution, while boxes shaded in yellow represent a significant contribution. Minor contributions are not shown.

The articles that were included in the AANEM review used a combination of clinical and radiological findings as a comparison. The 9 studies they cited in their final review revealed overall sensitivity of needle EMG in the diagnosis of cervical radiculopathy to be between 50% and 71%, which they described as having moderate diagnostic sensitivity. Studies that reported more motor deficits clinically had higher reported sensitivities in their review. Based on these reported sensitivities, it is important to understand that a negative EMG study for cervical radiculopathy does not rule out the presence of disease.

Appropriate EMG Study Design

Following the publication of the AANEM practice parameter, Dillingham and colleagues[15] published an article discussing the sensitivity of needle EMG screening in diagnosing cervical radiculopathies. The main question tackled in this study was how many muscles should be sampled to provide good sensitivity in detecting radiculopathy. Most electromyographers would agree sampling a few muscles is not sufficient to detect radiculopathy, but it is important to define the minimum number of muscles needed to ensure a quality examination. The study looked at 101 patients with cervical radiculopathy and tested 10 muscles in each patient. Analysis revealed that testing 6 muscles including the cervical PSPs achieved a sensitivity of 94% to 98% for the presence of radiculopathy. If PSPs were not tested, they recommend testing of 8 limb muscles to achieve a sensitivity of 92% to 95%.

PSP Findings

While the presence of fibrillations and positive sharp waves (PSWs) in the limb muscles of normal subjects is considered very unusual, the documentation of these waveforms in the PSP muscles of normal subjects is more controversial. Two studies showed presence of PSWs in the cervical PSPs in normal subjects without neck pain or radicular arm pain. The first study found PSWs in 92% of PSPs in subjects older than 40 years old and fibrillations in 8% of subjects greater than 40 years old. They found no PSPs or fibrillations in patients under 40 years old.[16] The second study noted PSWs in 12% of the PSP muscles tested on asymptomatic subjects.[17] These studies illustrate some of the caveats of diagnosing radiculopathy based primarily on PSP findings, particularly in an older population.

However, such studies do not negate the importance of the PSP examination. As mentioned previously, Dillingham found that testing PSPs adds significant sensitivity to the needle examination for cervical radiculopathy. The presence of PSP abnormalities in combination with limb findings makes radiculopathy a more likely diagnosis. Lack of PSP findings may indicate a more distal lesion localized to the brachial plexus or peripheral nerve. The pattern of EMG abnormalities and nerve conduction study findings would help also to differentiate nerve root- from nonroot-level causes of upper extremity nerve dysfunction.

There are also other limitations to PSP muscle sampling. The proximity of the PSP to the nerve root means it may be the first abnormality detected in an early acute radiculopathy (as soon as 7 days), but also it may be the first muscle to return to normal. So based on the timing of the electrodiagnostic examination, a patient may have clear upper extremity myotomal EMG pattern with absent or subtle PSP abnormalities. It is also important to note that PSPs can also be positive in other diseases not related to nerve root compression. For example, patients with both motor neuron disease and inflammatory myopathies such as polymyositis may demonstrate PSWs in the PSP muscles. Finally, PSPs may exhibit both PSWs and fibrillations many years following any posterior approach spinal surgery. Some have also expressed concern of seeing some PSP abnormalities related to muscle trauma from repeated epidural steroid injections.

SPECIFICITY OF NEEDLE EMG

While sensitivity is a critical component in determining the utility of a test, a test must also have good specificity to ensure low false-positive results. Anecdotal evidence, clinical experience, and published studies involving normal subjects confirm high specificity of needle EMG in diagnosis of radiculopathy. A recent study looking at EMG patterns in the lower extremities showed no false-negative diagnoses of radiculopathy (ie, 100% specificity) when a pattern of acute changes was shown in 2 limbs and the PSP muscles.[18] Using less strict criteria of greater than 30% polyphasia in the same muscle groups, specificity was still excellent, at 87% to 97%.

NERVE CONDUCTION STUDIES

The primary role of nerve conduction studies in patients with symptoms of cervical radiculopathy is to determine if other neurologic processes exist as an explanation for a patient's clinical picture, or if another process coexists with a root level problem. The AANEM's 1999 practice parameter recommends performing at least 1 motor and sensory study when evaluating a patient for cervical radiculopathy. In pure radiculopathy, the sensory nerve studies should be normal. As described in detail previously, the pathologic lesion in radiculopathy typically occurs proximal to the DRG. Since the DRG houses the cell bodies for the sensory nerves, the sensory nerve studies should be normal. Marked abnormalities in sensory studies should prompt the electromyographer to look for disease processes that occur distal to the DRG, such as plexopathy, generalized peripheral neuropathy, or peripheral nerve entrapments. The motor nerve conduction studies are also typically normal in cervical radiculopathy unless there is severe axon loss or multilevel disease.

The extent of the nerve conduction studies performed needs to be determined by the clinical scenario, and the differential diagnosis should be generated following the history and physical examination performed by the electromyographer. It is very common for patients who present with neck pain and radicular symptoms to also have symptoms that affect the hand, such as numbness. While neuropathic pain, numbness, and/or paresthesias could be related to cervical radiculopathy, in these cases, one must look more thoroughly for common nerve entrapments such as median neuropathy at the wrist or ulnar neuropathy at the elbow. If trauma has occurred or patients present with sudden shoulder pain followed by weakness, additional nerve conduction studies would also be considered to look for brachial plexus-level issues related to trauma or an idiopathic acute brachial neuritis.

Ulnar neuropathy can mimic symptoms of C8/T1 radiculopathy. Ulnar motor studies should be performed in patients presenting for evaluation of cervical radiculopathy who also have paresthesias or symptoms in typical ulnar innervated areas. In patients with predominantly median distribution symptoms or more diffuse sensory complaints, nerve conduction studies looking for carpal tunnel syndrome are indicated. Median motor studies and thorough sensory comparison evaluations such as the Robinson Index should be considered to ensure accurate diagnoses.[19]

Nerve conduction studies are also important for patients who may have symptoms of more generalized peripheral neuropathy. If the patient has symptoms of diffuse paresthesias (upper and lower extremities) or other neuropathic risk factors such as diabetes or alcohol use, the electromyographer may need to expand the electrodiagnostic study to include the contralateral limb, as well as potential nerve conduction studies in the lower extremity. In an appropriately designed study, the nerve conduction studies should be able to differentiate between peripheral nerve entrapment and a generalized process. The exception to this is when there is a severe peripheral neuropathy with many absent responses.

LATE RESPONSES

The utility of late responses such as F-waves and H-reflexes in diagnoses of cervical radiculopathy is debated. While H-reflexes can be useful in diagnosing S1 radiculopathies, there is less evidence to support use of late responses in the upper extremity. The 1999 AAEM practice parameter considers testing for F-waves and H-reflexes as optional studies when considering the diagnosis of cervical radiculopthy. F-waves are not sensitive in diagnosing radiculopathy and tend to be abnormal in severe disease. Like EMG, F-wave study only tests motor fibers. Furthermore, it is not useful to localize lesions. For example, F-waves recorded from the abductor pollicis brevis or abductor digiti minimi are evaluating both C8 and T1 pathways, so abnormalities do not single out a nerve root. Also, abnormalities of F-waves can be consistent with lesions in the peripheral nerve, plexus, or nerve root. A more recent study, published in 2007, suggested that various F-wave parameters may improve the diagnostic yield for cervical radiculopathy when combined with needle EMG. However, the study also noted that F-wave abnormalities could not localize a lesion to a specific cervical level.[20] It is also important to note that F-waves tend not to be well tolerated by patients, since they require supramaximal stimulation. This, combined with questionable diagnostic utility, contributes to the low use of these studies to diagnose cervical radiculopathy.

H-reflex study recording over the gastrocnemius or soleus muscle is commonly performed when considering an S1 radiculopathy. In the upper extremities, C6/C7 levels can also be evaluated by stimulating the median nerve at the elbow to obtain an H-reflex to the flexor carpi radialis. It is reported that this response is obtainable in 90% of normal subjects but may require facilitation techniques.[21] Two more recent studies reported that the upper extremity H-reflex can add utility in the diagnosis of cervical radiculopathies, especially in cases when clinical symptoms are less clear and needle EMG is normal.[22,23]

SOMATOSENSORY EVOKED POTENTIALS

There is conflicting evidence on the utility of somatosensory evoked potentials (SEPs) in the diagnosis of cervical radiculopathy. Mixed nerve studies of the tibial, median, and ulnar nerves may be useful in assessing patients with cervical myelopathy or other central causes of neurologic symptoms (ie, multiple sclerosis). Dermatomal SEPs, in theory, should provide information on single-root sensory nerve root dysfunction for patients with cervical radiculopathy; however, review of clinical studies does not provide clear evidence to support routine use of SEPs in the diagnoses of cervical radiculopathy.[24]

SUMMARY

Referral for evaluation for cervical radiculopathy is a common request in electrodiagnostic laboratories. To properly diagnose cervical radiculopathy, a combination of clinical signs/symptoms, imaging, and electrodiagnostic studies should be used. It is crucial to generate a differential diagnosis to consider various causes of neuropathic and musculoskeletal pain that may be affect the upper extremity. Based on these findings, the provider can design an appropriate study based on the differential diagnoses.

It is also critical to understand the spinal anatomy of the cervical region, both with regards to the orientation of the spinal roots, as well as the location of the dorsal root ganglion. Needle EMG is the most useful electrodiagnostic technique, and it provides moderate sensitivity in the diagnosis of cervical radiculopathy. Appropriate sampling of muscle must be done including PSPs, if possible, to ensure a diagnostically accurate study. Nerve conduction studies are often needed to rule out peripheral nerve entrapments or atypical presentations for peripheral neuropathies.

Electrodiagnosis provides moderate sensitivity in diagnosing cervical radiculopathy. With good specificity, it is useful in confirming disease, excluding other diseases, and helping to localize lesions. It is critical to remember that a normal study does not rule out the presence of cervical radiculopathy. Electrodiagnostic findings can be particularly useful for patients with atypical symptoms, potentially pain-mediated weakness, and nonfocal imaging findings.

REFERENCES

1. Radhakrishnan K, Litchy WJ, O'Fallon WM, et al. Epidemiology of cervical radiculopathy. A population-based study from Rochester, Minnesota, 1976 through 1990. Brain 1994;117(2):325–35.
2. Schoenfeld AJ, George AA, Bader JO, et al. Incidence and epidemiology of cervical radiculopathy in the United States military: 2000 to 2009. J Spinal Disord Tech 2012;25(1):17–22.
3. Yabuki S, Kikuchi S. Positions of dorsal root ganglia in the cervical spine. An anatomic and clinical study. Spine (Phila Pa 1976) 1996;21:1513.
4. Ellenberg MR, Honet JC, Treanor WJ. Cervical radiculopathy. Arch Phys Med Rehabil 1994;75:342.

5. Carette S, Fehlings MG. Clinical practice. Cervical radiculopathy. N Engl J Med 2005;353:392.
6. Yoss RE, Corbin KB, McCarthy CS, et al. Significance of symptoms and signs and localization of involved root in cervical disc protrusion. Neurology 1957;7:673–83.
7. Spurling R, Scoville W. Lateral rupture of the cervical intervertebral discs: a common cause of shoulder and arm pain. Surg Gynecol Obstet 1944;78:350.
8. Rubinstein SM, Pool JJ, van Tulder MW, et al. A systematic review of the diagnostic accuracy of provocative tests of the neck for diagnosing cervical radiculopathy. Eur Spine J 2007;16:307.
9. Pyhtinen J, Laitinen J. Cervical intervertebral foramen narrowing and myelographic nerve root sleeve deformities. Neuroradiology 1993;35:596–7.
10. Kaiser JA, Holladn BA. Imaging of the cervical spin. Spine 1998;148:233–6.
11. Bartlett RJ, Hill CR, Gardiner E. A comparison of T2 and gadolinium enhanced MRI with CT myelography in cervical radiculopathy. Br J Radiol 1998;71:11.
12. Houser OW, Onofrio BM, Miller GM, et al. Cervical neural foraminal canal stenosis: computerized tomographic myelography diagnosis. J Neurosurg 1993;79:84.
13. Matsumoto M, Okada E, Ichihara D, et al. Age-related changes of thoracic and cervical intervertebral discs in asymptomatic subjects. Spine (Phila Pa 1976) 2010;35(14):1359–64.
14. AAEM. Practice parameter for needle electromyographic evaluation of patients with suspected cervical radiculopathy. Muscle Nerve 1999;(Suppl 8):s209–21.
15. Dillingham TR, Lauder TD, Andary M, et al. Identification of cervical radiculopathies: optimizing the electromyographer screen. Am J Phys Med Rehabil 2001; 80:84–91.
16. Gilad R, Dabby M, Boaz M, et al. Cervical paraspinal electromyography: normal values in 100 control subjects. J Clin Neurophysiol 2006;23:573–6.
17. Date ES, Kim B, Yoon JS, et al. Cervical paraspinal spontaneous activity in asymptomatic subjects. Muscle Nerve 2006;34:361–4.
18. Tong HC. Specificity of needle electromyography for lumbar radiculopathy in 55- to 79-yr-old subjects with low pain and sciatica without stenosis. Am J Phys Med Rehabil 2011;90:233–42.
19. Robinson LR, Micklesen PJ, Wang L. Strategies for analyzing nerve conduction data; superiority of a summary index over single tests. Muscle Nerve 1998;21: 1166–71.
20. Lo YL, Chan LL, Leoh T, et al. Diagnostic utility in F waves in cervical radiculopathy: electrophysiological and magnetic resonance imaging correlation. Clin Neurol Neurosurg 2008;110:58–61.
21. Jabre JF. Surface recording of the H-reflex of the flexor carpi radialis. Muscle Nerve 1981;4:435–8.
22. Miller TA, Pardo R, Yaworski R. Clinical utility of reflex studies in assessing cervical radiculopathy. Muscle Nerve 1999;22:1075–9.
23. Eliaspour D, Sanati E, Moqadam M, et al. Utility of flexor carpi radialis H-reflex in diagnosis of cervical radiculopathy. J Clin Neurophysiol 2009;26:458–60.
24. Aminoff MJ, Eisen AA. AAEM minimonograph 19: somatosensory evoked potentials. Muscle Nerve 1998;21:277–90.

Electrodiagnosis of Brachial Plexopathies and Proximal Upper Extremity Neuropathies

Zachary Simmons, MD*

KEYWORDS

- Brachial plexus • Brachial plexopathy • Axillary nerve • Musculocutaneous nerve
- Suprascapular nerve • Nerve conduction studies • Electromyography

KEY POINTS

- The brachial plexus provides all motor and sensory innervation of the upper extremity.
- The plexus is usually derived from the C5 through T1 anterior primary rami, which divide in various ways to form the upper, middle, and lower trunks; the lateral, posterior, and medial cords; and multiple terminal branches.
- Traction is the most common cause of brachial plexopathy, although compression, lacerations, ischemia, neoplasms, radiation, thoracic outlet syndrome, and neuralgic amyotrophy may all produce brachial plexus lesions.
- Upper extremity mononeuropathies affecting the musculocutaneous, axillary, and suprascapular motor nerves and the medial and lateral antebrachial cutaneous sensory nerves often occur in the context of more widespread brachial plexus damage, often from trauma or neuralgic amyotrophy but may occur in isolation.
- Extensive electrodiagnostic testing often is needed to properly localize lesions of the brachial plexus, frequently requiring testing of sensory nerves, which are not commonly used in the assessment of other types of lesions.

INTRODUCTION

Few anatomic structures are as daunting to medical students, residents, and practicing physicians as the brachial plexus. Yet, detailed understanding of brachial plexus anatomy is central to electrodiagnosis because of the plexus' role in supplying all motor and sensory innervation of the upper extremity and shoulder girdle. There also are several proximal upper extremity nerves, derived from the brachial plexus,

Conflicts of Interest: None.
Neuromuscular Program and ALS Center, Penn State Hershey Medical Center, Penn State College of Medicine, PA, USA
* Department of Neurology, Penn State Hershey Medical Center, EC 037 30 Hope Drive, PO Box 859, Hershey, PA 17033.
E-mail address: zsimmons@psu.edu

which are not commonly tested in most electrodiagnostic evaluations but knowledge of which is important to any electromyographer involved in brachial plexus studies.

Patients commonly are referred to the electromyographer because of weakness, pain, or numbness of an upper limb, with a request to assess for brachial plexopathy. A properly trained electromyographer can combine sensory and motor nerve conduction studies with a detailed needle electromyographic examination to differentiate brachial plexopathy from radiculopathy, mononeuropathy, or mononeuropathy multiplex and then to localize the lesion within the brachial plexus. In this way, the electromyographer provides essential input, which the referring clinician can use for diagnosis, treatment, and prognosis.

ANATOMY OF THE BRACHIAL PLEXUS AND ITS MAJOR BRANCHES

The brachial plexus has 5 components: roots, trunks, divisions, cords, and terminal branches (**Fig. 1**). It runs behind the scalene muscles proximally and then behind the clavicle and pectoral muscles more distally as it courses from the neck into the shoulder girdle and arm. Proximal to the clavicle are the roots and trunks. Beneath it are the divisions. Distal to it are the cords and terminal nerve branches. In addition to providing the motor nerve supply to all muscles of the upper extremities and shoulder girdle, the brachial plexus supplies upper extremity cutaneous sensation (**Fig. 2**). The major clinically significant terminal branches of the brachial plexus and their origins from the plexus are summarized in **Table 1**. The components of the brachial plexus each have specific anatomic details with which the electromyographer should become familiar:

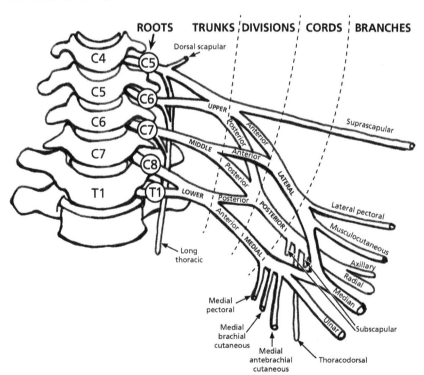

Fig. 1. Brachial plexus. The components shown are the roots, trunks, divisions, cords, and the major terminal branches.

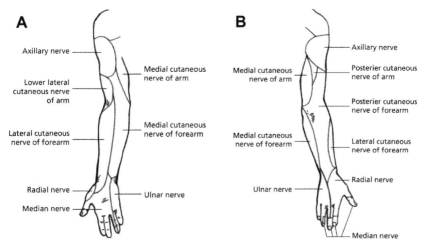

Fig. 2. Cutaneous innervation of the upper extremities. (*A*) Right upper extremity, anterior aspect; (*B*) right upper extremity, posterior aspect.

Roots

The brachial plexus arises from the spinal cord at the C5 through T1 levels. Each of these levels gives rise to dorsal (sensory) and ventral (motor) rootlets, which then merge to form a short spinal nerve. This in turn divides into anterior and posterior primary rami (**Fig. 3**). The anterior primary rami are often referred to as the roots of the brachial plexus and are located immediately external to the intervertebral foramina. There is anatomic variation. The term "prefixed plexus" is used when there is a contribution from C4 and the T1 contribution is minimal. In such cases, all the nerve contributions to the brachial plexus are shifted one level superiorly. In a postfixed

Table 1	
Major upper extremity nerves	
Nerve	**Origin**
Dorsal scapular	C5 ($\pm$C4) root
Long thoracic	C5, C6 ($\pm$C7) roots
Suprascapular	Upper trunk
Lateral pectoral	Lateral cord
Musculocutaneous/lateral antebrachial cutaneous	Lateral cord
Medial pectoral	Medial cord
Medial brachial cutaneous	Medial cord
Medial antebrachial cutaneous	Medial cord
Ulnar	Medial cord
Median	Lateral and medial cords
Upper subscapular	Posterior cord
Lower subscapular	Posterior cord
Thoracodorsal	Posterior cord
Axillary	Posterior cord
Radial	Posterior cord

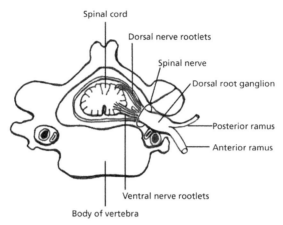

Spinal cord

Dorsal nerve rootlets

Spinal nerve

Dorsal root ganglion

Posterior ramus

Anterior ramus

Ventral nerve rootlets

Body of vertebra

Fig. 3. Details of the anatomy at a cervical spinal cord level. The dorsal and ventral rootlets combine to form a spinal nerve, which then divides into anterior and posterior primary rami.

plexus, there is a minimal contribution from C5 and a more substantial contribution from T2, resulting in the plexus being shifted one root level inferiorly. At times, the plexus may be expanded, with contributions from C4 through T2. Two branches originate directly at the root level: (1) the dorsal scapular nerve is derived from the C5 root, sometimes with a contribution from C4, and provides innervation to the major and minor rhomboid muscles and (2) the long thoracic nerve comes directly off the C5, C6, and sometimes the C7 anterior primary rami, innervating the serratus anterior muscle. Electromyographers should bear in mind that the cervical paraspinal muscles are innervated by the posterior primary rami and, therefore, can also be considered to have their innervation arise directly at the root level.

Trunks

There are 3 trunks. The upper trunk is formed by merger of the C5 and C6 roots. The middle trunk is the continuation of the C7 root. The C8 and T1 roots merge to form the lower trunk. One major branch and one minor one arise from the upper trunk. The suprascapular nerve, derived from the C5 and C6 roots, is the major terminal branch originating at the trunk level, coming off the upper trunk to provide innervation to the supraspinatus and infraspinatus muscles. It passes through the suprascapular notch of the scapula, an area covered by the transverse scapular ligament, and supplies motor branches to the supraspinatus muscle. Then, it continues around the spinoglenoid notch of the scapular spine (bounded by the scapula spine medially and the spinoglenoid ligament [inferior transverse scapular ligament] laterally) to supply motor branches to the infraspinatus muscle. The nerve to the subclavius is the minor branch of the upper trunk, which cannot be tested easily by physical examination or electrodiagnosis. There are no significant terminal branches arising directly from the middle or lower trunk.

Divisions

Each of the 3 trunks divides into an anterior and a posterior division, situated behind the clavicle. No terminal branches arise directly from the divisions.

Cords

The 3 cords are formed from the 6 divisions. The anterior divisions of the upper and middle trunks form the lateral cord, whereas the anterior division of the lower trunk continues as the medial cord. All 3 posterior divisions merge to form the posterior cord. Several terminal branches arise at the cord level.

Branches of the lateral cord: (1) The lateral pectoral nerve is derived from the C5-C7 spinal nerve levels and innervates the pectoralis major muscle. (2) The musculocutaneous nerve is derived from the C5-C6 spinal levels, sometimes with a contribution from C7. It innervates the coracobrachialis, biceps brachii, and brachialis muscles and gives rise to the lateral antebrachial cutaneous nerve (lateral cutaneous nerve of the forearm), which provides cutaneous sensation to the lateral forearm from wrist to elbow.

Branches of the medial cord: (1) The medial pectoral nerve is formed from C8 and T1 spinal nerves. It innervates the pectoralis minor muscle and the inferior portions of the pectoralis major muscle. (2) The medial brachial cutaneous nerve (medial cutaneous nerve of the arm) provides cutaneous sensation to the medial arm proximal to the elbow. (3) The medial antebrachial cutaneous nerve (medial cutaneous nerve of the forearm) provides cutaneous sensation to the medial forearm between the wrist and elbow. (4) The ulnar nerve arises from spinal levels C8-T1 primarily, usually with a contribution from C7. It supplies many forearm and hand muscles and provides cutaneous sensation over the medial hand, part of the ring finger, and all of the little finger.

Branch of both the lateral and medial cords: The median nerve is derived from spinal levels C6-T1. The motor fibers are derived from all these levels, whereas sensory fibers are derived primarily from C6-C7. Occasionally C5 contributes. Sensory fibers travel through the upper and middle trunks to the lateral cord. Motor fibers travel through all trunks to the lateral and medial cords. The different spinal level origins, and the different trunk and cord pathways, of the motor and sensory fibers, has meaningful clinical and electrodiagnostic implications for localization. The median nerve supplies forearm and hand muscles and cutaneous sensation over part of the hand.

Branches of the posterior cord: (1) The upper subscapular nerve is derived from the C5-C6 spinal levels and innervates the upper portion of the subscapularis muscle. (2) The lower subscapular nerve is derived from the C5-C6 spinal levels and innervates the lower portion of the subscapularis muscle and the teres major muscle. (3) The thoracodorsal nerve arises between the upper and lower subscapular nerves, derives from the C5-C7 spinal levels, and innervates the latissimus dorsi muscle. (4) The axillary nerve is derived from spinal levels C5-C7. It supplies the teres minor muscle and then terminates by innervating the deltoid muscle. It also supplies cutaneous sensation to the lateral aspect of the upper arm overlying the deltoid muscle. (5) The radial nerve arises from spinal levels C5-C8, occasionally with a T1 contribution. It supplies the triceps muscle, anconeus muscle, and muscles of the forearm and hand. It also provides cutaneous sensation to the arm, forearm, and hand as the posterior cutaneous nerve of the arm, lower lateral cutaneous nerve of the arm, posterior cutaneous nerve of the forearm, and superficial radial sensory nerve.

CAUSES OF BRACHIAL PLEXOPATHY

There are many causes of brachial plexopathy, and these may result in lesions at many levels. A listing of the most common causes is provided in **Box 1**. A few of these merit more detailed discussion.

Traction

Traction injuries are common. There are many causes, including a fall onto the shoulder from a height, traction to a limb when it is pulled severely, sports injuries (particularly in football), and closed traction during motor vehicle accidents.[1] Traction

---

Box 1
Common causes of brachial plexopathy

- Traction
  - Fall from a height, particularly onto shoulder
  - Trauma in which the arm is pulled down, damaging the upper plexus
  - Trauma in which the arm is pulled up, damaging the lower plexus
  - Sports injuries, especially football
  - Motor vehicle accidents and other trauma
  - Obstetric paralysis
  - Surgery, particularly during median sternotomy
- Compression
  - Supraclavicular plexopathy from pack straps
  - Infraclavicular plexopathy from crutches
  - Hematoma, aneurysm, arteriovenous malformations
- Lacerations from penetrating injuries
  - Gunshot or other missile
  - Knife or other penetrating sharp object
  - Neurovascular injury, particularly during trauma
- Ischemia
- Neoplastic infiltration
- Radiation therapy
- Thoracic outlet syndrome
- Neuralgic amyotrophy (Parsonage-Turner syndrome)
- Iatrogenic injury
  - Direct injury during surgery

---

during surgery may result in postoperative brachial plexopathy. This plexopathy most commonly occurs after chest surgeries due to stretch injuries to the plexus from chest wall retraction. The lower trunk or medial cord usually is involved, with the expected clinical presentation as described later in this article. Recovery depends on the severity of axonal injury. Obstetric paralysis typically has been attributed to traction on the neck by the clinician during passage in the birth canal.[2] However, it now appears that some of these injuries develop prenatally or are due to propulsive forces over which the birth attendant does not have control.[1,3] Upper or upper and middle plexus involvement are most common, although about 23% of infants sustain pan-plexus injuries.[4]

Neoplastic and Radiation-induced Brachial Plexopathy

Radiation-induced brachial plexopathy is most commonly a delayed syndrome, occurring from a few weeks to many years after radiation. The higher the radiation dose, the higher the risk of developing a radiation-induced brachial plexopathy.[5] The electromyographer is most often called on to distinguish a radiation-induced plexopathy from one due to neoplastic infiltration. Radiation-induced plexopathy is less likely to be painful, and more likely to be characterized by progressively evolving sensory disturbances. Electrodiagnostically, myokymic discharges and fasciculation potentials are more likely to be present in radiation-induced plexopathy. In contrast, neoplastic brachial plexopathy usually is characterized by prominent pain, more rapidly developing symptoms, often accompanied by a Horner syndrome, and rarely associated with fasciculation potentials or myokymia.[1,6] Tumors at the lung apex (Pancoast tumors) most commonly invade the lower portion of the plexus, but metastases from other types of malignancies or direct infiltration of the nerves or nerve sheaths can also occur at any level of the plexus.

Thoracic Outlet Syndrome

This syndrome has been the subject of extensive review, to which the interested reader is referred.[1,7–9] True neurogenic thoracic outlet syndrome is rare. Most are caused by a fibrous band from a rudimentary cervical rib to the first thoracic rib, which entraps the lower trunk of the brachial plexus. Thus, the clinical presentation and the electrodiagnostic findings are those of a lower trunk brachial plexopathy, the exception being that the T1 fibers usually are preferentially affected, resulting in greater atrophy of the thenar than hypothenar mucles.[7] Sensory loss parallels that seen in lower trunk plexopathies.

Neuralgic Amyotrophy (Parsonage-Turner Syndrome)

Also termed immune brachial plexus neuropathy, this condition is most commonly sporadic, although it may be familial. First described in detail in the modern era by Parsonage and Turner in 1948[10] and then described in detail with respect to its natural history more than 20 years later,[11] this condition is now well recognized by most neurologists, but often unknown to nonneurologists and confused with cervical radiculopathy. Individuals of all ages may be affected, and there is a male predominance. The symptoms are widely varied, as has been well described.[12,13] Most commonly, the initial symptom is pain of abrupt onset, often severe, usually in the shoulder or periscapular region. Pain generally begins to improve in 2 to 3 weeks, in association with the development of weakness. The weakness may involve the brachial plexus in a patchy fashion, for example affecting one or more trunks or single peripheral nerves, most commonly the long thoracic, suprascapular, or axillary nerves. Bilateral involvement occurs in about one-third of patients, usually asymmetrically. It may be preceded by a flulike or other febrile illness. Reports of this syndrome following a variety of conditions (immune, infectious, neoplastic, traumatic, etc) have been reported, suggesting that a variety of events can trigger an immune-mediated attack on the brachial plexus.[14] Electrodiagnostic studies may reveal a pattern of brachial plexus involvement not readily localizable to one or more specific trunks, divisions, cords, or peripheral nerves. This patchy or multifocal involvement is common and is a hallmark of this syndrome. Pathogenetically, this condition appears to be an inflammatory, immune-mediated process.[15]

CAUSES OF PROXIMAL UPPER EXTREMITY NEUROPATHIES
Medial Antebrachial Cutaneous (MAC) Nerve

Lesions generally arise from lesions that affect the lower trunk or medial cord of the brachial plexus. Several causes of brachial plexopathy are particularly likely to affect the lower trunk or medial cord and thus the MAC nerve: (1) trauma in which the arm and shoulder are pulled up; (2) invasion of the plexus by a Pancoast tumor at the lung apex; (3) stretch injuries of the lower plexus during chest surgery such as coronary artery bypass surgery; and (4) thoracic outlet syndrome entrapping the lower trunk of the plexus.

Musculocutaneous Nerve

Lesions are most commonly caused by trauma to the shoulder and upper arm, especially factures of the proximal humerus from falls or sports injuries. In such cases, other nerves usually are damaged as well. For example, primary shoulder dislocations or fractures of the humeral neck may result in injuries to several nerves, including the axillary, suprascapular, radial, and musculocutaneous nerves.[16] Other forms of trauma, including gunshot wounds and lacerations, also may produce musculocutaneous nerve lesions. Isolated nontraumatic lesions of the musculocutaneous nerve are rare, usually occurring as it passes through the coracobrachialis muscle. Causes include weightlifting or other vigorous physical exercises,[17,18] as well as surgery, pressure during sleep, and malpositioning during anesthesia.[19,20] Rare cases of musculocutaneous nerve compression have included repeated carrying of items on the shoulder with the arm curled around the item, or osteochondroma of the humerus compressing the musculocutaneous nerve.[21] The musculocutaneous nerve may also be involved in neuralgic amyotrophy.

Lateral Antebrachial Cutaneous (LAC) Nerve

Injuries can occur in isolation without involvement of the main portion of the musculocutaneous nerves. The LAC nerve may be entrapped, usually at the elbow, where it is compressed by the biceps aponeurosis and tendon against the brachialis muscle.[19,22] Other causes of isolated LAC injury include hyperextension injury of the elbow, such as during sports, and antecubital phlebotomy.[23]

Axillary Nerve

This is most commonly damaged by trauma, including shoulder dislocations, fractures of the humeral neck,[16] blunt trauma to the shoulder in contact sports,[24] gunshot wounds, and injections. Compression may produce an axillary neuropathy during general anesthesia or by sleeping with the arms above the head. The nerve may be entrapped within the quadrilateral space (formed by the humerus, teres minor muscle, teres major muscle, and long head of the triceps muscle) by muscular hypertrophy and repetitive trauma in athletes such as tennis players and baseball pitchers.[25–27] As for other upper extremity neuropathies, neuralgic amyotrophy may be a cause.

Suprascapular Nerve

This may be entrapped as it passes through the suprascapular notch, or, less commonly, as it passes through the spinoglenoid notch.[28,29] Causes of suprascapular nerve entrapment also include mass lesions such as ganglion cysts, sarcomas, and metastatic carcinomas.[30–33] Traumatic causes of suprascapular neuropathy include shoulder dislocation or protraction or scapular fracture,[34,35] as well as injuries that generally produce more widespread damage to the brachial plexus such as stretch, gunshot, and penetrating injuries. Weightlifters may suffer suprascapular neuropathies, probably due to repetitive movement of the scapula. Other athletic activities involving overhand activities can predispose individuals to suprascapular entrapment, particularly at the spinoglenoid notch. Such injuries are particularly common in professional volleyball players[36,37] but also are seen in baseball pitchers and dancers.[38,39] As with many other upper extremity neuropathies, the suprascapular nerve also may be affected in neuralgic amyotrophy.

CLINICAL PRESENTATIONS OF BRACHIAL PLEXOPATHY

Familiarity with the clinical features of brachial plexopathies at the trunk and cord levels facilitates more targeted and clinically useful electrodiagnostic evaluations.

Upper Trunk Plexopathy

Weakness will be seen in muscles innervated at the C5-C6 levels such as the spinati (arm external rotation), deltoid (arm abduction), biceps, and brachioradialis (elbow flexion). Some muscles are partially innervated from the upper trunk, and may be partially affected, such as the pronator teres (forearm pronation), flexor carpi radialis (wrist flexion), and triceps (elbow extension). The biceps and brachioradialis reflexes are decreased or absent. Sensory loss is expected to be over the lateral upper arm in the distribution of the axillary nerve, in the lateral hand and digits 1 to 3 (median and radial sensory branches), and in the distribution of the lateral antebrachial cutaneous nerve over the lateral forearm.

Middle Trunk Plexopathy

Isolated lesions of the middle trunk are rare and usually occur in conjunction with more widespread brachial plexus lesions. The middle trunk is formed from the C7 anterior primary ramus, and so has the same clinical features as a C7 radiculopathy, with weakness of elbow, wrist, and finger extension, as well as weakness of the flexor carpi radialis (wrist flexion) and pronator teres (forearm pronation) muscles. The triceps reflex is decreased or absent. Sensory loss is over the distribution of the posterior cutaneous nerve of the forearm and in the hand over the middle finger and to a lesser degree index and ring fingers.

Lower Trunk Plexopathy

The lower trunk is formed from the C8-T1 spinal levels. Lesions involve all ulnar-innervated muscles and also C8-T1 median-innervated muscles, such as the flexor pollicis longus, pronator quadratus, and intrinsic hand muscles, and C8-innervated radial muscles, such as the extensor indicis, extensor digitorum, and extensor carpi ulnaris, resulting in weakness of grip due to weakness of hand muscles, inability to fully flex the fingers and thumb, and partial weakness of finger and wrist extension. No upper extremity reflex abnormalities are present. Sensory abnormalities occur in the medial arm, medial forearm, medial hand, and digits 4 to 5.

Lateral Cord Plexopathy

Lesions at this level result in weakness of C6-C7 innervated median muscles such as the pronator teres and flexor carpi radialis (wrist flexion) and in weakness of elbow flexion due to involvement of the biceps brachii muscle. The biceps reflex is decreased or absent, but the brachioradialis and triceps reflexes are normal. Sensory loss occurs over the lateral forearm and hand and digits 1 to 3.

Posterior Cord Plexopathy

Weakness occurs in all muscles innervated by the radial nerve, resulting in finger extension weakness, wrist drop, and arm extension weakness at the elbow. There is weakness of shoulder abduction (deltoid) and adduction (latissimus dorsi). The triceps and brachioradialis reflexes are decreased or absent, although the biceps reflexes is preserved. There is sensory loss in the distributions of the axillary nerve, posterior cutaneous nerve of the arm, and superficial radial nerve.

Medial Cord Plexopathy

This lesion results in the same clinical deficits as a lower trunk lesion, except for preservation of radial-innervated C8 fibers. Patients demonstrate weakness of all ulnar-innervated muscles and C8-T1-innervated median muscles, leading to weakness of grip due to weakness of hand muscles and to inability to fully flex the fingers and thumb. However, finger and wrist extensors are spared. There is sensory loss in the same distribution as for lower trunk lesions: medial arm, medial forearm, medial hand, and digits 4 to 5. There are no reflex abnormalities.

Panplexopathy

Widespread lesions of this type cause weakness of the upper extremity except for remaining function of the rhomboids and serratus anterior muscles. Reflexes are all decreased or absent. There is widespread sensory loss.

CLINICAL PRESENTATIONS OF PROXIMAL UPPER EXTREMITY NEUROPATHIES

The *MAC nerve* is exclusively a sensory nerve, supplying cutaneous sensation over the medial portion of the forearm. Lesions of this nerve result in sensory loss in this distribution, without weakness and without reflex changes. As noted earlier, lesions of this nerve often occur in association with lesions of the lower trunk or medial cord of the brachial plexus.

Patients with *musculocutaneous neuropathies* present with weakness of elbow flexion, an absent biceps reflex, and sensory alteration in the distribution of the *LAC nerve* (lateral forearm), whereas those with an isolated LAC neuropathy demonstrate the sensory alteration, but with normal muscle strength and reflexes. Patients in whom the *LAC nerve* is entrapped at the elbow present with pain in the anterolateral aspect of the elbow region, which is worsened by pronation of the arm and extension at the elbow.[19,22,40]

Axillary nerve lesions result in partial weakness of shoulder abduction and external rotation, motions that are partially maintained by the supraspinatus and infraspinatus muscles, respectively. Atrophy of the deltoid region of the upper arm may result. There is sensory loss over the lateral aspect of the upper arm.

Entrapment of the *suprascapular nerve* at the suprascapular notch usually is accompanied by pain, most prominently along the superior aspect of the scapula and radiating to the posterior and lateral shoulder. The pain may be referred to arm, neck, or upper anterior chest wall[21,29] and may be exacerbated by shoulder movements. The suprascapular notch may be tender to palpation. When suprascapular nerve is injured or when it is entrapped at the suprascapular notch, the clinical manifestation is primarily weakness of shoulder external rotation (infraspinatus muscle weakness). Shoulder abduction (supraspinatus muscle) is weakened only slightly because of preservation of the deltoid muscle. Atrophy may be noted, particularly of the infraspinatus muscle, which is only partly covered by the overlying trapezius muscle. If entrapment occurs at the spinoglenoid ligament, then only infraspinatus weakness results, resulting in weakness of shoulder external rotation but no weakness of shoulder abduction. There is no cutaneous sensory alteration.

ELECTRODIAGNOSIS OF BRACHIAL PLEXOPATHIES

As is generally the case with electrodiagnosis, the electromyographer's role is one of localization and assessment of severity, than determination of causes. It is important for the electromyographer to have a good understanding of the history and examination findings of the patient being studied, of course, because this information, in conjunction with information about localization and severity, is the key in narrowing down the range of possible causes and in permitting the electromyographer to use his or her knowledge to function as a true electrodiagnostic consultant and partner in the diagnosis and care of the patient, than simply as a technical proceduralist. There are few types of disorders in which electrodiagnosis is more important than in brachial plexopathies, which can be due to a wide variety of causes and present and evolve in many different ways. Electrodiagnostic evaluations of brachial plexopathies are generally complex, involving the study of multiple nerves and muscles to permit accurate localization. General principles that guide the performance of the electrodiagnostic evaluation of brachial plexopathies, are provided in **Boxes 2–4** and **Table 2**.

Upper Trunk Plexopathy

Sensory studies will reveal abnormalities in the following nerves: LAC, median sensory (particularly to the thumb), and radial sensory (particularly to the thumb) nerves. Routine studies of the median and ulnar motor nerves are normal, but studies of the suprascapular, axillary, and musculocutaneous nerves, if performed, may be abnormal. Needle examination is expected to demonstrate abnormalities in the supraspinatus, infraspinatus, deltoid, biceps brachii, and brachioradialis muscles. The pronator teres, flexor carpi radialis, triceps, and extensor carpi radialis muscles may show abnormalities. C5-C6 muscles innervated at the root level will be spared, including the cervical paraspinal, serratus anterior, and rhomboid muscles.

Middle Trunk Plexopathy

The median sensory response is expected to be abnormal when recording from the middle finger. Routine studies of the median and ulnar motor nerves are normal.

Box 2
Guidelines for sensory nerve studies in brachial plexopathy

- Sensory nerve studies are a key feature in distinguishing brachial plexopathies from radiculopathies. In radiculopathy, because the lesion occurs proximal to the dorsal root ganglion, sensory nerve conduction studies are NORMAL, even in the distribution of the numbness, because the sensory nerve is intact from the level of its cell body (the dorsal root ganglion) to the level of the skin. In plexopathies (or in peripheral neuropathies), the lesion occurs at or distal to the dorsal root ganglion so that the sensory nerve conduction studies are ABNORMAL because of axon loss from the level of the cell body to the skin.

- Beginning with standard median, ulnar, and radial sensory studies usually is most helpful.

- It is often helpful to perform extensive sensory nerve studies, including some uncommonly studied nerves, to distinguish a brachial plexopathy from radiculopathy or from multiple mononeuropathies and to more precisely localize the plexopathy. Medial and lateral antebrachial cutaneous nerve studies are particularly useful for distinguishing plexopathy from radiculopathy.

- Side-to-side comparisons of sensory amplitudes are helpful, particularly when assessing uncommonly studied nerves, for which normal values may be less well established. A sensory nerve action potential amplitude on the symptomatic side that is less than half of that on the asymptomatic side is considered to be abnormal, even if the absolute value of the amplitude falls within the normal range.

- Careful selection of the digit used when recording a median or radial sensory response can improve sensitivity and specificity. **Table 2** lists some sensory studies, which are particularly useful in the electrodiagnostic assessment of brachial plexopathies.

Box 3
Guidelines for motor nerve studies in brachial plexopathy

- Beginning with standard median, ulnar, and (in selected instances) radial motor studies usually is most helpful.

- Suprascapular, axillary, and musculocutaneous nerve studies should be considered in selected cases. These studies are not commonly performed because the needed information often is obtained through needle examination of the muscles supplied by these motor nerves. However, nerve conduction studies should be considered if the needle examination cannot be performed or is limited. These nerve studies can provide useful information regarding upper trunk, posterior cord, and lateral cord plexopathies.

Needle examination generally reveals abnormalities in C7-innervated muscles, such as the pronator teres, flexor carpi radialis, triceps, extensor carpi radialis, and extensor digitorum communis muscles. C7 muscles innervated at the root level will be spared, such as the cervical paraspinal and serratus anterior muscles.

Lower Trunk Plexopathy

Several sensory studies will be abnormal, including the studies of MAC nerve, the median sensory to the ring finger, the ulnar sensory to the little finger, and the dorsal ulnar cutaneous sensory nerve. In testing of motor nerves, if there is sufficient axon loss, then the median and ulnar motor studies may be abnormal, with the degree of abnormality being determined by the severity of the axon loss. Partial axon loss may reveal low compound muscle action potential (CMAP) amplitudes, mildly to moderately prolonged distal motor latencies, and mildly to moderately slowed conduction velocities. Severe axon loss could result in absent responses. On needle examination, abnormalities are expected in C8-T1-innervated muscles, including all ulnar-innervated muscles and selected median and radial muscles. Of the radial-innervated muscles, the extensor indicis is a particularly useful muscle to test. Median-innervated muscles, which are likely to be abnormal, are the flexor pollicis longus, pronator quadratus, and intrinsic hand muscles. Of course, cervical paraspinal muscles will be spared.

Lateral Cord Plexopathy

Abnormalities are expected in the LAC nerve and the median sensory nerve, recording from the thumb, index, or middle finger. Routine studies of the median and ulnar motor

---

Box 4
Guidelines for the needle examination in brachial plexopathy

- The needle examination in brachial plexopathies often will need to be extensive if it is to result in accurate localization.

- The presence or absence of axonal continuity often is of great value to the surgeon. So it is important to search carefully for voluntary motor unit action potential firing in weak muscles. If axonal continuity is present, surgical exploration may be postponed.

- Keep in mind those muscles that are innervated at the root level, proximal to the brachial plexus. Those muscles will be abnormal in some radiculopathies but normal in brachial plexopathies.

- There are variations in the spinal levels supplying the various portions of the plexus. Denervation in unexpected muscles or the absence of denervation in muscles expected to be affected may represent not only the patchy nature of some brachial plexopathies, but also the anatomic variations that may occur.

Clinical Finding	Clinical Considerations	Sensory Nerve to Study	Localization When Abnormal
Table 2			
Median and radial sensory studies of importance in assessment of brachial plexopathy			
Sensory loss lateral forearm and hand	• Upper trunk plexopathy • Lateral cord plexopathy • C6 radiculopathy	Median sensory to the thumb	Upper trunk or lateral cord plexopathy or median neuropathy
		Radial sensory to the thumb	Upper trunk or posterior cord plexopathy or radial neuropathy
		Lateral antebrachial cutaneous nerve	Upper trunk or lateral cord plexopathy
Sensory loss medial forearm and hand	• Lower trunk plexopathy • Medial cord plexopathy • C8-T1 radiculopathy	Ulnar sensory to the little finger	Lower trunk or medial cord plexopathy or ulnar neuropathy
		Dorsal cutaneous ulnar sensory nerve	Lower trunk or medial cord plexopathy or ulnar neuropathy proximal to the wrist
		Medial antebrachial cutaneous nerve	Lower trunk or medial cord plexopathy

nerves are normal. Needle examination reveals abnormalities in the biceps brachii and median-innervated forearm muscles (pronator teres, flexor carpi radialis), with sparing of the more distal median-innervated muscles such as the flexor pollicis longus and median-innervated hand muscles. Cervical paraspinal muscles and other muscles innervated at the root level are spared.

Posterior Cord Plexopathy

The radial sensory study is abnormal. Routine studies of the median and ulnar motor nerves are normal. When studying the radial motor nerve, if there is sufficient axon loss, then the radial motor studies may be abnormal, with the degree of abnormality being determined by the severity of the axon loss. Partial axon loss may reveal low CMAP amplitudes, mildly to moderately prolonged distal motor latencies, and mildly to moderately slowed conduction velocities. Severe axon loss could result in absent responses. Needle examination is expected to show abnormalities in all radial-innervated muscles and in the deltoid, teres minor, and latissimus dorsi muscles.

Medial Cord Plexopathy

Electrodiagnostic testing is expected to produce the same findings as for a lower trunk lesion, but with sparing of C8 muscles innervated by the radial nerve. Abnormalities are expected on testing of the MAC nerve, the median sensory to the ring finger, the ulnar sensory to the little finger, and the dorsal ulnar cutaneous sensory nerve. On motor nerve testing, if there is sufficient axon loss, then the median and ulnar motor studies may be abnormal, with the degree of abnormality being determined by the severity of the axon loss. Partial axon loss may reveal low CMAP amplitudes, mildly to moderately prolonged distal motor latencies, and mildly to moderately slowed conduction velocities. Severe axon loss could result in absent responses. Needle examination should reveal abnormalities in C8-T1-innervated muscles supplied by the ulnar and median nerves, including all ulnar-innervated muscles and selected median-innervated muscles such as the flexor pollicis longus, pronator quadratus, and intrinsic hand muscles. As noted earlier, radial-innervated C8 muscles are spared. The extensor indicis is a particularly useful muscle to test. Once again, cervical paraspinal muscles are spared, as with all plexus lesions.

Panplexopathy

As expected, the abnormalities here are widespread. Median, ulnar, and radial sensory responses are abnormal, as are the MAC and LAC nerve studies. If there is sufficient axon loss, then the median, ulnar, and radial motor studies may be abnormal, as may the suprascapular, axillary, and musculocutaneous nerve studies, with the degree of abnormality being determined by the severity of the axon loss. Partial axon loss may reveal low CMAP amplitudes, mildly to moderately prolonged distal motor latencies, and mildly to moderately slowed conduction velocities. Severe axon loss could result in absent responses. On needle examination, abnormalities are expected in all muscles of the upper extremity and shoulder girdle except for those innervated directly at the root level, specifically the cervical paraspinal, rhomboid, and serratus anterior muscles.

ELECTRODIAGNOSIS OF PROXIMAL UPPER EXTREMITY NEUROPATHIES
Medial Antebrachial Cutaneous Nerve

Recording electrodes (**Fig. 4**)
- Active electrode (E1): On the medial forearm, 12 cm distal to the stimulation site, on a line between the stimulation site and the ulnar aspect of the wrist.
- Reference electrode (E2): 3 to 4 cm distal to E1.

Stimulator
- In the medial portion of the antecubital fossa, midway between the tendon of the biceps brachii muscle and medial epicondyle.

Normal values[21]
- Amplitude greater than or equal to 5 μV
- Conduction velocity greater than or equal to 50 m/s
- Distal peak latency less than or equal to 3.2 ms

Alternative normal values[41]
- Amplitude greater than or equal to 10 μV
- Conduction velocity greater than or equal to 41.7 m/s

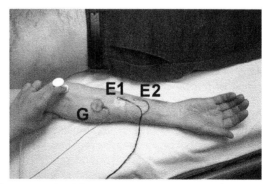

Fig. 4. Nerve conduction study of the medial antebrachial cutaneous nerve. Stimulation is at the medial portion of the antecubital fossa. Recording is from the medial forearm. E1, active electrode; E2, reference electrode; G, ground.

- Distal peak latency mean 2.1 ms

Notes

- The nerve is superficial, and maximal responses usually are obtained at low levels of stimulation.
- Side-to-side comparisons of the symptomatic and asymptomatic side are more useful than absolute values.

Musculocutaneous Nerve

Recording electrodes (**Fig. 5**)

- Active electrode (E1): Over the biceps, just distal to the midpoint of the muscle.
- Reference electrode (E2): Distally to E1 in the antecubital fossa, over the biceps tendon.

Stimulator

- Erb point

Normal values[21]

- Latency less than or equal to 5.7 ms at distance 23 to 29 cm, using calipers

Alternative normal values[42,43]

- Latency less than or equal to 5.7 ms at distance of 23.5 to 29 cm (calipers), 28 to 41.5 cm (tape, arm at side), or 26 to 35.5 cm (tape, arm abducted 90°)
- Latency 5.5 ms to 6.7 ms at distance of 25 to 33 cm, using calipers

Notes

- Supramaximal stimulation is difficult to achieve. Best to compare symptomatic to asymptomatic side.

Lateral Antebrachial Cutaneous Nerve

Recording electrodes (**Fig. 6**)

- Active electrode (E1): On the lateral forearm, 12 cm distal to the stimulation site, on a line between the stimulation site and the radial pulse.
- Reference electrode (E2): 3 to 4 cm distal to E1

Stimulator

- Lateral portion of the antecubital fossa, just lateral to the tendon of the biceps brachii muscle.

Normal values[21]

- Amplitude greater than or equal to 10 μV
- Conduction velocity greater than or equal to 55 m/s

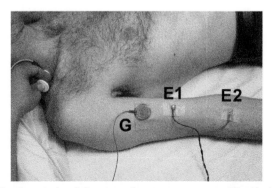

Fig. 5. Nerve conduction study of the musculocutaneous nerve. Stimulation is at Erb point. Recording is from the biceps, just distal to the midpoint. E1, active electrode; E2, reference electrode; G, ground.

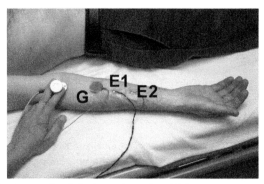

Fig. 6. Nerve conduction study of the lateral antebrachial cutaneous nerve. Stimulation is at the lateral portion of the antecubital fossa. Recording is from the lateral forearm. E1, active electrode; E2, reference electrode; G, ground.

- Peak latency less than or equal to 3.0 ms
Alternative normal values[44]
- Amplitude greater than or equal to 12 μV
- Conduction velocity greater than or equal to 57.8 m/s
- Distal peak latency less than or equal to 2.5 ms
Notes
- The nerve is superficial, and maximal responses usually are obtained at low levels of stimulation.
- Side-to-side comparisons of the symptomatic and asymptomatic side are more useful than absolute values.

Axillary Nerve

Recording electrodes (**Fig. 7**)
- Active electrode (E1): Middle deltoid
- Reference electrode (E2): Distally to E1, over the deltoid tendon.
Stimulator
- Erb point
Normal values[42]

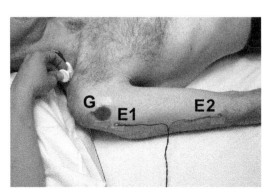

Fig. 7. Nerve conduction study of the axillary nerve. Stimulation is at Erb point. Recording is from the middle deltoid. E1, active electrode; E2, reference electrode; G, ground.

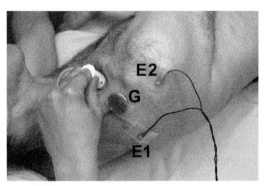

Fig. 8. Nerve conduction study of the suprascapular nerve, recording from the supraspinatus muscle. A needle than a surface-recording electrode would be used. Stimulation is at Erb point. E1, active electrode; E2, reference electrode; G, ground.

- Latency less than or equal to 5.0 ms at a distance of 14.8 to 21 cm (calipers), 20 to 26.5 cm (tape, arm at side), or 17.5 to 25.3 cm (tape, arm abducted 90°).
Notes
- Compare symptomatic to asymptomatic side.
- May be technically difficult to obtain supramaximal stimulation.

Suprascapular Nerve

Recording electrodes (**Figs. 8** and **9**)
- Active electrode (E1): A monopolar needle in the supraspinatus or infraspinatus muscle. Do NOT use a surface electrode because the trapezius muscle is more superficial and covers the intended muscles.
- Reference electrode (E2): Distally over shoulder joint.
Stimulator
- Erb point.
Normal values[42]
- Recording from supraspinatus muscle: Latency less than or equal to 3.7 ms at a distance of 7.4 to 12 cm (calipers) or 9 to 13.8 cm (tape, arm at side or abducted 90°)

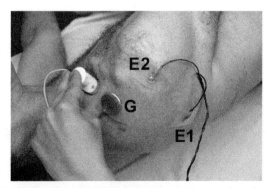

Fig. 9. Nerve conduction study of the suprascapular nerve, recording from the infraspinatus muscle. A needle than a surface-recording electrode would be used. Stimulation is at Erb point. E1, active electrode; E2, reference electrode; G, ground.

- Recording from infraspinatus muscle: Latency less than or equal to 4.2 ms at a distance of 10 to 15 cm (calipers) or 15 to 19.5 cm (tape, arm at side or abducted 90°).

Notes
- Compare symptomatic to asymptomatic side.
- May be technically difficult to obtain supramaximal stimulation.

SUMMARY

Although initially intimidating to many electromyographers, the brachial plexus is a highly organized structure, knowledge of which will, in conjunction with familiarity with proximal upper extremity nerves, permit logical clinical and electrodiagnostic evaluations that result in useful conclusions regarding localization and severity of abnormalities. A willingness to take the time to perform some additional electrodiagnostic evaluation beyond the "standard" studies generally will be rewarded with information that is helpful to the referring clinician. When combined with knowledge of possible causes of brachial plexus lesions, the electrodiagnostic evaluation will truly function as an extension of the clinical examination.

REFERENCES

1. Wilbourn AJ. Brachial plexus lesions. In: Dyck PJ, Thomas PK, editors. Peripheral neuropathy. 4th edition. Philadelphia: Elsevier Saunders; 2005. p. 1339–73.
2. Dodds SD, Wolfe SW. Perinatal brachial plexus palsy. Curr Opin Pediatr 2000;12: 40–7.
3. Sandmire HF, DeMott RK. Erb's palsy: concepts of causation. Obstet Gynecol 2000;95:941–2.
4. Gilbert A. Long-term evaluation of brachial plexus surgery in obstetrical palsy. Hand Clin 1995;11:583–94.
5. Johansson S, Svensson H, Larsson L-G, et al. Brachial plexopathy after postoperative radiotherapy of breast cancer patients. Acta Oncol 2000;39:373–82.
6. Olsen NK, Pfeiffer P, Johannsen L, et al. Radiation-induced brachial plexopathy: neurological follow-up in 161 recurrence-free breast cancer patients. Int J Radiat Oncol Biol Phys 1993;26:43–9.
7. Levin KH, Wilbourn AJ, Maggiano HJ. Cervical rib and median sternotomy-related brachial plexopathies. Neurology 1998;50:1407–13.
8. Sanders RJ, Hammond SL, Rao NM. Thoracic outlet syndrome: a review. Neurologist 2008;14:365–73.
9. Ozoa G, Alves D, Fish DE. Thoracic outlet syndrome. Phys Med Rehabil Clin N Am 2011;22:473–83.
10. Parsonage M, Turner J. Neuralgic amyotrophy: the shoulder-girdle syndrome. Lancet 1948;1:973–8.
11. Tsairis P, Dyck PJ, Mulder DW. Natural history of brachial plexus neuropathy. Arch Neurol 1972;27:109–17.
12. England JD, Sumner AJ. Neuralgic amyotrophy: an increasingly diverse entity. Muscle Nerve 1987;10:60–8.
13. England JD. The variations of neuralgic amyotrophy. Muscle Nerve 1999;22: 435–6.
14. Suarez GA. Immune brachial plexus neuropathy. In: Dyck PJ, Thomas PK, editors. Peripheral neuropathy. 4th edition. Philadelphia: Elsevier Saunders; 2005. p. 2299–308.

15. Suarez GA, Giannini C, Bosch EP, et al. Immune brachial plexus neuropathy: suggestive evidence for an inflammatory-immune pathogenesis. Neurology 1996;46:559–61.
16. De Laat EA, Visser CP, Coene LN, et al. Nerve lesions in primary shoulder dislocations and humeral neck fractures: a prospective clinical and EMG study. J Bone Joint Surg Br 1994;76:381–3.
17. Braddom RL, Wolfe C. Musculocutaneous nerve injury after heavy exercise. Arch Phys Med Rehabil 1978;59:290–3.
18. Mastaglia FL. Musculocutaneous nerve injury after strenuous physical activity. Med J Aust 1986;145:153–4.
19. Davidson JJ, Bassett FH, Nunley JA. Musculocutaneous nerve entrapment revisited. J Shoulder Elbow Surg 1998;7:250–5.
20. Dumitru D, Zwarts MJ. Brachial plexopathies and proximal mononeuropathies. In: Dumitru D, Amato AA, Zwarts M, editors. Electrodiagnostic medicine. 2nd edition. Philadelphia: Hanley & Belfus; 2002. p. 777–836.
21. Preston DC, Shapiro BE. Electromyography and neuromuscular disorders. Philadelphia: Elsevier; 2005.
22. Bassett FH, Nunley JA. Compression of the musculocutaneous nerve at the elbow. J Bone Joint Surg Am 1982;64:1050–2.
23. Sander HW, Conigliari M, Masdeu JC. Antecubital phlebotomy complicated by lateral antebrachial cutaneous neuropathy. N Engl J Med 1998;339:2024.
24. Perlmutter GS, Leffert RD, Zarins B. Direct injury to the axillary nerve in athletes playing contact sports. Am J Sports Med 1997;25:65–8.
25. Cahill BR, Palmer RE. Quadrilateral space syndrome. J Hand Surg 1983;8:65–9.
26. Redler MR, Ruland LJ, McCue FC. Quadrilateral space syndrome in a throwing athlete. Am J Sports Med 1986;14:511–3.
27. McKowen HC, Voorhies RM. Axillary nerve entrapment in the quadrilateral space. J Neurosurg 1987;66:932–4.
28. Aiello I, Serra G, Traina GC, et al. Entrapment of the suprascapular nerve at the spinoglenoid notch. Ann Neurol 1982;12:314–6.
29. Post M, Mayer J. Suprascapular nerve entrapment: diagnosis and treatment. Clin Orthop 1987;223:126–36.
30. Ganzhorn RW, Hocker JT, Horowitz M, et al. Suprascapular nerve entrapment: a case report. J Bone Joint Surg Am 1981;63:492–4.
31. Thomason RC, Schneider W, Kennedy T. Entrapment neuropathy of the inferior branch of the suprascapular nerve by ganglia. Clin Orthop 1982;166:185–7.
32. Moore TP, Fritts HM, Quick DC, et al. Suprascapular nerve entrapment caused by supraglenoid cyst compression. J Shoulder Elbow Surg 1997;6:455–62.
33. McCluskey L, Feinberg D, Dolinskas C. Suprascapular neuropathy related to glenohumeral joint cyst. Muscle Nerve 1999;22:772–7.
34. Zoltan JD. Injury to the suprascapular nerve associated with anterior dislocation of the shoulder: case report and review of the literature. J Trauma 1979;19:203–6.
35. Toon TN, Bravois M, Guillen M. Suprascapular nerve injury following trauma to the shoulder. J Trauma 1981;21:652–5.
36. Antoniadis G, Richter HP, Rath S, et al. Suprascapular nerve entrapment: experience with 28 cases. J Neurosurg 1996;85:1020–5.
37. Ferreti A, DeCarli A, Fontana M. Injury of the suprascapular nerve at the spinoglenoid notch: the natural history of infraspinatus atrophy in volleyball players. Am J Sports Med 1998;26:759–63.
38. Ringel SP, Treihaft M, Carry M, et al. Suprascapular neuropathy in pitchers. Am J Sports Med 1990;18:80–6.

39. Kukowsky B. Suprascapular nerve lesion as an occupational neuropathy in a semiprofessional dancer. Arch Phys Med Rehabil 1993;74:768–9.

40. Felsenthal G, Mondell DL, Reischer MA, et al. Forearm pain secondary to compression syndrome of the lateral cutaneous nerve of the forearm. Arch Phys Med Rehabil 1984;65:139–41.

41. Pribyl R, You SB, Jantra P. Sensory nerve conduction velocity of the medial antebrachial cutaneous nerve. Electromyogr Clin Neurophysiol 1979;19:41–6.

42. Kraft GH. Axillary, musculocutaneous and suprascapular nerve latency studies. Arch Phys Med Rehabil 1972;53:383–7.

43. Oh SJ. Clinical electromyography: nerve conduction studies. 3rd edition. Philadelphia: Lippincott Williams & Wilkins; 2003.

44. Spindler HA, Felsenthal G. Sensory conduction in the musculocutaneous nerve. Arch Phys Med Rehabil 1978;59:20–3.

Anatomical, Clinical, and Electrodiagnostic Features of Radial Neuropathies

Leo H. Wang, MD, PhD[a],*, Michael D. Weiss, MD[b]

KEYWORDS

- Radial • Posterior interosseous • Neuropathy • Electrodiagnostic study

KEY POINTS

- The radial nerve subserves the extensor compartment of the arm.
- Radial nerve lesions are common because of the length and winding course of the nerve.
- The radial nerve is in direct contact with bone at the midpoint and distal third of the humerus, and therefore most vulnerable to compression or contusion from fractures.
- Electrodiagnostic studies are useful to localize and characterize the injury as axonal or demyelinating.
- Radial neuropathies at the midhumeral shaft tend to have good prognosis.

INTRODUCTION

The radial nerve is the principal nerve in the upper extremity that subserves the extensor compartments of the arm. It has a long and winding course rendering it vulnerable to injury. Radial neuropathies are commonly a consequence of acute traumatic injury and only rarely caused by entrapment in the absence of such an injury. This article reviews the anatomy of the radial nerve, common sites of injury and their presentation, and the electrodiagnostic approach to localizing the lesion.

ANATOMY OF THE RADIAL NERVE
Course of the Radial Nerve

The radial nerve subserves the extensors of the arms and fingers and the sensory nerves of the extensor surface of the arm.[1–3] Because it serves the sensory and motor

Disclosures: Dr Wang has no relevant disclosures. Dr Weiss is a consultant for CSL-Behring and a speaker for Grifols Inc. and Walgreens. He has research support from the Northeast ALS Consortium and ALS Therapy Alliance.
^a Department of Neurology, University of Washington Medical Center, University of Washington, Box 356465, 1959 Northeast Pacific Street, Seattle, WA 98195, USA; ^b Department of Neurology, University of Washington Medical Center, 1959 Northeast Pacific Street, Seattle, WA 98195, USA
* Corresponding author.
E-mail address: leowang@uw.edu

Phys Med Rehabil Clin N Am 24 (2013) 33–47
http://dx.doi.org/10.1016/j.pmr.2012.08.018
1047-9651/13/$ – see front matter © 2013 Elsevier Inc. All rights reserved.

nerves of the dorsal arm, it derives innervation from most-to-all of the spinal roots that participate in the brachial plexus (C5–C8 with inconstant T1 contribution), and all three derived trunks. The three trunks divide into the anterior and posterior division. The recombined posterior division continues on as the posterior cord. Both the posterior division and posterior cord serve the posterior "extensor" compartment.[4] The posterior cord follows posterior to the axillary artery and divides into two terminal branches, the axillary nerve and the radial nerve. The axillary nerve lies lateral to the radial nerve and winds around the surgical neck of the humerus. The radial nerve continues posteriorly following the axillary artery and subsequently the deep brachial artery. From the medial side of the humerus, the radial nerve quickly winds back posteriorly around the spiral groove of the humerus.

In the spiral groove, it passes through the medial and lateral heads of the triceps. After it turns in the spiral groove to the dorsal side and becomes lateral to the humerus, it pierces the lateral intermuscular septum (around the distal one-third of the humeral length[5,6]) and courses around the lateral humeral condyle, entering the anterior compartment. At the elbow, it divides in the posterior interosseous nerve (PIN) and the superficial branch of the radial nerve. The superficial branch of the radial nerve goes under the brachioradialis and extends down the radius border only to emerge before the hand and the anatomic snuffbox. The PIN travels deep through the supinator muscle by the arcade of Frohse (a tendinous structure in one- to two-thirds of the population) into the middle of the forearm. In the forearm, it is in contact with the interosseous membrane.

Motor Innervation

The first two motor branches of the radial nerve innervate the forearm extensors, the triceps, and anconeus (**Fig. 1**). These branches come off within or proximal to the spiral groove. The radial nerve only innervates the lateral and medial heads of the triceps; the axillary nerve innervates the third (long) head.[7] After the spiral groove, the radial nerve gives off branches to the brachialis, brachioradialis, and extensor carpi radialis longus. The brachialis and brachioradialis are two of the three forearm flexors. The biceps brachii is the third forearm flexor. The biceps is usually innervated by the musculocutaneous nerve and flexes the forearm in supination. The brachialis is innervated by the musculocutaneous nerve with some contribution to the lateral part by the radial nerve,[8–13] and flexes the forearm in all positions. The brachioradialis is usually the sole radial-innervated forearm flexor and flexes the forearm midway between supination and pronation. The extensor carpi radialis longus is one of several wrist extensors. However, it is the only wrist extensor that is innervated by the radial nerve proximal to the elbow and the PIN and is spared in PIN lesions. The extensor carpi radialis longus is a wrist extensor when the hand is deviated radially.

The first muscle innervated by the PIN is the supinator. The PIN innervates the muscle before the nerve enters the arcade of Frohse.[14] The supinator rotates the forearm outward to result in the palm being face up. The next group of muscles innervated by the PIN is the superficial extensor group comprised of the two other wrist extensors (extensor carpi radialis brevis and extensor carpi ulnaris), and the finger extensors (extensor digitorum communis, extensor digiti minimi, extensor indicis, extensor pollicis longus, abductor pollicis longus, and extensor pollicis brevis). The extensor carpi ulnaris is a wrist extensor when the hand is deviated in the ulnar direction. The extensor digitorum communis extends the metacarpophalangeal joints of the second through fifth digits, whereas the extensor indicis and the extensor digiti minimi extend the same joint for the second and fifth digit, respectively. The extensor pollicis longus extends the thumb into the thumbs-up position. The extensor pollicis brevis extends the thumb at the metacarpophalangeal joint. The abductor pollicis longus abducts the thumb at the wrist.

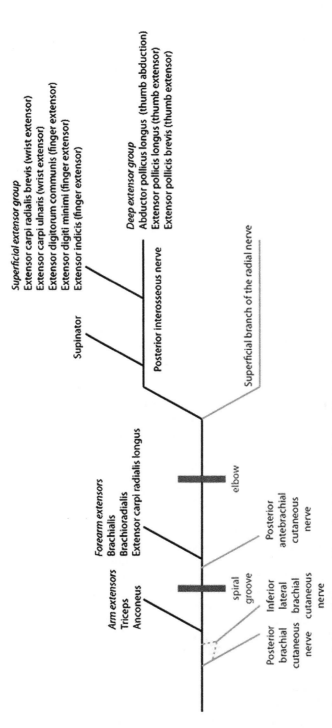

Fig. 1. Branches of the radial nerve. Motor branches are black and sensory branches are gray.

Sensory Innervation

The sensory branches of the radial nerve supply sensation to the dorsum of the arm, forearm, and hand. There are three major sensory branches: (1) the posterior brachial cutaneous nerve, (2) the posterior antebrachial cutaneous nerve, and (3) the superficial branch of the radial nerve. There is great variation in the sensory area innervated by the radial nerve primarily because of overlapping contributions from other nerves.

The posterior brachial cutaneous nerve (posterior cutaneous nerve of arm) originates before the nerve branch to the triceps. This sensory branch covers the midline posterior arm. The inferior lateral brachial cutaneous nerve supplies the lateral arm below the shoulders and may be a separate sensory branch off the main radial nerve or the posterior brachial cutaneous nerve. The sensory territory of the arm is shared with the superior lateral brachial cutaneous nerve, which arises from the axillary nerve, and the intercostobrachial and medial brachial cutaneous nerves.

The posterior antebrachial cutaneous nerve (posterior cutaneous nerve of the forearm) originates between the nerve branch to the triceps and the spiral groove. This sensory branch covers the midline posterior forearm. The sensory territory of the forearm is shared with the medial antebrachial cutaneous nerve and the lateral antebrachial cutaneous nerve that is the terminal branch of the musculocutaneous nerve.

The superficial branch of the radial nerve is a terminal branch of the radial nerve along with the PIN. This sensory branch covers the lateral two-thirds of the dorsum of the hand, extending up to the proximal first 3.5 digits. The sensory territory of the hand is shared with the median nerve that wraps over the palmar surface to cover the tips of the first 3.5 digits and the dorsal ulnar cutaneous nerve from the ulnar nerve. The PIN is mainly a terminal motor branch, but contains few sensory fibers that innervate the ligaments of the radiocarpal, intercarpal, and carpometacarpal joints.[15]

The overlapping contributions from other nerves are important,[16,17] because this may explain why radial nerve lesions are not always accompanied by sensory deficits. These findings may be confounded by the hirsute nature of the dorsal surface of the arm.

ETIOLOGY AND CLINICAL PRESENTATION

Radial nerve lesions are commonly caused by traumatic injury from the length and winding course of the radial nerve about the humerus and uncommonly from entrapment in the absence of acute trauma. Lesions can occur anywhere along its course. Etiologies can include direct external nerve compression or contusion from trauma. Common lesions involve contusion from humeral fractures or external compression affecting the nerve at the mid-arm, contusions from proximal radial fractures, or inflammation around the elbow affecting the PIN. The nerve was the most commonly injured peripheral nerve during World War I, accounting for around one-fourth of peripheral nerve injuries.[18] One conjecture is that the nerve was injured when arms were raised in shock to protect the body or head from flying bullets. In the current era, combat-related wounds are more complicated; however, there was still a significant increase in radial nerve lesions when the US military entered into the Iraq conflicts.[19]

Lesions in the Axilla

Lesions in the axilla affecting the posterior cord or the radial nerve are uncommon. These lesions can result from compression by crutches of the nerve against the humerus or muscles of the axilla ("crutch paralysis"), missile injuries, shoulder dislocation, or proximal humeral fracture. Such lesions would result in weakness of all radial-innervated muscles (most prominently a wrist drop); loss of the triceps and brachioradialis reflexes; and loss of sensation along the dorsum of the arm.

Lesions in the Arm

Lesions in the arm are the most common causes of radial nerve lesions. There are two areas where the radial nerve is in direct contact with the humeral bone without any interposing muscle or fascial tissue as protection and therefore the most vulnerable.[20] One such area is the distal third of the humeral bone where the nerve lies directly lateral to the bone, which is the reason why fracture of the humerus at the supracondylar humeral shaft is the most common cause of a radial nerve lesion in the upper arm. The second area where the radial nerve is in direct contact with the humerus is approximately 6 cm centered around the midshaft of the humerus where the potentially palpable deltoid tuberosity is situated. Here the radial nerve lies posterior to the bone and is especially susceptible to injury in midshaft fractures (occurring in about 12% of such fractures[21]) and iatrogenic injury after operative fixation of such fractures. Tardy radial neuropathies also result from the nerve being compressed or engulfed by callus formed over time after fractures.

The midshaft segment of the radial nerve directly behind humerus is also susceptible to direct compressive lesions. This area is commonly thought to be associated with the "spiral groove." However, this may be more of a conceptual term than a real structural entity.[20] Compressive lesions in this area are responsible for the most classical radial nerve injury, often called "Saturday night palsy" or "sleep paralysis." The common folklore is that such palsies affect patients who drape their arm over a hard chair or sofa edge after deep sleep made deeper by imbibing alcohol or sedatives. However, intense interrogation does not always elicit a history of inebriation or draping the arm over a hard object. Other possible compressive methods can include compressing the arm against the head or body of the patient or his or her partner during sleep. Such similar pathogenesis also explains why radial nerve palsies occur as a consequence of arm positioning during anesthesia.[22] This site is also susceptible to compressive neuropathies in patients with hereditary neuropathy with liability to pressure palsies.[23]

Other rare manifestations include compression by tendinous fibers of the lateral head of the triceps, tourniquets, and arm muscles during vigorous or repetitive arm exercise. Patients with such lesions usually present with wrist and finger drops. There is variable sparing of muscles innervated by the radial nerve above the elbow depending on the location of the lesion and differential fascicular involvement. Lesions at the "spiral groove" tend to have weakness of radial-innervated muscles except for arm extension because the motor branch to the triceps and anconeus splits off before the midshaft area. Weakness of the brachialis muscle may or may not be present (depending on differential fascicular involvement). Because the posterior brachial cutaneous nerve also splits off before the midshaft area, if sensation is lost, it only affects the forearm or hand. The triceps reflex is spared. Lesions distal to the "spiral groove" above the elbow may spare the brachioradialis or extensor carpi radialis longus muscles.

Lesions at the Elbow

Lesions at the elbow mainly affect muscles innervated by the PIN. Traumatic contusions to the nerve can be the result of fractures of the proximal radius or midarm fractures of the radius or ulna and iatrogenic injury during repair of such fractures and arthroscopic elbow procedures. Nerve entrapment can occur at the tendinous edge of the extensor carpi radialis, the distal edge of the supinator, and the arcade of Frohse. Compressive lesions to the nerve can be caused by inflamed hypertrophied synovium in rheumatoid arthritis and soft tissue masses and tumors, such as lipomas, myoxmas, ganglia from the elbow joints, neurofibromas, schwannomas, chondromas, traumatic aneurysms of the posterior interosseous artery, and hemangiomas.[24–34] A tardy posterior interosseous neuropathy can also occur after unreduced radial head dislocation and proximal ulnar fractures.[35]

The radial tunnel and its associated syndrome seem to be orthopedic concepts that engender much skepticism from neurologists. The radial tunnel is located anterior to the proximal radius after the radial capitulum and before the PIN travels below the superficial portion of the supinator muscle at the arcade of Frohse. The brachioradialis, extensor carpi brevis, and longus form the lateral border and the biceps tendon and brachialis muscle form the medial border. Fibrous bands, muscles, or blood vessels within this area have been implicated in PIN entrapment.[36] Other noncompressive causes of posterior interosseous neuropathy are acute brachial plexus neuropathy (brachial neuritis) or multifocal motor neuropathy.

The radial tunnel syndrome is associated with chronic pain without any significant motor deficits. It is mainly characterized by localized tenderness over the lateral part of the proximal forearm, an area distal to the lateral epicondyle, and worsened by supination or finger and wrist extension. Pain may confound the exact degree of weakness. The crux of the controversy is whether neurologists believe there is true involvement of the PIN because there is usually none of the expected finger greater than wrist extensor weakness. Proponents believe that chronic damage and inflammation of the extensor muscle attachment to the epicondyle by the supinator, extensor carpi radialis brevis, extensor digitorum, extensor digiti minimi, and extensor carpi ulnaris as a consequence of overuse cause an entrapment of the PIN in the radial tunnel and argue that the pain is from impingement of the PIN pain fibers to the bone, joint, or muscle. There is significant overlap clinically between the radial tunnel syndrome and lateral epicondylitis, also known as tennis elbow, lateral tennis elbow, or lateral tendinosis, which is the result of overuse of the extensor and supinator muscles, especially with playing tennis. Radial tunnel syndrome is thought to be the reason why patients have resistant, chronic, and persistent tennis elbow. Neurologists tend to be skeptical that radial tunnel release relieves pain because of direct decompression of the PIN and believe that the division of the superficial portion of the supinator muscle itself relieves tension on the lateral epicondyle.[36] It is the contention of the authors that entrapment of the radial nerve at the radial tunnel is a rare occurrence and cannot be clearly established without electrophysiologic confirmation.

Typically, supination and sensation are spared in posterior interosseous neuropathies. Finger extension is more affected than wrist extension weakness, because the motor branch to the extensor carpi radialis splits off before the elbow. Therefore, the wrist deviates radially, especially when forming a fist or extending. An important examination point is that examination of ulnar-innervated muscles (while in the dropped wrist position) may demonstrate a pseudoulnar palsy as the ulnar-innervated intrinsic hand muscles insert on the extensor muscles and require coactivation of radial-innervated finger extensors.[37] This can be more apparent in patients with chronic radial nerve palsies where there is loss of intrinsic hand muscle strength because of prolonged disuse. Some patients with nontraumatic posterior interosseous neuropathy may complain of pain,[38] possibly caused by injury to the sensory fibers of the PIN that innervate the ligaments of the radiocarpal, intercarpal, and carpometacarpal joints.[15]

Lesions of the Superficial Branch of the Radial Nerve

Lesions of the superficial branch of the radial nerve cause a pure sensory syndrome known as cheiralgia paresthetica or Wartenberg disease. Traumatic contusions caused by crush or twisting injuries of the wrist or forearm can cause such a neuropathy. Entrapments are rare. Compressive lesions can be secondary to repetitive occupational pronation-supination movements, wristwatch bands, casts, or even handcuffs. Similar to "Saturday night palsy," many patients with handcuff neuropathies are inebriated.[39,40] Patients typically describe pain or burning over the sensory area of the superficial branch of the radial nerve centered around the anatomic snuffbox. This can be exacerbated by pinching and gripping activities or hyperpronation provocative testing (ie, pronation of the forearm while the wrist is in ulnar flexion).

Differential Diagnosis

The differential diagnosis for radial nerve palsies includes other lesions along the motor pathway that subserve the activation of extensor compartment muscles of the forearm. Distally to proximally, such sites include the posterior cord, brachial plexus, cervical roots, and the cerebral cortex. Typically, there are other clues to distinguish among these sites of injury. Posterior cord lesions typically also involve deltoid weakness and sensory loss in the shoulder region. Although a C7 radiculopathy may mimic a proximal radial neuropathy, including mild sensory symptoms and signs in the radial sensory distribution in the dorsum of the hand, the usual finding also of sensory loss involving the palmar aspect of the third finger would not be seen with a radial neuropathy. When a C7 nerve root lesion is severe enough to cause muscle weakness, median-innervated muscles supplied by the C7 nerve root, such as the pronator teres and flexor carpi radialis, may also be affected excluding the diagnosis of radial neuropathy. Cerebral cortical infarcts located in the precentral "hand knob" area may cause an isolated wrist drop but are usually accompanied with signs of upper motor neuron dysfunction, such as hyperreflexia. The differential diagnosis for a partial PIN lesion may include rupture of thumb and finger extensors that can occur in rheumatoid arthritis and a focal myopathy of the finger extensors.[41] Rheumatologic diseases may also mimic neuromuscular weakness of the forearm extensor compartment. For instance, de Quervain tenosynovitis can cause pain in the distribution of the superficial branch of the radial nerve and is in the differential diagnosis of lesions affecting that nerve.

ASSESSMENT
Electrodiagnostic Testing

Electrodiagnostic testing is often the key to confirming a radial mononeuropathy and localizing the area of injury, and is considered an extension of the neurologic examination. It should involve radial sensory nerve conduction, radial motor nerve conduction, including segments in the proximal arm, and needle electromyography (EMG) study of relevant muscles (see **Fig. 1**; **Fig. 2**). Testing should also be performed to rule out other disorders that may mimic a radial neuropathy, such as C7 radiculopathy, brachial plexopathy, or mononeuropathy multiplex.

Motor Nerve Conduction Studies

Motor nerve conduction study of the radial nerve is most helpful in identifying the demyelinating lesions in the "spiral groove." Motor nerve conduction study is usually performed by placing the active electrode over the belly of the extensor indicis proprius, three to four fingerbreadths from the distal ulna (**Fig. 3**A). The distal stimulation

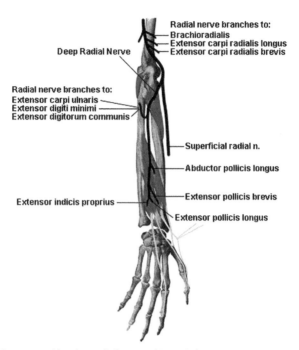

Radial nerve branches to:
Brachioradialis
Extensor carpi radialis longus
Extensor carpi radialis brevis

Deep Radial Nerve

Radial nerve branches to:
Extensor carpi ulnaris
Extensor digiti minimi
Extensor digitorum communis

Superficial radial n.

Abductor pollicis longus

Extensor pollicis brevis

Extensor indicis proprius

Extensor pollicis longus

Fig. 2. Muscles innervated by the radial nerve. (Copyright 2003–2004 University of Washington. All rights reserved including all photographs and images. No reuse, redistribution or commercial use without prior written permission of the authors and the University of Washington. *From* Teitz C, Graney D. Musculoskeletal atlas: a musculoskeletal atlas of the human body. Seattle (WA): University of Washington, http://depts.washington.edu/msatlas/127.html,2012; with permission.)

site is usually 4 to 8 cm proximal to the middle of the forearm. A second stimulation site is at the lateral epicondyle. A third stimulation site is around the "spiral groove." Onset latency for the distal compound muscle action potential (CMAP) is usually fast, as are conduction velocities, which can be as high as 75 m/s.[42] Other recording sites are the extensor digitorum communis, extensor carpi ulnaris, and brachioradialis muscles.[43]

Conduction block or temporal dispersion can occur proximal to midshaft. The key to localizing such an injury is stimulation proximal to the "spiral groove" to detect the conduction block. Axonal loss may be estimated from the decrease in the compound motor action potential and typically occurs between 5 and 7 days after an insult. In a case series of 21 patients with nontraumatic compression-related radial neuropathy at the spiral groove and radial motor nerve conduction studies performed 7 days or later, 10% had reduced distal radial CMAP amplitude and approximately 60% had conduction block or reduced conduction velocity in the spiral groove.[44] In the same case series, there was clinical follow-up on 23 patients, who all experienced complete recovery.[44] In a small case series of 33 patients with traumatic radial neuropathies presented by Malikowski and colleagues,[45] the absence of radial CMAP was associated with 65% partial or full recovery, and the presence of radial CMAP was associated with 85% partial or full recovery.

Sensory Nerve Conduction Studies

Sensory nerve conduction study of the radial nerve typically assesses just the superficial branch of the radial nerve and is recorded at the anatomic stuff box (see **Fig. 3**B)

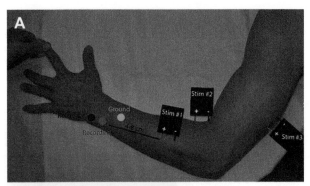

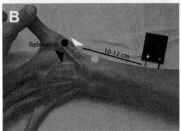

Fig. 3. Radial nerve conduction studies. (*A*) Radial motor nerve conduction study recorded from the extensor indicis proprius. The recording electrode is placed two fingerbreadths or approximately 4 cm proximal to the ulnar styloid over the motor point of the extensor indicis proprius. The first stimulation point (Stim #1) is 4 to 8 cm proximal to the recording electrode in the forearm. The second stimulation point (Stim #2) is in the groove between the biceps and brachioradialis muscles in the elbow. The third stimulation point (Stim #3) is around the spiral groove. (*B*) Sensory nerve conduction study of the superficial branch of the radial nerve recorded from the anatomic snuffbox. The anatomic snuffbox is best shown by extending and abducting the thumb. The *black arrowhead* shows the medial border formed by the tendon of the extensor pollicis longus. The *white arrowhead* shows the lateral border formed by tendons of the extensor pollicis brevis and abductor pollicis longus.

with stimulation 10 cm proximally at the lateral border of the forearm along the radius. Therefore, the study is only able to document abnormalities in that region. The study may be normal in proximal demyelinating lesions (in approximately 75%–80% of the studies in Mondelli and colleagues[46] and Arnold and colleagues[44]), or demonstrate a prolonged distal motor latency and reduced prolonged conduction velocity if demyelination affects a more distal portion of the nerve.

Axonal loss of sensory nerves is seen more commonly in traumatic radial neuropathies.[46] Axonal loss of sensory nerves, if shown, can be documented by a decrease in the sensory nerve action potential amplitude after 7 to 10 days. If still within the normal range, mild axonal injury may be demonstrated by comparing the sensory nerve action potential amplitude with the normal side to demonstrate a greater than 50% reduction in the side-to-side amplitudes. The absence or presence of the sensory response typically has no bearing on the prognosis of recovery in traumatic radial neuropathies.[45] However, posterior brachial cutaneous sensory nerve conduction studies may have some prognostic value in midforearm lesions.[47] For these studies, the nerve is stimulated at the elbow 2 cm medial to the lateral epicondyle, between the triceps and biceps muscles. The recording electrode is placed 12 cm distal to the stimulating electrode along a line between the stimulation electrode and the mid-dorsum of the wrist.

Needle EMG

The needle EMG examination is as equally important as nerve conduction in localizing the lesion. Muscles typically studied during needle EMG include, from proximal to distal, the triceps brachii (**Fig. 4**A), brachioradialis (see **Fig. 4**B), extensor carpi radialis (see **Fig. 4**C), extensor digitorum communis (see **Fig. 4**D), extensor carpi ulnaris

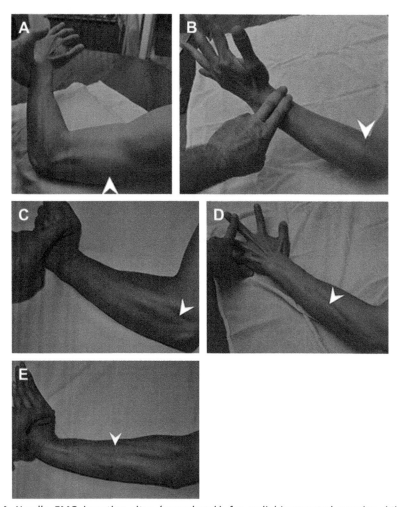

Fig. 4. Needle EMG insertion sites (*arrowheads*) for radial-innervated muscles. (*A*) The triceps brachii is tested by extension of the arm against the hand. The insertion site is shown for the lateral head of the triceps. (*B*) The brachioradialis is tested by flexing the forearm midway between supination and pronation. The insertion site is at the level of the antebrachial cubital fossa. (*C*) The extensor carpi radialis longus is tested by extending the hand at the wrist while the hand is deviated toward the radius. Flexing or relaxing the fingers and thumb minimizes participation of the digit extensors. The insertion site is two finger-breadths distal to the lateral epicondyle. (*D*) The extensor digitorum communis is tested by extension of the middle finger. The insertion site is a third way down the radius and ulna and midpoint between the two. (*E*) The extensor carpi ulnaris is tested by extending the hand at the wrist while the hand is deviated toward the ulna. The insertion site is at the level of the mid-ulna above its shaft.

(see **Fig. 4E**), and extensor indicis proprius. Needle EMG of these muscles helps localize the lesion along the radial nerve. The anconeus is also an easily examined muscle but is an extension of the triceps. Because the differential diagnosis includes posterior cord or C7 nerve root lesions, examination of the deltoid, pronator teres, or flexor carpi radialis may also be helpful in localizing the lesions.

Axonal injuries may cause neurogenic findings in time. Demyelinating injuries, such as compression at the midhumeral shaft, cause a reduction in recruitment pattern. However, the distinction between axonal and demyelinating injuries may be best made approximately 4 weeks after the initial injury. As such, a repeat EMG study may be necessary if the initial study was done too early. In one study by Arnold and colleagues,[44] the authors found abnormal spontaneous activity in all patients at least 3 weeks after symptom onset, despite prominent demyelinating features. Mondelli and colleagues[46] also showed abnormal spontaneous activity in 50% of nontraumatic cases and 72% of traumatic cases. In traumatic cases, assessing recruitment in the EMG examination of the brachioradialis may be the most predictive of recovery. In one study, only 33% of patients with absent recruitment had good outcomes, 67% of patients with discrete recruitment had good outcomes, and 92% of patients with full, central, or reduced recruitment had good outcomes.[45] Posterior interosseous neuropathies are better identified by EMG than nerve conduction studies. Interestingly, partial denervation of the extensor carpi radialis can be seen.[38]

ALTERNATIVE TESTING MODALITIES

Ultrasound is a newer imaging modality that can be useful in localizing lesions, especially compressive masses.[48–51] There are small case series that report ultrasonographic localization of radial nerve swelling in traumatic and nontraumatic radial neuropathy at the spiral groove.[50] Most promising was the ability to diagnose the lesion rapidly after symptom onset. However, these studies are small and require considerable technical expertise. Magnetic resonance neurogram may be another imaging modality that is useful; however, no dedicated studies have been published.

TREATMENT AND PROGNOSIS

The main management goal of radial neuropathies is to improve hand function. Radial neuropathies at the midhumeral shaft tend to have good prognosis regardless of whether they are demyelinating or axonal. Demyelinating lesions usually improve in 3 months and have an approximately 67% to 100% rate of full recovery.[44,52,53] Axonal injuries caused by closed fracture of the humerus also have a recovery rate around 90%.[21] Therefore, in patients with radial neuropathies associated with fracture of the humeral shaft, the recommendation is to wait for clinical improvement for 2 to 6 months before exploratory surgery of the radial nerve.[21] The recovery of the nerve is similar with early or late repair. A similar approach is recommended for posterior interosseous neuropathies secondary to forearm fractures or orthopedic procedures of the arm or elbow.[54] In these cases, compressive masses deserve surgical exploration.

In severe cases of radial neuropathy where there is no recovery of radial nerve function, tendon transfers or median to radial nerve transfers[55] have been documented to be of benefit. Tendon transfers usually involve transposition of volar-sided tendons to the dorsal compartment through subcutaneous tunnels, and usually involve the pronator teres, flexor carpi ulnaries, palmaris longus, or flexor digitorum communis with the idea of restoring wrist, finger, or thumb extension along with thumb abduction.[56–62]

The main treatment of wrist drop is to provide dorsal wrist cock-up splints with or without dynamic finger extensions. This maintains some hand function, especially ulnar-innervated finger abduction and adduction. Splinting remains the most important intervention, especially because most radial palsies have a good prognosis.

SUMMARY

Radial neuropathy is a common mononeuropathy of the upper extremity and may be encountered as the result of acute traumatic injuries or fractures, surgical intervention, or compression, which are increased in wartime and inebriation. Clinically, posterior cord plexopathy, cervical radiculopathies, cortical strokes in the precentral "hand knob" area, and focal myopathies may present with similar findings of wrist or finger drop. Electrodiagnostic studies are useful to determine the location and pathologic nature (ie, axonal or demyelinating) of the injury. Electrodiagnostic testing should include motor nerve conduction studies to the extensor indicis proprius, sensory nerve conduction studies of the superficial branch of the radial nerve, and needle EMG of radial-innervated muscles and nonradial muscles supplied by the C7 nerve root. Radial neuropathies associated with humeral mid-shaft fractures or compression lesions in particular generally have a good prognosis.

ACKNOWLEDGMENTS

The authors thank Carol Teitz, MD, and Dan Graney, PhD, for permission to use their illustration from the University of Washington "Musculoskeletal Atlas: A Musculoskeletal Atlas of the Human Body". They also thank William T. Kidder for expert help with photography and Dr Glenn Lopate for reviewing the manuscript.

REFERENCES

1. Radial nerve [online]. Available at: http://en.wikipedia.org/wiki/Radial_nerve.
2. Brazis P, Masdeu J, Biller J. Localization in clinical anatomy. Philadelphia: Lippincott Williams & Wilkins; 2007.
3. Fisch A. Neuroanatomy: draw it to know it. New York: Oxford University Press; 2009.
4. Moore K, Dalley A, AMR A. Clinically oriented anatomy. 6th edition. Baltimore (USA): Lippincott Williams & Wilkins; 2009.
5. Cox CL, Riherd D, Tubbs RS, et al. Predicting radial nerve location using palpable landmarks. Clin Anat 2010;23:420–6.
6. Fleming P, Lenehan B, Sankar R, et al. One-third, two-thirds: relationship of the radial nerve to the lateral intermuscular septum in the arm. Clin Anat 2004;17: 26–9.
7. de Seze MP, Rezzouk J, de Seze M, et al. Does the motor branch of the long head of the triceps brachii arise from the radial nerve? An anatomic and electromyographic study. Surg Radiol Anat 2004;26:459–61.
8. Blackburn SC, Wood CP, Evans DJ, et al. Radial nerve contribution to brachialis in the UK caucasian population: position is predictable based on surface landmarks. Clin Anat 2007;20:64–7.
9. Ip MC, Chang KS. A study on the radial supply of the human brachialis muscle. Anat Rec 1968;162:363–71.
10. Ji H, Chung I. The muscular branch of the radial nerve to the brachialis muscle in Korean. Korean J Phys Anthropol 2002;15:127–31.

11. Mahakkanukrauh P, Somsarp V. Dual innervation of the brachialis muscle. Clin Anat 2002;15:206–9.
12. Puffer RC, Murthy NS, Spinner RJ. The spectrum of denervation patterns on MRI reflects the dual innervation of the brachialis. Clin Anat 2011;24:511–3.
13. Sunderland S. The intraneural topography of the radial, median and ulnar nerves. Brain 1945;68:243–99.
14. Tubbs RS, Salter EG, Wellons JC III, et al. Superficial surgical landmarks for iden-tifying the posterior interosseous nerve. J Neurosurg 2006;104:796–9.
15. Dellon AL, Seif SS. Anatomic dissections relating the posterior interosseous nerve to the carpus, and the etiology of dorsal wrist ganglion pain. J Hand Surg 1978;3:326–32.
16. Loukas M, Louis RG Jr, Wartmann CT, et al. The clinical anatomy of the commu-nications between the radial and ulnar nerves on the dorsal surface of the hand. Surg Radiol Anat 2008;30:85–90.
17. Marathe R, Mankar S, Joshi M, et al. Communication between radial nerve and medial cutaneous nerve of forearm. J Neurosci Rural Pract 2010;1:49–50.
18. Pollack L, Davis L. Peripheral nerve injuries. New York: Paul B. Hoeber; 1933.
19. Brininger TL, Antczak A, Breland HL. Upper extremity injuries in the U.S. mili-tary during peacetime years and wartime years. J Hand Ther 2008;21:115–22 [quiz: 123].
20. Carlan D, Pratt J, Patterson JM, et al. The radial nerve in the brachium: an anatomic study in human cadavers. J Hand Surg 2007;32:1177–82.
21. Shao YC, Harwood P, Grotz MR, et al. Radial nerve palsy associated with frac-tures of the shaft of the humerus: a systematic review. J Bone Joint Surg Br 2005;87:1647–52.
22. Tuncali BE, Tuncali B, Kuvaki B, et al. Radial nerve injury after general anaes-thesia in the lateral decubitus position. Anaesthesia 2005;60:602–4.
23. Mouton P, Tardieu S, Gouider R, et al. Spectrum of clinical and electrophysio-logic features in HNPP patients with the 17p11.2 deletion. Neurology 1999;52:1440–6.
24. Ganapathy K, Winston T, Seshadri V. Posterior interosseous nerve palsy due to intermuscular lipoma. Surg Neurol 2006;65:495–6 [discussion: 496].
25. Jou IM, Wang HN, Wang PH, et al. Compression of the radial nerve at the elbow by a ganglion: two case reports. J Med Case Rep 2009;3:7258.
26. Malipeddi A, Reddy VR, Kallarackal G. Posterior interosseous nerve palsy: an unusual complication of rheumatoid arthritis: case report and review of the litera-ture. Semin Arthritis Rheum 2011;40:576–9.
27. Nishida J, Shimamura T, Ehara S, et al. Posterior interosseous nerve palsy caused by parosteal lipoma of proximal radius. Skeletal Radiol 1998;27:375–9.
28. Steiger R, Vogelin E. Compression of the radial nerve caused by an occult ganglion. Three case reports. J Hand Surg 1998;23:420–1.
29. Valer A, Carrera L, Ramirez G. Myxoma causing paralysis of the posterior inter-osseous nerve. Acta Orthop Belg 1993;59:423–5.
30. Loh YC, Stanley JK, Jari S, et al. Neuroma of the distal posterior interosseous nerve. A cause of iatrogenic wrist pain. J Bone Joint Surg Br 1998;80:629–30.
31. Bowen TL, Stone KH. Posterior interosseous nerve paralysis caused by a ganglion at the elbow. J Bone Joint Surg Br 1966;48:774–6.
32. Cravens G, Kline DG. Posterior interosseous nerve palsies. Neurosurgery 1990;27:397–402.
33. Dharapak C, Nimberg GA. Posterior interosseous nerve compression. Report of a case caused by traumatic aneurysm. Clin Orthop Relat Res 1974;101:225–8.

34. Lallemand RC, Weller RO. Intraneural neurofibromas involving the posterior interosseous nerve. J Neurol Neurosurg Psychiatr 1973;36:991–6.
35. Fernandez E, Pallini R, Lauretti L, et al. Neurosurgery of the peripheral nervous system: the posterior interosseous nerve syndrome. Surg Neurol 1998;49:637–9.
36. Campbell WW, Landau ME. Controversial entrapment neuropathies. Neurosurg Clin N Am 2008;19:597–608, vi–vii.
37. Sadeh M, Gilad R, Dabby R, et al. Apparent weakness of ulnar-innervated muscles in radial palsy. Neurology 2004;62:1424–5.
38. Fardin P, Negrin P, Sparta S, et al. Posterior interosseous nerve neuropathy. Clinical and electromyographical aspects. Electromyogr Clin Neurophysiol 1992;32:229–34.
39. Grant AC, Cook AA. A prospective study of handcuff neuropathies. Muscle Nerve 2000;23:933–8.
40. Scott TF, Yager JG, Gross JA. Handcuff neuropathy revisited. Muscle Nerve 1989;12:219–20.
41. Erdem S, Demirci M, Tan E. Focal myopathy mimicking posterior interosseous nerve syndrome. Muscle Nerve 2001;24:969–72.
42. Trojaborg W, Sindrup EH. Motor and sensory conduction in different segments of the radial nerve in normal subjects. J Neurol Neurosurg Psychiatr 1969;32:354–9.
43. Negrin P, Fardin P. The electromyographic prognosis of traumatic paralysis of radial nerve. Study of its myelinic and axonal damage. Electromyogr Clin Neurophysiol 1984;24:481–4.
44. Arnold WD, Krishna VR, Freimer M, et al. Prognosis of acute compressive radial neuropathy. Muscle Nerve 2012;45:893–5.
45. Malikowski T, Micklesen PJ, Robinson LR. Prognostic values of electrodiagnostic studies in traumatic radial neuropathy. Muscle Nerve 2007;36:364–7.
46. Mondelli M, Morana P, Ballerini M, et al. Mononeuropathies of the radial nerve: clinical and neurographic findings in 91 consecutive cases. J Electromyogr Kinesiol 2005;15:377–83.
47. Lo YL, Prakash KM, Leoh TH, et al. Posterior antebrachial cutaneous nerve conduction study in radial neuropathy. J Neurol Sci 2004;223:199–202.
48. Bodner G, Buchberger W, Schocke M, et al. Radial nerve palsy associated with humeral shaft fracture: evaluation with US. Initial experience. Radiology 2001;219:811–6.
49. Jacobson JA, Fessell DP, Lobo Lda G, et al. Entrapment neuropathies I: upper limb (carpal tunnel excluded). Semin Musculoskelet Radiol 2010;14:473–86.
50. Lo YL, Fook-Chong S, Leoh TH, et al. Rapid ultrasonographic diagnosis of radial entrapment neuropathy at the spiral groove. J Neurol Sci 2008;271:75–9.
51. Bodner G, Huber B, Schwabegger A, et al. Sonographic detection of radial nerve entrapment within a humerus fracture. J Ultrasound Med 1999;18:703–6.
52. Escolar DM, Jones HR Jr. Pediatric radial mononeuropathies: a clinical and electromyographic study of sixteen children with review of the literature. Muscle Nerve 1996;19:876–83.
53. Watson BV, Brown WF. Quantitation of axon loss and conduction block in acute radial nerve palsies. Muscle Nerve 1992;15:768–73.
54. Stewart J. Focal peripheral neuropathies. 4th edition. West Vancouver (Canada): JBJ Publishing; 2010.
55. Lowe JB III, Tung TR, Mackinnon SE. New surgical option for radial nerve paralysis. Plast Reconstr Surg 2002;110:836–43.
56. Chuinard RG, Boyes JH, Stark HH, et al. Tendon transfers for radial nerve palsy: use of superficialis tendons for digital extension. J Hand Surg 1978;3:560–70.

57. Kozin SH. Tendon transfers for radial and median nerve palsies. J Hand Ther 2005;18:208–15.
58. Reid RL. Radial nerve palsy. Hand Clin 1988;4:179–85.
59. Riordan DC. Tendon transfers for nerve paralysis of the hand and wrist. Curr Pract Orthop Surg 1964;23:17–40.
60. Riordan DC. Tendon transfers in hand surgery. J Hand Surg 1983;8:748–53.
61. Tsuge K. Tendon transfers for radial nerve palsy. Aust N Z J Surg 1980;50:267–72.
62. Krishnan KG, Schackert G. An analysis of results after selective tendon transfers through the interosseous membrane to provide selective finger and thumb extension in chronic irreparable radial nerve lesions. J Hand Surg 2008;33:223–31.

Clinical Features and Electrodiagnosis of Ulnar Neuropathies

Mark E. Landau, MD[a],*, William W. Campbell, MD, MSHA[b]

KEYWORDS

- Ulnar neuropathy • Electrodiagnosis • EMG • Sensitivity • Specificity

KEY POINTS

- The most common locations for ulnar mononeuropathy are at the retroepicondylar (RTC) groove and the humeroulnar arcade.
- Precise localization of the ulnar nerve below and above the elbow with submaximal stimulations improves accuracy of the distance measurement.
- The factors that can lead to spuriously low nerve conduction velocity (NCV) across the elbow include a cold elbow and falsely low distance measurements.
- Multiple internally consistent abnormalities should be present to ensure accurate diagnosis of ulnar neuropathy at the elbow.
- In the setting of ulnar mononeuropathies, when routine electrodiagnostic studies fail to demonstrate focal slowing of NCV across the elbow, short-segment techniques should be done.
- The electromyographer should ascertain the specific point of abnormality (ie, the RTC groove, humeroulnar arcade, or other location) prior to surgical referrals.

INTRODUCTION

The ulnar nerve may be compressed at several sites. Ulnar neuropathy at the elbow (UNE) is the second most frequent upper extremity compression neuropathy. There are 4 different sites of potential compression in the region of the elbow. The nerve may also sustain focal injury in the wrist and hand and even less frequently in the axilla, upper arm, or forearm. Distinguishing between these different compression sites is not

Disclaimer: The views expressed are those of the authors and do not reflect the official policies of the Department of the Army, the Department of Defense, or the US Government.
[a] Department of Neurology, Walter Reed National Military Medical Center, 8900 Wisconsin Ave, Bethesda, MD 20815, USA; [b] Department of Neurology, Uniformed Services University of the Health Sciences, Bethesda, MD 20814, USA
* Corresponding author.
E-mail address: Mark.Landau@med.navy.mil

Phys Med Rehabil Clin N Am 24 (2013) 49–66
http://dx.doi.org/10.1016/j.pmr.2012.08.019   pmr.theclinics.com
1047-9651/13/$ – see front matter Published by Elsevier Inc.

always straightforward. In most cases, the earliest electrodiagnostic findings are demyelinating. Early diagnosis and management can prevent secondary axonal damage and permanent disability.

RELEVANT ANATOMY

Anatomic details are important in understanding focal ulnar mononeuropathies.[1,2] The ulnar nerve branches from the medial cord of the brachial plexus and courses in the forearm just medial to the brachial artery. It passes between the medial intermuscular septum (MIS) and the medial head of the triceps prior to reaching the medial epicondyle. The existence of the arcade of Struthers between the MIS and medial head of the triceps is debatable.[3] The nerve then passes just dorsal to the ME, and into the ulnar groove, ventral to the olecranon process (OP). It subsequently passes beneath the humeroulnar aponeurotic arcade (HUA), a dense aponeurosis between the tendinous attachments of the flexor carpi ulnaris (FCU) muscle typically 1.0 cm to 2.5 cm distal to the ME.[2] The nerve then runs through the belly of the FCU and exits from the muscle through the deep flexor pronator aponeurosis.

In elbow extension, the medial epicondyle and OP are juxtaposed, with the HUA slack and the nerve lying loosely in the groove. With elbow flexion, the OP moves forward and away from the ME. The humeral head of the FCU, attached to the ME, and the ulnar head, attached to the OP, are pulled apart, progressively tightening the HUA across the nerve, resulting in pressure increases up 19 mm Hg in the ulnar groove.[4] In addition, with elbow flexion, the ulnar collateral ligament bulges into the floor of the groove and the medial head of the triceps may be pulled into the groove from behind.[1] In extension, the ulnar groove is smooth, round, and capacious, but in flexion the nerve finds itself in inhospitable surroundings, in a flattened, tortuous, and narrow canal with the HUA pulled tightly across it. In full flexion, the nerve partially or completely subluxes out of its groove in many normal individuals.[5]

The only motor branches in the forearm are those to the FCU and flexor digitorum profundus (FDP). The palmar ulnar cutaneous branch (PUC) separates from the main trunk in the mid to distal forearm, and enters the hand superficial to the Guyon canal, supplying sensation to the skin of the hypothenar region. The dorsal ulnar cutaneous (DUC) branch leaves the main trunk 5 cm to 10 cm proximal to the wrist, arcs around the ulna, and innervates the dorsal skin of the medial hand and fingers. The ulnar nerve then enters the hand through the Guyon canal.

The transverse carpal ligament, which arches over and forms the roof of the carpal tunnel, dips downward to form the floor of the Guyon canal. The roof, lateral, and medial boundaries of the canal are formed by the volar carpal ligament and the thin palmaris brevis muscle, hook of the hamate, and the pisiform bone, respectively. Just beyond the transverse carpal ligament, the pisohamate ligament runs from the pisiform bone to the hook of the hamate and forms the distal part of the floor of the canal. The nerve exits the Guyon canal by passing beneath the pisohamate ligament.

In the hand, the nerve bifurcates into the superficial terminal division and the deep palmar division. The superficial terminal portion supplies sensation to the small finger and ulnar half of the ring finger. The deep palmar branch subserves no cutaneous sensation but innervates all of the hypothenar muscles, the third and fourth lumbricals, all of the palmar and dorsal interossei, the adductor pollicis, the deep head of the flexor pollicis brevis, and the first dorsal interosseous (FDI). There are frequent anatomic variations.

Anatomic factors account for much of the susceptibility of the ulnar nerve to injury at the elbow. The lack of protective covering over the nerve in its course through the ulnar groove accounts for its susceptibility to external pressure. Repetitive elbow flexion and extension may predispose to UNE because of the dynamic changes in the nerve's passageway with motion. With elbow joint derangement due to trauma or arthritic changes, the nerve's vulnerability increases even further. Valgus deformities increase the stretch on the nerve with elbow flexion, and osteophytic overgrowth further narrows an often already narrow passageway. Most ulnar neuropathies occur at the level of the RTC groove. The nerve may also be entrapped at the HUA or at the point of exit from the FCU.[6–10]

The internal architecture of the ulnar nerve, particularly the fascicular arrangement, has an important impact on the clinical and electrodiagnostic findings.[11] The fibers destined for the FCU, the PUC, and DUC lie in individual fascicles at the elbow and in a deep dorsolateral position, rendering them less susceptible to damage with UNE. This can create difficulty differentiating UNE from ulnar neuropathy at the wrist (UNW).

CLINICAL FEATURES

In the majority of patients with UNE, the initial symptoms are typically intermittent numbness and tingling in the ulnar nerve distribution, often associated with elbow flexion, particularly at night. These intermittent symptoms may occur over months or years, although in patients with more severe entrapment, permanent symptoms may develop more rapidly. The amount of pain and paresthesia varies, and for some patients the sensory loss is not bothersome. In contrast to carpal tunnel syndrome, where pain is usually a prominent feature, UNE tends to cause numbness and paresthesias and pain is less prominent, often absent. Vanderpool and colleagues[1] state that subjective motor loss may not be noted for months or years, depending on the degree of compression. In contrast, pain and dysesthesias are more frequent components with acute injury to the elbow, pain and dysesthesias are more frequent components. Elbow pain is rare except in acute focal injury.

The sensory abnormalities in ulnar neuropathies do not always conform to the expected distribution due to anatomic variations. Splitting sensory symptoms of the ring finger is highly specific for ulnar neuropathy. C8 radiculopathy and brachial plexopathy are more likely to affect the entire ring finger or spare it completely. In UNE, paresthesias typically involve the digits to a greater extent than the dorsal and palmar aspects of the medial hand, due to relative sparing of the DUC and PUC.[11] The cutaneous field of the ulnar nerve does not extend more than a few centimeters proximal to the wrist crease. Sensory abnormalities in the forearm should raise the suspicion for plexus or nerve root lesions.

The motor disability from ulnar nerve palsy is related to 4 components[1]: strength of pinch between the thumb and adjacent digits,[2] coordination of thumb and digits in tasks requiring precision,[3] synchrony of digital flexion during grasp, and[4] strength of power grasp. Wrist flexion weakness is rarely significant due to normal function of the flexor carpi radialis.

Froment sign is due to weakness of the adductor policus and FDI, with compensation provided by the flexor pollicis longus. The lumbricals flex the metacarpophalangeal joints and extend the interphalangeal joints. In ulnar lesions, unopposed extensor tone at the fourth and fifth metacarpophalangeal joints and unopposed flexor tone at the interphalangeal joints produces the ulnar griffe or claw deformity. Clawing varies, depending on the amount of muscle weakness. A distal ulnar lesion that spares the FDP induces more clawing than more proximal lesions due to greater flexion of the interphalangeal joints of the fourth and fifth digits. The palmaris brevis (PB) sign is a wrinkling of the skin over the hypothenar eminence during 5th digit abduction. This is due to contraction of the PB which is spared with UNW. The elbow flexion test is analogous to the carpal compression test and the Phalen test seeking to elicit ulnar paresthesias on forcefully flexing the elbow and applying pressure over the ulnar groove. Tinel sign is sometimes useful. But some patients have generally mechano-sensitive nerves, and only a disproportionately active Tinel sign over the suspect ulnar nerve has any significance. Both have a high incidence of false positives.

The forearm muscles, FCU and FDP, are frequently spared in UNE, so the lack of clinical or electromyographic abnormality in these muscles in no way excludes a lesion at the elbow.[11,12] Abnormalities of these muscles are more common in lesions in the ulnar groove than compression at the HUA. Sparing seems related to either the redundant innervation via several branchlets from the main ulnar trunk or relative differences in fascicular vulnerabililty. Branches to the FCU do not arise from the ulnar nerve proximal to the elbow.[2]

One of the earliest signs of UNE is weakness of the third palmar interosseous, sometimes manifested by an abducted posture of the small finger (Wartenberg sign). The FDI is easily observed, and the bulk can be palpated and compared with the opposite side. It is particularly useful to test small hand muscles against the strength of an examiner's like muscles, after the methods described by Wolf.[13] Demonstrating weakness in muscles outside the ulnar nerve distribution is vital for recognizing lower brachial plexopathies, C8 radiculopathies, and motor neuron diseases.

Ulnar nerve lesions in the wrist and hand can cause a confusing array of clinical findings, ranging from a pure sensory deficit to pure motor syndromes with weakness, which may or may not involve the hypothenar muscles. Of the different lesions of the ulnar nerve near the wrist, the most common and extensively reported is a compression of the deep palmar branch. In their now classic article, Shea and McClain[14] classified ulnar compression syndromes of the wrist and hand into 3 types. In type I, the lesion is proximal to or within Guyon canal, involves both the superficial and deep branches, and causes a mixed motor and sensory deficit, with weakness involving all the ulnar hand muscles. In type II, the lesion is within Guyon canal or at the pisohamate hiatus, involves the deep branch, and causes a pure motor deficit with a variable pattern of weakness depending on the precise site of compression. A type III lesion is in Guyon canal or in the palmaris brevis, involves the superficial branch only and causes a purely sensory deficit. In the type I and III lesions, sensory loss should spare the dorsum of the hand, innervated by the DUC branch, and should also largely spare the hypothenar eminence because its innervation is via the palmar cutaneous branch, which arises proximal to the wrist. Other proposed UNW classification schemes add nominal value.

TERMINOLOGY

Careless use of terms, such as tardy ulnar palsy and cubital tunnel syndrome, has resulted in a nosologic quagmire. In 1878, Panas first described UNE developing long after an elbow injury, and the term, *tardy ulnar palsy*, was later applied to UNE after remote elbow trauma, generally after an old fracture or dislocation.[15] The term soon degenerated into a nonspecific, generic term for any UNE, on the weak presumption that trauma must have occurred but patients simply could not recall it. The HUA as a site of ulnar compression was first described in 1916 by the British neurologist Dr F. Buzzard[16] and his surgical colleague, Mr P. Sargent. The observation was lost until the 1950s when Osborne, Fiendel, and Stratford rediscovered it.

Osborne referred to the condition as spontaneous ulnar paresis.[17] The HUA is sometimes referred to as Osborne band.

Feindel and Stratford[10] introduced the term, *cubital tunnel syndrome*, to refer to patients with compression of the nerve by the HUA. They were attempting to define a subgroup of patients who suffered from a focal entrapment at the origin of the FCU and who could be spared a transposition procedure and managed with simple release of the aponeurotic arcade. The title of their article is illuminating, *The Role of the Cubital Tunnel in Tardy Ulnar Palsy.* As with tardy ulnar palsy, the term, cubital tunnel syndrome, soon degenerated into a useless, nonspecific, generic label for any UNE. Most physicians believed *cubital tunnel* refers to the nerve's subcutaneous passage through the ulnar groove and that cubital tunnel syndrome is synonymous with UNE, a serious misperception of the original intent. The authors restrict the use of the term to cases due to constriction by the HUA.

ETIOLOGY

There are 4 locations in the region of the elbow where the ulnar nerve may suffer compression: at the MIS, in the RTC groove, at the HUA, and at the point of exit from the FCU. Lesions in the RTC groove account for the vast majority of cases, but HUA compression is also common. In the 2 studies that have convincingly addressed the issue, there is remarkable concordance in the incidence of RTC abnormalities (69% and 62%) and HUA abnormalities (ie, cubital tunnel syndrome [23% and 28%]) and changes in both the RTC and HUA (8% and 10%).[18,19] Other investigators disagree. Kline and colleagues[21] reported 460 cases of ulnar entrapment at the elbow localized with intraoperative NAP inching. Conduction abnormalities always lay just proximal to and through the ulnar groove; there were only 8 cases of HUA entrapment.[20,21] The exit compression syndrome is infrequent but turns up regularly if examiners are sensitive to its existence.[6,9] The nerve can rarely be compressed by the MIS or arcade of Struthers proximal to the elbow.

Lesions occur in the RTC groove for several reasons, including acute or chronic external pressure, bony or scar impingement, anomalous muscles or bands, chronic stretch, particularly in the presence of a valgus deformity, and, rarely, mass lesions. In 30% to 50% of cases, no specific cause is discovered in spite of careful investigation, including surgical exposure.[22]

Causes of UNW include extrinsic compressive neuropathy, fractures of the wrist, thrombosis of the ulnar artery secondary to trauma, and masses within Guyon canal, such as a ganglion.

RECURRENT SUBLUXATION OF THE ULNAR NERVE

Subluxation is often listed as a cause of UNE, but its role is far from clear. Childress[5] examined 1000 normal, asymptomatic people and found an incidence of ulnar nerve subluxation of 16%. All these patients were asymptomatic, and the majority had the condition bilaterally. The incidence of subluxation in patients with UNE and how it compares with that in the general population is unknown. It is not clear by any means that subluxation predisposes to UNE and could help prevent UNE by allowing the nerve to escape from a narrow groove during flexion. If subluxation does predispose to UNE, it could be a result of the repetitive rubbing of the nerve across the epicondyle causing a RTC neuropathy (friction neuritis). Just as plausibly, subluxation could cause angulation of the nerve under the HUA during elbow flexion and result in HUA compression.

ELECTROPHYSIOLOGIC EVALUATION

Electrodiagnosis can play several roles in the evaluation of ulnar neuropathies. It can document the presence of a mononeuropathy; localize the lesion to any of several locations in the wrist, forearm, or elbow; and distinguish a mononeuropathy from a plexopathy, radiculopathy, polyneuropathy, or motor neuron disease. An abnormality can be confirmed prior to surgery and can be used to quantitate recovery following treatment. There are, however, limited data relating quantitative results of studies with prognosis after surgery. Electrodiagnosis of the ulnar nerve at the elbow is not nearly as straightforward as that of the median nerve at the wrist. The diagnostic yield is less and the interpretations of the data often more difficult. There are many possible techniques to use, and several studies have suggested useful approaches that are not commonly used in EMG laboratories.

NERVE CONDUCTION STUDIES
Ulnar Neuropathy at the Elbow

There have been several problem areas in the electrodiagnosis of UNE. These include controversy over the best elbow position, the ideal length of the across-elbow segment, and the value of absolute slowing in the above elbow (AE) to below elbow (BE) segment in contrast to a relative slowing of the AE-BE segment compared with the BE-wrist segment.

Technical errors are a major source of misdiagnosis. Care should be taken to insure supramaximal stimulation, especially at the BE site where the ulnar nerve lies deep in the FCU distal to the HUA. A common error is to stimulate too far posteriorly for the AE site, which can significantly alter the latency. The nerve curves acutely around the elbow and moves quickly toward the biceps, not the triceps. To minimize error, the AE and BE nerve locations can be mapped with submaximal stimulations before carrying out the conduction studies. It is frequently difficult to accurately measure around the curved elbow with a standard flat tape measure. A useful trick is to use a more flexible electrode wire lead to measure, marking the distance from the end of the wire placed at the AE site down to the point of BE stimulation, then laying the wire atop a tape measure to get the distance. The elbow should be in the same position used to obtain the reference values, and no change in position should be permitted between stimulation and measurement.

The difficulties with elbow position relate to the discrepancies between true nerve length and measured skin distance in different elbow positions. In extension, the nerve has redundancy, which progressively plays out with flexion. In extreme flexion, the nerve begins to stretch and slide distally and may partially or completely sublux. In extension, skin distance is falsely short compared with true nerve length, causing spurious and artifactual conduction slowing. In extreme flexion, if subluxation occurs, the skin distance is falsely long, causing spurious quickening.

Checkles and colleagues,[23] in a now classic article, first pointed out the remarkable difference in CV between an extended and a flexed position. Absolute AE-BE NCVs in the range of 35 m/s to 38 m/s and differences in the range of 20 m/s to 30 m/s between the AE-BE segment compared with the BE-wrist segment have been regularly reported in controls studied with the elbow extended.[10] This position-related, artifactual slowing likely explains the high incidence of subclinical UNE reported by some investigators.[24] It is not clear that there is any difference in the relative diagnostic sensitivity of the different elbow positions in detecting abnormalities in patients with clinically defined UNE, as long as appropriate reference values are used. It is clear that consistency is paramount. A standard position must be used for stimulation as well as for the measurement of distance, and this must be the same position used for obtaining the reference values. The American Association of Neuromuscular and Electrodiagnostic Medicine (AANEM) practice parameter on the electrodiagnosis of UNE concluded the most logical elbow position for ulnar conduction studies was moderate flexion, 70° to 90° from horizontal (**Box 1**).[8]

The ADM or the FDI for recording may be used; the latter is also useful for identifying lesions of the deep palmar branch. There is value in doing NCV while recording from both the FDI and ADM in order to detect lesions causing selective damage.[25,26] Although the ADM is more commonly studied, the motor fibers to the FDI are more likely to be abnormal in a lesion at the elbow, and conduction studies are more likely to show conduction block (CB).[10]

After Maynard and Stolov's[27] influential article on experimental error, a minimum 10 cm across-elbow distance became standard. This article showed specifically how errors in measurement of latency and distance affect calculation of NCV, with errors in latency measurement accounting for 89% of the error, and error from distance measurement accounting for only 11%. A repeat of the same study using computer-automated equipment demonstrated an improvement in latency measurements errors.[28] This improvement in latency measurement, however, did not offset the significantly worsened error, resulting from distance measurements across a nonlinear surface.[29] The distance measurement error for the curved across-elbow segment can be 3 times higher than for a straight-line segment of comparable length. A decrease of greater than 10 m/s between the distal and proximal segments can occur from distance measurement error alone.

Although accepted that longer distance measurements are used to lessen experimental error and improve specificity for diagnosis, focal nerve injuries typically cause

---

Box 1
Synopsis of the recommendations of the AAEM practice parameter on ulnar neuropathy at the elbow

1. When using moderate-elbow flexion (70°–90° from horizontal), a 10-cm across-elbow distance, and surface stimulation and recording, the following abnormalities suggest a focal lesion involving the ulnar nerve at the elbow:

   a. Absolute motor NCV from AE to BE of less than 50 m/s

   b. An AE to BE segment greater than 10 m/s slower than the BE-wrist segment

   c. A decrease in compound muscle action potential (CMAP) negative peak amplitude from BE to AE greater than 20%

   d. A significant change in CMAP configuration at the AE site compared with the BE site

   e. Multiple internally consistent abnormalities

2. If routine motor studies are inconclusive, the following procedures may be of benefit:

   a. NCS recorded from the FDI muscle

   b. An inching study

3. Needle examination should include the FDI, the most frequently abnormal muscle, and ulnar innervated forearm flexors. If ulnar innervated muscles are abnormal, the examination should be extended to include nonulnar C8/medial cord/lower trunk muscles to exclude brachial plexopathy, and the cervical paraspinals to exclude radiculopathy

Data from Campbell WW, Carroll DJ, Greenberg MK, et al. Literature review of the usefulness of nerve conduction studies and electromyography in the evaluation of patients with ulnar neuropathy at the elbow. Muscle Nerve 1999;22(Suppl 8):S175–205.

abnormalities of nerve conduction over a 1-cm segment.[18] Studying long nerve segments may mask focal slowing by including lengths of normally conducting nerve. Thus, shorter distances are necessary to improve sensitivity. Two independently conducted studies, that equally weighted sensitivity and specificity, concluded that optimal distance to detect focal lesions is approximately 5 cm to 6 cm.[30,31]

The technical and biologic factors that affect determination of ulnar forearm and across-elbow NCV are different. Technically, the distance measurement for the across-elbow segment is nonlinear and shorter than the forearm segment. Two important biologic variables are body mass index (BMI) and temperature. Each effects NCV determination, but the effects on the across-elbow and forearm segment are different. The across-elbow segment NCV directly correlates with BMI, but the forearm segment does not.[32,33] As BMI increases, the distance measurement increases and dissociates from the actual nerve distance. Thus, demonstrating a difference in the NCV between the 2 segments is more difficult in those with high BMIs (possible false-negative study) and is easier in those with low BMIs (possible false-positive study).

Ambient temperatures also affect ulnar forearm and across-elbow NCV differently. Low skin temperature causes no appreciable change in forearm NCV but significantly lower across-elbow NCV.[34,35] The deep location of the forearm segment presumably insulates this segment from surface temperature fluctuations, whereas the superficial location of the across-elbow segment makes it more susceptible to temperature effects. This discrepancy can be seen when there are no other indications from other nerve conduction studies of cool temperature effects (eg, prolonged peak latencies of sensory potentials). Failure to maintain adequate temperature of the across-elbow segment may, therefore, lead to false-positive studies and should be warmed particularly when there are no other clinical or electrodiagnostic findings that support the diagnosis of UNE (cold elbow syndrome). The continued use of the forearm NCV as an internal control variable for diagnosis of UNE should be reconsidered.

All or most cases of UNE demonstrate demyelinating abnormalities. Focal demyelination at the elbow leads to an excessive dispersal of conduction velocities of the motor axons, which produces a low amplitude, long duration, fragmented CMAP on stimulation proximal to the elbow compared with stimulation distal to the elbow. A decline in total area under the CMAP curve correlates better with true CB, but temporal dispersion (TD) is just as suggestive of focal demyelination.[36,37] A reduction in amplitude of more than 20% or a significant change in CMAP configuration between the BE and AE sites is suggestive of UNE. A reduction in amplitude of more than 25% was the best criterion for localization in one study.[38]

Some patients with UNE have no or minimally detectable conduction velocity abnormalities, the so-called pure axon loss ulnar neuropathy.[39] Sensory and motor studies demonstrate decreased amplitudes and slowing of NCV consistent with axonal loss but no differences between across-elbow and forearm NCVs. In nearly all cases, however, if other muscles are used to measure NCV (ie, FCU or FDI) or short-segment studies are performed, focal demyelination can be disclosed.[18]

The distal sensory nerve action potential (NAP) is a sensitive indicator of ulnar nerve function. Most patients with UNE have a low amplitude or absent NAP, although it is a nonspecific, nonlocalizing, finding.[7,24] A lesion at the elbow can sometimes be identified by sensory studies using needle electrodes to record possible focal slowing and NAP dispersion at the elbow, especially in patients with only sensory symptoms. Such NAP studies have significant pitfalls and limitations and should only be used if the examiner is fully aware of the technical details and the applicable literature.[8]

Motor conduction studies in patients have shown localizing abnormalities in symptomatic elbows with a sensitivity of 37% to 100%.[38,40–45] Eisen[24] demonstrated 53%

sensitivity in severe cases and 27% in mild cases. In general, change in the absolute CV is a more sensitive indicator of abnormality than is abnormality of the relative CV. The results of various studies are reviewed in detail by Campbell and colleagues.[8]

An ancillary technique measures ulnar nerve conduction to the FCU.[46,47] Benecke and Conrad[47] found the technique equally sensitive to motor conduction to the ADM.[48] Payan was able to localize the lesion to the elbow in another 10 of his 50 cases with this method.[40] The technique is limited by the nerve fibers to the FCU tending to be spared in UNE.

Ulnar Neuropathy at the Wrist

Assessment of conduction to the FDI muscle, in addition to the routine motor latencies to the ADM, is integral to the evaluation of distal ulnar neuropathies.[48] Olney and Wilbourn[49] studied conduction to the FDI and ADM in 373 nerves, determining absolute distal motor latency (DML) to the FDI as well as differences between the latency to FDI and the ADM on the same side and differences in the side-to-side FDI latencies.[49] With stimulation at the proximal wrist crease, 5.5 cm to 6.5 cm proximal to the ADM recording site, the upper limit of normal for DML was 3.4 ms to the ADM and 4.5 ms to the FDI. There was an increase of approximately 0.5 ms per decade in the DML to each muscle, but advancing age did not significantly alter the side-to-side latency difference or ipsilateral muscle-to-muscle difference. According to this study, the side-to-side difference in DML should not exceed 1.0 ms for the ADM or 1.3 ms for the FDI. The ipsilateral difference in DML to the ADM versus FDI should not exceed 2.0 ms. A CMAP amplitude less than 6 mV for the FDI and less than 5 mV for the ADM was considered abnormal.

A lesion of the deep palmar branch, beyond the branches to the hypothenar muscles, causes prolongation of the DML to the FDI in the face of a normal motor latency to the ADM and normal sensory studies. Even if the DML is not prolonged, the CMAP may demonstrate fragmentation, dispersion, or CB. Needle electrode examination (NEE) typically shows denervation in all the ulnar intrinsic hand muscles except those of the hypothenar eminence. A sequential assessment of the first through the fourth dorsal interossei can sometimes provide precise localization. When the lesion involves the volar sensory branch alone, only the distal sensory action potentials are abnormal.

As with carpal tunnel syndrome, some ulnar lesions at the wrist cause mild secondary slowing of motor conduction velocity in the forearm segment. Care must be taken in the final assessment to determine the site of most significant slowing, and the final electrophysiologic diagnosis should reflect the perspective of the entire picture.

SHORT-SEGMENT STUDIES

Precise localization of demyelinating ulnar neuropathies at the elbow or wrist region can often be achieved by inching or short-segment incremental studies (SSISs)— monitoring the CMAP while moving the stimulator in discrete, small steps.[7,18–20,50,51] When there is definitive CB or TD, precise measurements between the stimuli are not necessary. Movement of the stimulator along the course of the nerve discloses the exact location of demyelinating injury with a sudden change in amplitude or configuration of the CMAP. There are at least 6 reported short-segment techniques for evaluation of the ulnar nerve, 5 for the elbow and 1 for the wrist region. Although these techniques have not been systematically compared with more routine techniques, it is possible that the use of short distances between stimulation points increases sensitivity for detection.

Irrespective of which technique is chosen, limiting technical error is of utmost importance. The elbow should be maintained in a fixed position throughout the study. Submaximal stimulations should be applied to the ulnar nerve to accurately determine its location prior to making any measurements. The nerve location is defined by where a submaximal stimulation produces the largest CMAP response. This is particularly important for detecting partial or complete subluxation of the nerve. When attempting to detect focal slowing without CB/TD, precise measurements are necessary. The authors recommend using calipers preset at 1 cm or 2 cm to determine stimulation points and minimize experimental error. During testing of each segment, maximal, but not excessively supramaximal, stimulations should be given to avoid inadvertent stimulus spread more distally.

Short-segment studies can be time consuming when meticulously performed. There are, however, multiple situations when SSISs can be useful. SSISs can differentiate lesions at the HUA from the RTC groove and potentially have an impact on determining which surgical technique is most suitable for an individual patient. The AANEM practice parameter recommended that multiple internally consistent abnormalities be present to make a diagnosis of UNE.[8] In patients with an isolated abnormality of decreased across-elbow NCV on routine NCS, SSISs can provide another abnormality to ensure accurate diagnosis. In cases of pure axon loss UNE, SSISs can demonstrate focal slowing, confirming localization in the elbow region. A completely normal SSISs in this situation suggests the possibility of a lesion elsewhere. In patients with persistent symptoms after ulnar nerve transposition, a modified short-segment study can be performed.[52]

The use of SSISs in mildly symptomatic patients to detect subtle abnormalities otherwise not seen on routine conduction studies is debatable. The results will not likely change conservative management. The mere diagnosis, however, may prevent ordering other unnecessary diagnostic tests or incorrectly attributing symptomatology to a different cause (eg, a cervical radiculopathy).

The CMAP can be recorded from any muscle with SSISs. FDI might be expected to yield the highest results followed be ADM and then, lastly, FCU. One study, however, demonstrated that recording over FCU was more sensitive than ADM for detecting focal slowing.[53]

ELECTROMYOGRAPHY

Although NEE is not as sensitive as nerve conduction studies for detecting UNE, denervation of ulnar-innervated hand muscles is commonly seen.[11,26,39] The FDI is the most frequently involved muscle, followed by the ADM, FDP, and FCU, respectively.[11] NEE can localize a lesion to the elbow only if ulnar-innervated forearm muscles are also involved, but they are spared in many patients (vida supra). Pickett and Coleman[38] found NEE abnormalities in two-thirds of their UNE patients, but the abnormalities localized the lesion to the elbow in only 1 of 5. Kimura[41] found NEE abnormalities were most frequent in patients with absent SNAPs; Eisen[24] found the incidence of NEE abnormalities correlated with the severity of motor conduction slowing. NEE is necessary in UNE diagnosis to exclude abnormalities in nonulnar innervated muscles.

AN APPROACH TO THE PATIENT

There are several regularly recurrent problem scenarios in dealing with suspected UNE:

1. Isolated slowing of NCV in the across-elbow segment of the ulnar nerve: When there are no other corroborating electrodiagnostic abnormalities, and the finding

does not correlate well with the clinical assessment, it is possibly artifactual, although some investigators have argued this represents subclinical ulnar neuropathy. The authors suspect that in many instances, this finding represents a technical error or the effects of cold temperatures.[27,33,35] This situation requires utmost care. The dictum, "never underestimate the ability of the EMG report to bring the knife down on the patient," applies.

2. Lesions of the ulnar nerve not at the elbow: An ulnar nerve lesion at the wrist can be identified by more significant slowing of nerve conduction across the wrist than across the elbow and by lack of denervation in the forearm. The NAP of the dorsal cutaneous branch is normal, with lesions at the wrist even if the NAP of the PUC or digital sensory branches is reduced, whereas all are usually abnormal with lesions at the elbow.[54,55] Rarely, ulnar entrapment occurs proximal to the elbow or in the forearm segment. These localizations should always be considered when no definitive slowing of conduction is noted in the elbow segment.

3. The pure axon loss lesion at the elbow: In some patients with UNE, it is difficult to demonstrate focal slowing across the elbow. When the forearm flexors are involved, probable localization to the elbow is still possible by NEE, although it is impossible to exclude a more proximal lesion in the axilla or upper arm. Helpful ancillary techniques in this situation include recording from the FDI, which may demonstrate focal slowing or CB even though fibers to the ADM do not, and/or SSISs, which can often demonstrate focal slowing missed when studying longer segments. Abnormality of the DUC can at least place the lesion proximal to its takeoff, but the DUC can occasionally be spared in elbow lesions. Many cases of pure axon loss UNE are likely due to lesions in unusual locations.

4. Patients with purely sensory symptoms and normal routine motor studies. Such patients usually have a mild or early UNE, and an adequate evaluation may well be to exclude other pathology, such as brachial plexopathy or cervical radiculopathy, and manage patients conservatively. To localize the lesion more confidently, FDI recording or SSISs may be useful. NAP recording, either surface or near nerve, across the elbow is technically difficult and the results should be interpreted cautiously.

5. Patients with forearm sparing: When conduction studies place the lesion at the elbow, sparing of the forearm muscles should be no deterrent to localization.

6. Wallerian degeneration with confusing distal abnormalities: When severe UNE causes major axon loss distal to the lesion, there may be secondary slowing of the entire distal ulnar nerve and prolongation of the DML, usually with an absent sensory potential and abundant denervation. In lesions of this severity, NEE abnormalities are usually present in the forearm muscles and FDI recording or SSISs often place the lesion at the elbow, even if routine studies are equivocal. An occasional error is to diagnose a second lesion at the wrist. If the CMAPs measured at the ADM or FDI are so small as to hinder accurate NCV determinations, recording over the FCU can be performed (the only situation in which the authors use this particular methodology).

7. Failed ulnar nerve surgery. Unfortunately, patients present with persistent or recurrent symptoms after an unsuccessful operation on the ulnar nerve. Sometimes there are no preoperative studies for comparison, in which case the electromyographer is reduced to guesswork. The first order of business should be to establish with certainty that no other process, such as plexopathy or radiculopathy, was responsible for the symptoms initially. One patient with persistent symptoms following two decompression surgeries for UNE was eventually found to have Ewing sarcoma in the axilla. Then the course of the nerve should be mapped to

determine whether or not transposition was done. This procedure alone may sometimes establish, by showing abrupt changes in nerve course, that kinking has occurred due to inadequate distal (more rarely proximal) release. After mapping the course of the nerve, an SSISs study can establish whether there is persistent focal compression or fibrosis, potentially amenable to reoperation, or whether there has been devascularization of a long nerve segment, an essentially end-stage condition.

SURGERY

The electrophysiologic contribution to the decision whether or not to operate is to document quantitatively the clinical state. For patients with mild sensory symptoms who are not believed surgical candidates, the studies should confirm only minimal abnormalities of sensory conduction.[56] For patients with mild to moderate motor and sensory symptoms who are considered for operation, studies are useful to demonstrate the degree of abnormality, to confirm the localization of injury, and to serve as a baseline for postoperative evaluation. Marked prolongation of conduction across the elbow suggests a poorer prognosis. In addition, deterioration can be determined objectively in those cases being followed.[42,54] For patients with severe muscle atrophy who are believed inappropriate candidates for surgery, EMG can document the irreversible loss of muscle.

After successful ulnar nerve surgery there usually is electrophysiologic improvement.[57] The NCV in the elbow segment improves, but remyelination with short, thin internodes may prevent a return to normality despite a good clinical outcome. The motor NCV can improve, however, even with a poor result.[58] Subsequently the amplitude of the NAP recovers, accompanied by clinical improvement.[57]

OTHER DIAGNOSTIC METHODS

High-definition ultrasound and MRI are becoming increasingly more useful adjuncts in the diagnosis of UNE. In a small study of 4 patients with symptoms of UNE and normal electrodiagnosis, ultrasound demonstrated enlargement near the elbow as defined by cross-sectional area (CSA).[59] The extent of the electrodiagnostic testing was not provided but nonetheless showed how promising this technique could be. There are several advantages over electrodiagnosis, to include patient tolerability, real time observation of structure, and time requirements. Ultrasound can distinguish focal enlargements of the nerve as typically seen in compression mononeuropathies from abnormal masses. Ultrasound does not provide any functional information regarding nerve conduction.

Parameters of ultrasound evaluation include nerve echogenicity, diameter, and CSA. Normally the ulnar nerve is echogenic with parallel internal linear echoes.[60] At the level of the ME, the nerve is more hypoechoic. Due to the quantitative nature, diameter and CSA are usually used for diagnosis. One complex study assessed multiple methods for quantitating nerve echogenicity and concluded that this parameter could distinguish UNE subjects from a healthy control group.[61]

Diameter is measured on longitudinal imaging and CSA on transverse imaging. Much of the ongoing research attempts to define reference values for each. One difficulty is determining the optimal control for comparison. An internal control uses comparison to the homologous region on the contralateral limb or to a predefined segment of the ulnar nerve away from the elbow. Alternatively, values derived from a normal control population can be used. With elbow flexion at 90°, the ulnar nerve changes shape and the CSA decreases. A critical review suggested that the maximum diameter and CSA of the ulnar nerve at the elbow are 2.4 mm and 8 mm^2 to 10 mm^2, respectively. The sensitivity for detecting enlargement of the ulnar nerve using these parameters was approximately 80%.[60] This is approximately the same sensitivity as for routine conduction studies.

There are also few data about false-positive results using ultrasound. For example, a professional bowler found to have an enlarged nerve on MRI performed for medial elbow pain had medial epicondylitis clinically, with no evidence of UNE. Electrodiagnostic studies, including SSISs and FDI recording, were completely normal. The AANEM practice parameter emphasized the importance of multiple, internally consistent abnormalities in the electrodiagnosis of UNE. The same should be said about the clinical, ultrasound, and MRI aspects.

The findings on ultrasound have been correlated to the abnormalities seen in electrodiagnosis. Volpe and colleagues[62] demonstrated that the maximum CSA was 14.6 mm^2 ± 5.0 mm^2 in UNE subjects versus 7.1 mm^2 ± 2.1 mm^2 in controls. The upper limit of normal based on mean plus 2 SDs in this study is 11.3 mm^2, significantly higher than in Beekman and colleagues'[60] critical review. The severity of the electrodiagnostic findings were predefined as mild, moderate, or severe. The severe UNE cases had a mean CSA of 18.3 mm ± 5.1 mm compared with 11.1 mm ± 3.4 mm in the milder group. The investigators concluded that ultrasound can have a role in severity stratification in addition to diagnosis.

Won and colleagues[63] used ultrasound to demonstrate ulnar nerve subluxation in 9 patients with clinical UNE but a paucity of electrophysiological evidence. They proposed that subluxation resulted in spuriously high distance measurements between stimulation points of the ulnar nerve above and below the elbow. The length of the ulnar nerve segment was remeasured under ultrasound guidance. The newly attained smaller distances resulted in a mean decrease of the ulnar NCV across the elbow by 7.9 m/s from the initial studies; subjects now had abnormalities that met criteria for UNE. Spuriously fast conduction velocities due to subluxation have been recognized and commented in previous studies.[8] Mapping the nerve by using submaximal stimuli can also readily detect subluxation and avoid this error.

MRI is also useful in the evaluation of UNE. MRI is reliable in detecting structural abnormalities around the nerve as well as intrinsic abnormalities within the nerve. Vucic and colleagues[64] demonstrated a higher specificity of MRI in detecting UNE than conventional electrodiagnostic studies. The most frequent MRI changes included high signal intensity within the nerve, nerve enlargement, a combination of both, or nerve compression. MRI had a 90% sensitivity, whereas electrodiagnosis had a 65% sensitivity. The investigators used a distance of 13 cm between AE and BE stimulation points for motor nerve conduction studies, limiting the diagnostic sensitivity for focal demyelination. Furthermore, it was not disclosed whether SSISs or motor studies to the FDI were performed to potentially increase the diagnostic yield. Nonetheless, the MRI was particularly sensitive, without any false-positive errors. There were 15 control subjects with normal-appearing nerves. Additionally, there were 19 subjects with abnormal electrodiagnostic studies that did not definitively localized to the elbow region. In 16 of these subjects, MRI detected the abnormality at the elbow.

Bäumer and colleagues[65] assessed the role of magnetic resonance neurography in UNE. They demonstrated an increased nerve T2 signal as measured by a T2-weighted contrast-to-noise ratio in subjects with UNE compared to controls, with a sensitivity and specificity of 83% and 85%, respectively. This is a more realistic specificity than the 100% claimed by Vucic and colleagues.[64] Furthermore, they were able to distinguish mild cases of UNE from severe ones via nerve caliber measurements.

Researchers are also evaluating the potential use of diffusion-weighted MRI in UNE diagnosis.[66] In all 3 of these referenced studies, the RTC groove was incorrectly called *cubital tunnel*.

There is a trend in research, with many studies assessing the utility of MRI or ultrasound in UNE, to attempt to demonstrate superiority of the newer modalities over conventional electrodiagnostic studies. Each technique has specific advantages over electrodiagnosis, and it could be speculated that either may ultimately replace electrodiagnosis as the primary tool in the evaluation of ulnar neuropathies. Further studies that develop well-defined, universal parameters of high specificity will be essential to avoid overdiagnoses and unnecessary treatment interventions.

INTRAOPERATIVE ELECTRONEUROGRAPHY

Intraoperative electroneurography (IE) can help elucidate the precise point of abnormality and guide the type of surgical procedure that is performed. For instance, it may demonstrate focal slowing at the level of the HUA, suggesting a simple release of this structure will suffice. Alternatively, IE may demonstrate an abnormality at the level of the RTC groove supporting the need for either anterior transposition or medical epicondylectomy. Intraoperative studies are not technically difficult or especially time consuming.[67,68]

In performing IE, it is important to minimize dissection to minimize complications. The authors' technique involves exposing the nerve via a curvilinear incision passing anterior to the ME; then, releasing the HUA (required for both transposition and simple decompression); then, with a minimum of further dissection, performing direct epineural stimulation over successive 1-cm segments while recording the M wave from the ADM.[68] Latency changes in excess of 0.45 ms over a 1-cm distance are considered abnormal, assuming an otherwise normal nerve. In patients with focal accentuation of a generalized neuropathy, judgment is required to best identify the pathologic segments. If the maximal abnormalities center about the site of the HUA (now divided), the procedure is terminated as a simple decompression. If maximal abnormalities center about the ME, further mobilization is carried out and the nerve transposed. If no pathologic segments are identified, the incision is extended and electroneurography repeated. In one such instance, a novel site of entrapment was uncovered.[6] Direct epineural recording of NAPs requires some isolation and mobilization of the nerve to place electrodes. Because the authors prefer to minimize dissection, they have not used this technique. In summary, an operation for UNE could be tailored to the specific pathology present and transposition done only when truly necessary. IE can help guide the choice of procedure. The recent surgical literature increasingly favors simple decompression over transposition as the initial procedure, making precise localization less important.[69] IE may still have a role to play in those patients who fail the initial procedure.

SUMMARY

UNE results from focal compression of the ulnar nerve, primarily at the RTC groove or the humeroulnar arcade. In nearly all cases, focal slowing of nerve conduction can be demonstrated in the ulnar nerve segment across the elbow. When focal slowing cannot be demonstrated, other localizations for ulnar nerve compression must be considered. Electrodiagnosis is currently the primary tool for diagnosis. False-positive and false-negative errors occur, however, and are highly dependent on operator technique. False-positive errors are perhaps more damaging, because they can lead to unnecessary surgery. Among the many important procedural steps, the electromyographer needs to precisely measure the distance between stimulation points above and below the elbow. Additionally, the elbow region should be warmed in cases of isolated slowing of NCV across the elbow, particularly in patients with low BMI or with little subcutaneous tissue in the elbow region. In cases referred for surgical intervention, the electromyographer should ascertain the specific point of abnormality (ie, the RTC or HUA or other). Ideally, the type of surgery performed is dictated by this determination.

REFERENCES

1. Vanderpool DW, Chalmers J, Lamb DW, et al. Peripheral compression lesions of the ulnar nerve. J Bone Joint Surg Br 1968;50:792–803.
2. Campbell WW, Pridgeon RM, Riaz G, et al. Variations in anatomy of the ulnar nerve at the cubital tunnel: pitfalls in the diagnosis of ulnar neuropathy at the elbow. Muscle Nerve 1991;14:733–8.
3. von Schroeder HP, Scheker LR. Redefining the "Arcade of Struthers". J Hand Surg Am 2003;28:1018–21.
4. Werner CO, Ohlin P, Elmqvist D. Pressures recorded in ulnar neuropathy. Acta Orthop Scand 1985;56:404–6.
5. Childress HM. Recurrent ulnar-nerve dislocation at the elbow. J Bone Joint Surg Am 1956;38:978–84.
6. Campbell WW, Pridgeon RM, Sahni SK. Entrapment neuropathy of the ulnar nerve at its point of exit from the flexor carpi ulnaris muscle. Muscle Nerve 1988;11:467–70.
7. Miller RG. The cubital tunnel syndrome: diagnosis and precise localization. Ann Neurol 1979;6:56–9.
8. Campbell WW, Carroll DJ, Greenberg MK, et al. Literature review of the useful-ness of nerve conduction studies and electromyography in the evaluation of patients with ulnar neuropathy at the elbow. Muscle Nerve 1999;22(Suppl 8): S175–205.
9. Amadio PC, Beckenbaugh RD. Entrapment of the ulnar nerve by the deep flexor-pronator aponeurosis. J Hand Surg Am 1986;11:83–7.
10. Feindel W, Stratford J. The role of the cubital tunnel in tardy ulnar palsy. Can J Surg 1958;78:351–3.
11. Stewart JD. The variable clinical manifestations of ulnar neuropathies at the elbow. J Neurol Neurosurg Psychiatry 1987;50:252–8.
12. Campbell WW, Pridgeon RM, Riaz G, et al. Sparing of the flexor carpi ulnaris in ulnar neuropathy at the elbow [see comments]. Muscle Nerve 1989;12:965–7.
13. Wolf JK. Segmental neurology: a guide to the examination and interpretation of sensory and motor function. Baltimore (MD): University Park Press; 1981.
14. Shea JD, McClain EJ. Ulnar nerve compression syndrome at and below the wrist. J Bone Joint Surg Am 1969;51:1095–103.
15. Panas J. Sur une cause peu connue de paralysie du nerf cubital. Arch generales de med 1878;2:5.
16. Buzzard EF. Some varieties of toxic and traumatic ulnar neuritis. Lancet 1922;1: 317–9.
17. Osborne G. Spontaneous ulnar nerve paresis. Br Med J 1958;1:218.
18. Campbell WW, Pridgeon RM, Sahni KS. Short segment incremental studies in the evaluation of ulnar neuropathy at the elbow. Muscle Nerve 1992;15:1050–4.
19. Kanakamedala RV, Simons DG, Porter RW, et al. Ulnar nerve entrapment at the elbow localized by short segment stimulation. Arch Phys Med Rehabil 1988;69: 959–63.

20. Brown WF, Yates SK, Ferguson GG. Cubital tunnel syndrome and ulnar neuropathy. Ann Neurol 1980;7:289–90.
21. Kim DH, Han K, Tiel RL, et al. Surgical outcomes of 654 ulnar nerve lesions. J Neurosurg 2003;98(5):993–1004.
22. Chan RC, Paine KW, Varghese G. Ulnar neuropathy at the elbow: comparison of simple decompression and anterior transposition. Neurosurgery 1983;7: 545–50.
23. Checkles NS, Russakov AD, Piero DL. Ulnar nerve conduction velocity—effect of elbow position on measurement. Arch Phys Med Rehabil 1971;53:362–5.
24. Eisen A. Early diagnosis of ulnar nerve palsy. Neurology 1974;24:256–62.
25. Shakir A, Micklesen PJ, Robinson LR. Which motor nerve conduction study is best in ulnar neuropathy at the elbow? Muscle Nerve 2004;29:585–90.
26. Jabre JF, Wilbourn AJ. The EMG findings in 100 consecutive ulnar neuropathies. Acta Neurol Scand 1979;60(Suppl 73):91.
27. Maynard FM, Stolov WC. Experimental error in determination of nerve conduction velocity. Arch Phys Med Rehabil 1972;53:362–72.
28. Landau ME, Diaz MI, Barner KC, et al. Optimal distance for segmental nerve conduction studies revisited. Muscle Nerve, 2003 nerve conduction studies revisited. Muscle Nerve 2003;27:367–9.
29. Landau ME, Diaz MI, Barner KC, et al. Changes in nerve conduction velocity across the elbow due to experimental error. Muscle Nerve 2002;26:838–40.
30. van Dijk JG, Meulstee J, Zwarts MJ, et al. What is the best way to assess focal slowing of the ulnar nerve? Clin Neurophysiol 2001;112:286–93.
31. Landau ME, Barner KC, Campbell WW. Optimal screening distance for ulnar neuropathy at the elbow. Muscle Nerve 2003;27:570–4.
32. Simmons Z, Nicholson T, Wilde C, et al. Variation of calculated ulnar motor conduction velocity across the elbow with body mass index. Muscle Nerve 1997;20:1607–8.
33. Landau ME, Barner KC, Campbell WW. Effect of body mass index on ulnar nerve conduction velocity, ulnar neuropathy at the elbow, and carpal tunnel syndrome. Muscle Nerve 2005;32:360–3.
34. Rutkove SB, Geffroy MA, Lichtenstein SH. Heat-sensitive conduction block in ulnar neuropathy at the elbow. Clin Neurophysiol 2001;112:280–5.
35. Landau ME, Barner KC, Murray ED, et al. Cold elbow syndrome: spurious slowing of ulnar nerve conduction velocity. Muscle Nerve 2005;32:815–7.
36. Olney RK, Miller RG. Conduction block in compression neuropathy: recognition and quantification. Muscle Nerve 1984;7:662–7.
37. Oh SJ, Kim DE, Kuruoglu HR. What is the best diagnostic index of conduction block and temporal dispersion? Muscle Nerve 1994;17:489–93.
38. Pickett JB, Coleman LL. Localizing ulnar nerve lesions to the elbow by motor conduction studies. Electromyogr Clin Neurophysiol 1984;24:343–60.
39. Levin KH. Common focal mononeuropathies and their electrodiagnosis. J Clin Neurophysiol 1993;10:181–9.
40. Payan J. Electrophysiological localization of ulnar nerve lesions. J Neurol Neurosurg Psychiatry 1969;32:208–20.
41. Kimura I. Early electrodiagnostic measurement of ulnar entrapment neuropathy of the elbow. Rinsho Shinkeigaku 1984;24:945–50 [in Japanese].
42. Gilliatt RW, Thomas PK. Changes in nerve conduction with ulnar lesions at the elbow. J Neurol Neurosurg Psychiatry 1960;23:312–20.
43. Hawley J, Capobianco J. Localizing ulnar nerve lesions by motor nerve conduction study. Electromyogr Clin Neurophysiol 1987;27:385–92.

44. Bielawski M, Hallett M. Position of the elbow in determination of abnormal motor conduction of the ulnar nerve across the elbow. Muscle Nerve 1989;12:803–9.
45. Kothari MJ, Preston DC. Comparison of the flexed and extended elbow positions in localizing ulnar neuropathy at the elbow. Muscle Nerve 1995;18:336–40.
46. Felsenthal G, Brockman PS, Mondell DL, et al. Proximal forearm ulnar nerve conduction techniques. Arch Phys Med Rehabil 1986;67:440–4.
47. Benecke R, Conrad B. The value of electrophysiological examination of the flexor carpi ulnaris muscle in the diagnosis of ulnar nerve lesions at the elbow. J Neurol 1980;223:207–17.
48. Olney RK, Hanson M. AAEE case report:15: ulnar neuropathy at or distal to the wrist. Muscle Nerve 1988;11:828–32.
49. Olney RK, Wilbourn AJ. Ulnar nerve conduction study of the first dorsal interosseous muscle. Arch Phys Med Rehabil 1985;66:16–8.
50. Azrieli Y, Weimer L, Lovelace R, et al. The utility of segmental nerve conduction studies in ulnar mononeuropathy at the elbow. Muscle Nerve 2003;27:46–50.
51. McIntosh KA, Preston DC, Logigian EL. Short-segment incremental studies to localize ulnar nerve entrapment at the wrist. Neurology 1998;50:303–6.
52. Paternostro-Sluga T, Ciovika R, Turkof E, et al. Short segment stimulation of the anterior transposed ulnar nerve at the elbow. Arch Phys Med Rehabil 2001;82:1171–5.
53. Lo YL, Leoh TH, Xu LQ, et al. Short-segment nerve conduction studies in the localization of ulnar neuropathy of the elbow: use of flexor carpi ulnaris recordings. Muscle Nerve 2005;31:633–6.
54. Jabre JF. Ulnar nerve lesions at the wrist: new technique for recording from the dorsal sensory branch of the ulnar nerve. Neurology 1980;30:873–6.
55. Kim DJ, Kalantri A, Guha S, et al. Dorsal cutaneous ulnar nerve conduction: diagnostic aid in ulnar neuropathy. Arch Neurol 1981;38:321–2.
56. Eisen A, Danon J. The mild cubital tunnel syndrome. Neurology 1974;24:608–13.
57. Payan J. Anterior transposition of the ulnar nerve: an electrophysiologic study. J Neurol Neurosurg Psychiatry 1970;33:157–65.
58. Friedman RJ, Cochran TP. A clinical and electrophysiological investigation of anterior transposition for ulnar neuropathy at the elbow. Arch Orthop Trauma Surg 1987;106:375–80.
59. Yoon JS, Walker FO, Cartwright MS. Ulnar neuropathy with normal electrodiagnosis and abnormal nerve ultrasound. Arch Phys Med Rehabil 2010;91:318–20.
60. Beekman R, Visser LH, Verhagen WI. Ultrasonography in ulnar neuropathy at the elbow: a critical review. Muscle Nerve 2011;34:627–35.
61. Boom J, Visser LH. Quantitative assessment of nerve echogenicity: comparison of methods for evaluating nerve echogenicity in ulnar neuropathy at the elbow. Clin Neurophysiol 2012;123(7):1446–53.
62. Volpe A, Rossato G, Bottanelli, et al. Ultrasound evaluation of ulnar neuropathy at the elbow: correlation with electrophysiological studies. Rheumatology 2009;48:1098–101.
63. Won SJ, Yoon JS, Kim JY, et al. Avoiding false-negative nerve conduction study in ulnar neuropathy at the elbow. Muscle Nerve 2011;44:583–6.
64. Vucic S, Cordato DJ, Yiannikas C, et al. Utility of magnetic resonance imaging in diagnosing ulnar neuropathy at the elbow. Clin Neurophysiol 2006;117:590–5.
65. Bäumer P, Dombert T, Staub F, et al. Ulnar neuropathy at the elbow: MR neurography—nerve T2 signal increase and caliber. Radiology 2011;260:199–206.
66. Iba K, Wada T, Tamakawa M, et al. Diffusion-weighted magnetic resonance imaging of the ulnar nerve in cubital tunnel syndrome. Hand Surg 2010;15:11–5.

67. Kaeser HE. Erregungsleitungsstorungen bei ulnarlsparesen. Dtsch Z Nerven-heilkd 1963;185:231–43.

68. Campbell WW, Sahni SK, Pridgeon RM, et al. Intraoperative electroneurography: management of ulnar neuropathy at the elbow. Muscle Nerve 1988;11:75–81.

69. Caliandro P, La Torre G, Padua R, et al. Treatment for ulnar neuropathy at the elbow. Cochrane Database Syst Rev 2011;(2):CD006839.

Electrodiagnosis of Carpal Tunnel Syndrome

Leilei Wang, MD, PhD*

KEYWORDS

- Carpal tunnel syndrome • Electrodiagnosis • Combined Sensory Index
- Nerve conduction study

KEY POINTS

- Carpal tunnel syndrome (CTS) will likely continue to be a common problem encountered by the electrodiagnostician, given recent evidence suggesting an increasing incidence of the condition.
- New modalities, such as MRI and ultrasound, are being applied to CTS and can potentially add important information about the anatomy and morphology of the carpal tunnel, median nerve, and surrounding tissue.
- Although CTS is a condition that is relatively easy to recognize, investigations to improve early CTS detection and treatment outcomes are warranted.

INTRODUCTION

Carpal tunnel syndrome (CTS) is the most common and the best studied of all focal neuropathies.[1,2] CTS has provided an unmatched teaching and learning experience for generations of students, physicians, and scholars involved in patient care and electrodiagnostic testing (EDX). The EDX methodology for evaluating CTS has served as an example for the study of all focal neuropathies.[3,4]

It is estimated that one in five patients presenting with upper limb pain, numbness, tingling, and weakness have the diagnosis of CTS. CTS also accounts for 90% of all known compression or entrapment neuropathies.[5,6] A search on PubMed using the phrase "carpal tunnel syndrome" yields more than 7000 articles published in the English language literature alone in the new millennium, 2000 of which have been published since the beginning of this decade. This ongoing scholarly interest in CTS holds promise for further refinements to the diagnosis and treatment of the

Funding sources: Nil.
Conflict of interest: Nil.
Department of Rehabilitation Medicine, University of Washington, Seattle, WA, USA
* Department of Rehabilitation Medicine, University of Washington, School of Medicine, 1959 Northeast Pacific Street, Box 356157, Seattle, Washington 98195.
E-mail address: lw7@uw.edu

disorder and, it is hoped, will lead to effective ways to prevent this common human ailment.

Recent epidemiologic studies suggest the number of people afflicted by CTS is substantial in US and European populations.[7–11] The prevalence of self-reported CTS in the US adult population has been estimated to be as high as 5%.[12] New demographic data indicate an increasing trend.

CTS was initially defined as a clinical disorder diagnosed by pattern recognition of patients presenting with similar symptoms and careful clinical examination. Rudimentary EDX for CTS began in the mid-1950s[13] and continued to develop throughout subsequent decades. EDX has been regarded as an objective, reliable, and valid test for CTS. More recent advancements in technology have brought EDX to a level of performance and reliability unavailable to earlier clinicians. There have also been improvements in the speed in which the study can be conducted and comfort afforded to the patient.

This article discusses the historical aspects related to the understanding of CTS and its diagnosis, highlighting observations about this disease that have yet to be challenged. This is followed by a discussion regarding the use of EDX as a diagnostic tool for CTS, as well as the author's approach to making the diagnosis of CTS. Finally, conclusions about future directions in the diagnosis, treatment and research of this disorder are presented.

HISTORICAL ASPECTS OF CTS

Descriptions of CTS by surgeons treating traumatic upper limb injuries date back to at least the mid-1800s.[14] Brain's[15] 1947 landmark publication in the *Lancet* reported spontaneous CTS and summarized earlier published cases from 1909 to 1945. The term acroparesthesias, coined by Ormerod in 1833 to describe paresthesias in the extremities, was later used to refer to the nighttime burning and pins-and-needles sensation in the fingers of middle-aged women. Acroparesthesias in the median nerve distribution continue to be useful in evaluating CTS. Another feature noted in the early history of CTS was that of thenar eminence atrophy and hand weakness. However, an understanding that the sensory and motor symptoms were caused by a single median nerve lesion at the wrist was not appreciated until many years after the first clinical descriptions of the disease. Eventually the hypotheses that thenar neuritis, brachial plexus lesions, or an extra cervical rib could cause CTS were refuted, and focal median nerve compression at the carpal tunnel (CT) was identified as the sole cause for both the sensory and motor deficits.

The term carpal tunnel syndrome was said to appear in print for the first time in a paper published by Kremer and colleagues[16] in 1933. George Phalen, an American orthopedic surgeon at the Cleveland Clinic, was credited with popularizing the use of the contemporary term beginning in the 1950s.[17–20] Besides using the Tinel test to help support the diagnosis of CTS, Phalen also gave us the wrist flexion test that carries his name. Both the Tinel and Phalen tests have been widely used in clinical practice and for research. However, the lack of an agreed on standard method contribute to the variable sensitivity and specificity of the tests.[21]

Many risk factors for CTS have been recognized early on such as pregnancy, space-occupying tumor, trauma (especially crush injuries), and work activities. The long list of known CTS risk factors includes age, rheumatoid arthritis, diabetes, hypothyroidism, obesity, square-shaped wrist, and many others. These risks can be divided into intrinsic (ie, genetic, biologic) and extrinsic (ie, environmental, activity-related) factors.

The present day understanding of the diagnosis and treatment of CTS incorporates contributions by many medical and surgical specialties, including orthopedics, physiatry, neurology, rheumatology, neurosurgery, plastic surgery, chiropractic, osteopathy, and others.[22] This frequently encountered condition typically presents with a constellation of signs and symptoms. The underlying pathogenesis has been well proven and accepted. It is now known that focal compression of the median nerve at the CT results in the symptoms of CTS as a consequence of injury to the sensory and motor nerves. Use of EDX medicine has proved to be indispensible in confirming the diagnosis of CTS.

ANATOMY OF THE CT

The CT is a dumb-bell-shaped passage, with an estimated width of 25 mm at its entrance and exit and 20 mm at its narrowest.[23,24] The pathophysiology of CTS is closely related to the anatomy of the CT. The median nerve, which is derived from the lateral and the medial cord of the brachial plexus and C6 to T1 nerve roots, follows a path at the elbow close to the brachial artery. As the median nerve approaches the distal crease of the wrist, before entering the cephalic margin of the CT, it splits off the palmar cutaneous branch to provide sensation to the palmar skin over the thenar eminence. Inside the CT, the median nerve is accompanied by nine long flexor tendons, including the four tendons of the flexor digitorum superficialis, the four tendons of the flexor digitorum profundus, and the flexor pollicis longus tendon.

The walls of the CT are made of fibro-osseous tissue, which is inelastic and unyielding to pressure (**Fig. 1**). The dorsal and lateral aspects of the tunnel are formed by four carpal bone prominences, including the proximal lateral scaphoid, the proximal medial pisiform, the distal medial hook of the hamate, and the tubercle of the trapezium. The floor is formed by the lunate and capitate bones, and the volar side is formed by the fibrous transverse carpal ligament. The narrow space enclosed by

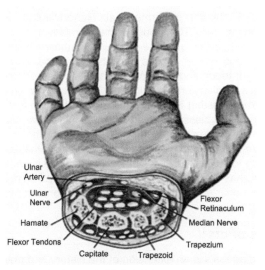

Fig. 1. The anatomy of the CT. (*From* Cobb TK, Cooney WP, An K. Pressure dynamics of the carpal tunnel and flexor compartment of the forearm. J Hand Surg Am 1995;20:193–8; with permission.)

the rigid wall and the crowded content make this segment of median nerve inside the CT particularly vulnerable to compression.

Intra-CT pressure plays a role in the pathophysiology of CTS. A recent study of fluid dynamics in CTS subjects demonstrated that intracarpal pressure is elevated and dissipation of this pressure is abnormally slow relative to controls.[25,26] CT pressure measured in CTS subjects had a mean of 32 mm Hg, compared with 2.5 mm Hg in the healthy control group.[27,28] Large myelinated nerve fibers in the CT are most susceptible to mechanical and ischemic damage. In CTS, microscopy has shown that disruption of myelin and the nodes of Ranvier results in conduction dysfunction and, when severe enough, axonal death.[29]

The severity and the rate of neuropathic changes correlate not only with the degree and duration of the compression, but also with the acuity of pressure elevation. The natural history of most spontaneous CTS is that of gradual onset and slow progression, often over months if not years. Acute CTS is less common and usually associated with traumatic injuries and bony fractures. Anticoagulation-related hemorrhages into the CT and prolonged mechanical drilling have been reported as causes of acute CTS. It is not entirely clear how much the mechanical force and ischemia from microvascular compromise contributes to the pathogenesis of CTS. Morphologically, the median nerve observed during CT surgery often has a flattened, pale, and edematous appearance. Pulsatile blood flow in the median nerve is restored within minutes after the release of the transverse carpal ligament. Symptomatic pain relief reported by patients also happens quickly, often within days after the surgery. The recovery of the median neuropathy may take weeks to months and is often incomplete, supporting the view that the cause of the symptoms in the patient with CTS is more complex than just demyelination and axonal loss of the median nerve.

CLINICAL EVALUATION OF CTS

A directed history and physical examination is essential for the diagnosis of CTS. Pain, tingling, numbness, relief with hand shaking, and the dropping of objects are common complaints. Thumb abduction weakness and atrophy of the thenar eminence are positive predictors of CTS. The self-performed Katz Hand Diagram drawing is useful in assessing some patients for CTS, though it has a relatively low sensitivity of 0.64 and specificity of 0.73 according to one study.[30] Numbness is typically appreciated in the thumb, index, and middle fingers but has been reported to be present in all fingers. Testing of light touch and pinprick sensation at the bedside typically demonstrates alterations in a median nerve distribution. Two-point discrimination or Semmes Weinstein monofilament testing is often used as well to help further define sensory deficits. Knowledge of the classic median nerve terminal branches serves to guide the physical examination. However, one should be aware that many variations and anomalies exist.[31] As mentioned previously, the Tinel and Phalen tests may also be of value in assessing for CTS. The flick sign or arm shaking is worthwhile mentioning because it reportedly has the best sensitivity and specificity.[32] In more severe cases of CTS, atrophy of the thenar eminence and thumb abduction and opposition weakness can be appreciated.

ELECTRODIAGNOSIS OF CTS

In essence, electrodiagnosis is an extension of the history and physical examination. The key finding for CTS is that of conduction slowing localized to the segment of the median nerve passing through the CT. Nerve conduction study (NCS) is more valuable than needle electromyography (EMG) study in general because of the underlying pathophysiology of focal demyelination in CTS. Both the distal location and relative ease of CTS study contribute to the reliable nature of EDX in the assessment of this disorder. Meticulous attention to electrode placement, distance measurements, stimulation intensity, skin temperature, and many others factors are important to prevent misdiagnosis of CTS. It is recommended that the temperature of the upper limb be maintained at 32°C for NCS. There is no uniform agreement on the best location for the temperature probe.

Sensory Conduction Studies

In early and mild CTS, mild sensory nerve conduction slowing across the CT is often the only abnormal finding. The peak latency of the median sensory nerve action potential (SNAP) is typically delayed or prolonged. The use of peak latency for detecting CTS, instead of the onset latency, has become increasingly embraced by many electrodiagnosticians because of the frequent challenge in identifying the onset of the SNAP in the presence of a large stimulus artifact. Sensory amplitudes vary greatly among individuals and offer limited diagnostic value until the amplitude becomes smaller than the range of normal reference values. As CTS progresses, sensory peak latency is progressively delayed and the amplitude becomes smaller. In more advanced CTS, there is often no recordable SNAP even with signal averaging and enhancement.

There are many different protocols for median nerve sensory conduction study to help diagnose CTS. Using antidromic techniques with stimulation applied to the wrist, median SNAPs can be recorded at the thumb, the index, the long, and the ring fingers. Median sensory fiber electrical signals can also be recorded in the long finger with the application of two stimuli, one at the wrist and one at the palm. When present, relative sensory nerve conduction slowing in the proximal segment can reveal focal median sensory nerve injury localized to the CT. Conduction block is suspected when the SNAP elicited with proximal stimulation is 50% or less in amplitude than that recorded with stimulation applied distal to the wrist. Proximal segmental conduction slowing relative to a more distal segment helps in differentiating CTS from length-dependent peripheral neuropathy. The method of sensory "inching" along the median nerve between the wrist and palm is not regularly used, but could potentially help localize conduction slowing to a short segment of the median nerve.[33]

Motor Conduction Studies

Median motor nerve conduction is usually obtained recording over the abductor pollicis brevis (APB) muscle. Delay of the distal motor latency (DML) supports the diagnosis of CTS. However, by itself, mild prolongation of the median DML does not absolutely suggest focal demyelination. The preferential loss of the large fast-conducting myelinated nerve fibers could also result in slower nerve conduction and delayed DML. It has been shown that mild proximal conduction slowing can occur in CTS and, therefore, a decreased median motor nerve conduction velocity in the forearm does not exclude the diagnosis of CTS. Comparing the conduction velocity and DML of the median nerve to that of the ulnar nerve, which travels outside the CT, helps to confirm CTS and differentiate it from length-dependent peripheral polyneuropathy.[34] One should also be aware of the possibility of anatomic variants such as a Martin-Gruber anastomosis in the forearm, but its presence generally does not cause confusion in the diagnosis of CTS in contrast to EDX for ulnar neuropathy at the elbow.

Short segment studies testing the recurrent median motor branch distal to the compression site have the potential for more precisely localizing a median neuropathy to the CT. In performing such testing, distal motor conduction block can sometimes be demonstrated as consequence of significant focal motor nerve demyelination.[35] However in practice, the short distance between stimulation and recording sites and the close proximity of the recurrent branch of the median motor nerve to the nearby ulnar motor nerve make such short segment testing challenging.

Needle EMG Studies

Needle EMG is often helpful in further characterizing the neuropathic insult, especially when the compound muscle action potential amplitude is reduced because this can be a consequence of either distal demyelination or denervation. Needle EMG can provide evidence of denervation by the presence of membrane instability, such as fibrillation potentials and positive sharp waves, and altered motor unit morphology. With severe CTS, electrodiagnostic evidence of axonal loss of motor nerves and subsequent motor unit reorganization can be seen in the intrinsic hand muscles innervated by the median nerve, including the APB, the superficial head of the flexor pollicis brevis, opponens pollicis, and the first and second lumbricals. However, axon loss of motor nerves is generally uncommon in CTS. Also, fibrillation potentials and positive sharp waves cannot be used to quantify the extent of motor axon loss. For most CTS cases, the use of needle EMG is debated.

Latency Differences in CTS

There are two methods to decide whether the median nerve latency is normal or prolonged, both of which require normal reference values obtained from healthy individuals without CTS. The first is the absolute latency method. Using this method, the median sensory or motor latency is compared against the normal reference value. Conduction slowing is determined if the latency exceeds the upper limit of normal. This absolute latency method has several drawbacks, especially for sensory conduction because the skin temperature effects and other factors. The recommendation is that each EDX laboratory establishes its own normal data. Unfortunately, this is not always achievable.

An increasing awareness of variation among normal reference values from laboratory to laboratory has led to the comparison reference value method. This newer method has been well described and was recommended for use in diagnosing CTS in a recent 2011 American Association of Neuromuscular and Electrodiagnostic Medicine (AANEM) monograph.[36] In this method, conduction study of the median nerve is compared with that of another nerve, usually in the same limb and typically the ulnar. Comparison reference values from different investigators show less variation, because of better built-in controls for differences in subjects, techniques, and equipments.

For instance, for the assessment of CTS, latency measurements can be compared using median–thenar and ulnar–hypothenar pairs.[37] With this protocol, a DML difference of greater than 1.2 to 1.8 ms is said to be significant.[2] This technique is especially useful when studying patients who have generalized peripheral polyneuropathy, most commonly from diabetes. As supporting evidence for probable CTS, this author uses a difference of greater than 2.0 ms comparing the median DML with the ipsilateral ulnar DML. When there are no sensory responses in the upper extremities of a diabetic patient who has additional unilateral hand paresthesias and weakness, such a motor comparison can be quite helpful to demonstrate evidence for CTS in the presence of diabetic peripheral neuropathy. Another useful technique in this setting of possible peripheral neuropathy and superimposed CTS is a comparison of the difference in DML between the median-innervated second lumbrical muscle and the ulnar-innervated first palmar interosseous muscle.[38] The author applies this approach in her laboratory but not routinely.

The Combined Sensory Index

Though the best electrodiagnostic test for CTS has yet to be determined, many studies for CTS have been designed over the last few years. For instance, using the absolute method, one can assess for CTS by obtaining median sensory latency recording from the thumb, and the index, long, and ring fingers. Using the comparison method, CTS can be diagnosed by determining median-radial sensory latency differences to the thumb, median-ulnar sensory differences to the ring finger, and transpalmar median-ulnar latency differences. An important question is whether one normal test is sensitive enough to refute the diagnosis of CTS. Because CT compression can affect some median nerve fascicles earlier or preferentially, one electrodiagnostic test may demonstrate CTS when another does not. Performing limited studies could reduce the sensitivity of EDX considerably, causing a false negative error. However, increasing the number of tests also likely increases the probability of reducing the specificity of testing, causing a false positive error in proportion to the number of tests performed. Although a false negative error may limit early detection and treatment, a false positive error could result in overtreatment, which has the potential to cause harm to the patient.[39]

The combined sensory index (CSI) is an attempt to maximize sensitivity for detecting CTS without reducing specificity by using a single score derived from multiple sensory tests. The CSI, sometimes called the Robinson index, is easy to obtain.[40] The CSI is the sum of comparisons of sensory latencies collected with three established sensory tests for the study of CTS using the following formula: CSI = ringdiff + thumbdiff + palmdiff. In this formula, ringdiff is the peak latency difference of the median and ulnar antidromic sensory nerve conduction to the ring finger stimulating 14 cm proximally, the thumbdiff is the peak latency difference of the median and radial antidromic sensory nerve conduction to the thumb stimulating 10 cm proximally, and the palmdiff is the transpalmar peak latency difference of the median and ulnar orthodromic conduction using a distance of 8 cm.[41] For example, if the latencies are 3.8 ms for median nerve conduction to the ring finger and 3.4 ms for ulnar nerve conduction to the ring finger, then the ringdiff is 0.4. If the median latency is 3.4 ms and the ulnar latency is 3.8 ms, then the ringdiff would be a negative number (−0.4). Using negative numbers helps to cancel random errors such as distance measurement and take into account of ulnar or radial sensory neuropathy if present.

The CSI has a high specificity (ie, few false positives), a high sensitivity (ie, few false negatives), and excellent test-retest reliability.[42] When the upper limit of the normal CSI is set at 0.9 ms, the test sensitivity is 0.83 and the specificity 0.95. If the normal upper limit for the CSI is raised from 0.9 ms to 1.1 ms, the sensitivity remains essentially the same at 0.82; however, the specificity increases to 1.00 indicating very low if any probability of false positive error. Generally, a CSI of 1.0 ms or greater would be consistent with CTS. The test and retest reliability for the CSI has been shown to be superior to that of other techniques in identifying CTS because of improved control for variables such as hand size, height, age, and temperature.

Study Approaches and Reporting of CTS

In the author's laboratory, CTS is considered with any clinical presentation of pain, numbness, paresthesias, and weakness in the upper extremities. Other potential diagnoses, such as arthritis, tendinopathy, polyneuropathy, brachial plexopathy, or cervical radiculopathy, are also entertained. Clinical impression of the likelihood of

CTS from history and physical examination is formed before EDX study. The author usually begins with median motor nerve conduction, followed by ulnar motor nerve conduction, and then the three sensory tests that form the CSI study. When bilateral CTS is suspected, the more symptomatic hand is studied first. If the median nerve is normal, the less symptomatic side is not always studied. The author does not perform NCS in the asymptomatic limb for the purpose of contralateral comparison of the median nerves given the significant incidence of bilateral EDX abnormalities in some asymptomatic population. This is in accordance with AANEM guidelines.

For most patients referred to our EDX laboratory with possible CTS, the author performs all three CSI sensory tests and reports the calculated CSI. The added time, cost, and discomfort to the patient of these studies are quite reasonable. The benefit of obtaining a complete CSI is its excellent reproducibility. Repeat CTS referrals on the same patients are fairly common in the author's institution. These patients have recurrent CTS after a period of satisfactory symptom relief using conservative treatments. Comparison of two CSI scores could provide information in regard to progression of CTS and is potentially of help to the patient and the treating physician in making treatment choices. A change of the CSI in such repeat studies of greater than 0.3 ms is considered to be statistically significant.[40] The author is occasionally asked to study the patient who has persistent hand pain and numbness after CT release surgery. The comparison of two CSI scores obtained before and after the operation, when available, is useful in differentiating residual median neuropathy versus incomplete release or recurrent CTS, which is rare.

For nerve conduction studies, the author prefers warming the upper limb rather than extrapolating using a latency or conduction velocity corrected for temperature. Individual thermostats in the study rooms help regulate room temperature to minimize skin temperature drop during the study, which is usually between 1°C and 2°C in our laboratory. Warming pads are used to maintain skin temperature, though a heat lamp or a hand-held hair dryer can also work. The author does not routinely perform needle EMG for CTS evaluation.

Needle EMG is performed if there is concern for the possibility of ulnar neuropathy, brachial plexopathy, cervical radiculopathy, or if there is a history of trauma. For example, non–median innervated C8 muscles, such as the first dorsal interosseus, abductor digiti minimus, or extensor indicis proprius, are examined in addition to the APB muscle if C8 radiculopathy is suspected. Needle EMG study of median-innervated forearm muscles, such as the pronator quadratus and pronator teres, help to differentiate CTS from less common median nerve entrapment syndromes that occur proximal to the wrist.

When providing the patient with CTS and the referring clinician with our EDX impression, the author confirms the localization of a median neuropathy at the wrist and comments on the electrodiagnostic evidence or sensory nerve involvement only or if there is focal demyelination of the motor nerve. The severity of the demyelination is also commented on in reference to the degree of conduction slowing and the presence or absence of motor conduction block. Denervation from CTS is rare, but when present, the extent and chronicity are also discussed in the report.

No matter the EDX protocol used, some patients with the clinical symptoms of CTS have negative findings. Conservative treatment (see later discussion) is a satisfactory approach for many of these patients. Conversely, EDX CTS in patients without clinical CTS symptoms should be reported with caution to referring clinicians to avoid the potential risk of overtreatment. A prevalence study of the Swedish general population found 18.4% of a control group to have abnormal EDX findings characteristic for CTS.[12]

TREATMENT OPTIONS FOR CTS

Acute CTS associated with trauma and bone fractures often requires timely open exploration and decompression, and EDX could be performed at the time of surgery or after the postoperational follow-up. For most subacute and chronic CTS, initial treatments are designed to relieve the uncomfortable and often disabling symptoms using nonsurgical methods. Early and mild symptoms of CTS are frequently self-limiting and often resolve within weeks. Simple and noninvasive treatments can provide significant symptomatic relief and protect the median nerve from further injury.[43] Pain in CTS can be alleviated with oral medications, such as Tylenol, nonsteroidal antiinflammatory medications, and gabapentin. Oral steroids are less commonly used. Treatment should be considered for underlying conditions that could predispose to CTS, such as diuretics for fluid retention, thyroid supplementation for hypothyroidism, insulin for diabetes, and immune modulating agents for rheumatoid arthritis. A nighttime wrist brace that reduces nocturnal wrist flexion is often of benefit. A recent prospective study showed that local steroid injections into the CT can be effective in treating CTS[44,45] and should be considered as an option. Educating the patient about avoiding overuse and activity modification is essential to prevent recurrence.

When pain persists and interferes with sleep and daily activities, the surgical option should be considered and supported. In reference to the CSI, outcomes of surgical release have been carefully examined in a few recent studies. Interestingly, patients with a CSI between 2.5 and 4.6 gain the most from carpal tunnel release (CTR).[46] However, improvement following CTR is also reported by many patients with a normal CSI and similarly in some patients with advanced chronic CTS. A decision to recommend CTR should be based not just on the electrodiagnostic abnormalities but also other physical and psychosocial and vocational factors that could play a role in the patient's functional recovery from such surgery. For instance, a recently published article reports that before surgery, whether or not and the duration of worker's compensation is a strong positive predictor for long-term disability related to CTS.[47]

SUMMARY

CTS will likely continue to be a common problem encountered by the electrodiagnostician, given recent evidence suggesting an increasing incidence of the condition. New modalities, such as MRI and ultrasound are being applied to CTS evaluation and can potentially add important information about the anatomy and morphology of the CT, median nerve, and nearby tissue.[48–50] With further refinement and higher resolution of imaging techniques, important information regarding median nerve, edema, inflammation, as well as the milieu of the surrounding CT, will be, it is hoped, provided, supplementing the EDX and clinical findings. Although CTS is a condition that is relatively easy to recognize, investigations aim for early detection, effective treatment including outcomes are warranted with the ultimate goals to alleviate suffering and disability.

REFERENCES

1. Entrapment Neuropathies, Chapter 3 Carpal Tunnel Syndrome. 3rd edition. In: Dawson DM, Hallett M, Wilbourn AJ, editors.
2. AANEM monograph Werner RA, Andary M. Electrodiagnostic evaluation of carpal tunnel syndrome. Muscle Nerve 2011;44:597–607.
3. Electrodiagnosis in diseases of nerve and muscle: principles and practice. 2nd edition. Jun Kimura. F.A. Davis Company. p. 501–5.

4. Electrodiagnostic Medicine. Daniel Dumitru. Philadelphia: Hanley & Belfus, Inc.; 1995. p. 867–8.
5. Schapper SM, Rechtsteiner EA. Ambulatory medicine car and utilization estimate for 2006. Natl Health Stat Report 2008;6:1–29.
6. Cullen KA, Hall MJ, Golosinskiy A. Ambulatory surgery in the United States, 2006. Natl Health Stat Report 2009;1–25.
7. Mondelli M, Giannni F, Giacchi M. Carpal tunnel syndrome incidence in a general population. Neurology 2002;58:289–94.
8. Nordstrom D, DeStefano F, Vierkant RA, et al. Incidence of diagnosed carpal tunnel syndrome in a general population. Epidemiology 1998;9:342–5.
9. Tanaka S, Wild DK, Seligman PJ, et al. The US prevalence of self-reported carpal tunnel syndrome. 1988 national health interview survey data. Am J Public Health 1994;84:1846–8.
10. Stevens JC, Sun S, Beard CM, et al. Carpal tunnel syndrome in Rochester, Minnesota, 1961–1980. Neurology 1988;38:134–8.
11. Aroori S, Spence RA. Carpal tunnel syndrome. Ulster Med J 2008;77:6–17.
12. Atroshi I, Gummesson C, Johnsson R, et al. Prevalence of carpal tunnel syndrome in a general population. JAMA 1999;281:153–8.
13. Jablecki CK, Andary MT, So YT, et al. Literature review of the usefulness of nerve conduction studies and electromyography in the evaluation of patients with carpal tunnel syndrome. Muscle Nerve 1993;16:1392–414.
14. Amadio PC. History of carpal tunnel syndrome, Chapter 1. In: Luchetti R, Amadio PC, editors. Carpal tunnel syndrome. Berlin: Springer; 2007. ISBN 978-3-540-22387-0.
15. Brain WR. Spontaneous compression of both median nerve in the carpal tunnel syndrome. Lancet 1947;1:277–82.
16. Kremer M, Gilliatt RW, Golding JS, et al. Acroparaesthesiae in the carpal-tunnel syndrome. Lancet 1953;2:590–5.
17. Phalen GS. Spontaneous compression of the median nerve at the wrist. JAMA 1951;145:1128–33.
18. Phalen GS, Kendrick JI. Compression neuropathy of the median nerve in the carpal tunnel. JAMA 1957;164:524–30.
19. Phalen GS. Reflection on 21 years' experience with the carpal-tunnel syndrome. JAMA 1970;212:1365–7.
20. Phalen GS. The birth of a syndrome, or carpal tunnel revisited. J Hand Surg Am 1981;6:109–10.
21. Alfonso MI, Dzwierzynski W. Hoffman-Tinel sign, the reality. Phys Med Rehabil Clin N Am 1998;9:721–36.
22. Russell BS. Carpal tunnel syndrome and the "double crush" hypothesis: a review and implications for chiropractic. Chiropr Osteopat 2008;16:2.
23. Robbins H. Anatomical study of the median nerve in the carpal tunnel and etiologies of the carpal-tunnel syndrome. J Bone Joint Surg Am 1963;45:953–66.
24. Yugueros P, Berger RA. Anatomy of the carpal tunnel, Chapter 2. In: Luchetti R, Amadio PC, editors. Carpal tunnel syndrome. Berlin: Springer; ISBN 978-3-540-22387-0. p. 10–2.
25. Cobb TK, Cooney WP, An K. Pressure dynamics of the carpal tunnel and flexor compartment of the forearm. J Hand Surg Am 1995;20:193–8.
26. Lundborg GN. Miniature compartment syndrome. J Neurol Neurosurg Psychiatr 1983;46:1119–24.
27. Szabo RM, Chidgey LK. Stress carpal tunnel pressure in patients with carpal tunnel syndrome and normal patients. J Hand Surg Am 1989;14:624–7.

28. Rempel D, Bach JM, Richmond CA, et al. Effects of forearm pronation/supination on carpal tunnel pressure. J Hand Surg Am 1998;23:38–42.
29. Sunderland S. Nerve and nerve injuries. Edinburgh (Scotland): Churchill Livingston; 1978.
30. Katz JN, Larson MG, Sabra A, et al. Carpal tunnel syndrome diagnostic utility of history and physical examination findings. Ann Intern Med 1990;112:321–7.
31. Lanz U. Anatomical variations of the median nerve in the carpal tunnel. J Hand Surg 1977;2:44–53.
32. Pryse-Phillips W. Validation of a diagnostic sign in carpal tunnel syndrome. J Neurol Neurosurg Psychiatry 1984;47:870–2.
33. Ross MA, Kimura J. AAEM case report #2: the carpal tunnel syndrome. Muscle Nerve 1995;18:567–73.
34. Sander HW, Quinto C, Saadeh PB, et al. Sensitive median—ulnar motor comparative techniques in carpal tunnel syndrome. Muscle Nerve 1999;22:88–98.
35. Lesser EA, Venkatesh S, Preston DC, et al. Stimulation distal to the lesion in patients with carpal tunnel syndrome. Muscle Nerve 1995;18:503–7.
36. AAEM. Practice parameter for electrodiagnostic studies in carpal tunnel syndrome: summary statement. Muscle Nerve 2002;25:918–22.
37. Boonyapisit K, Katirji B, Shapiro BE, et al. Lumbrical and interossei recording in severe carpal tunnel syndrome. Muscle Nerve 2002;25:102–5.
38. Preston DC, Logigian EL. Lumbrical and interossei recording in carpal tunnel syndrome. Muscle Nerve 1992;15:1253–7.
39. Robinson LR, Temkin NR, Fujimoto WY, et al. Impact of statistical methodology on normal limits in nerve conduction studies. Muscle Nerve 1991;14:1084–90.
40. Robinson LR, Micklesen PJ, Wang L. Optimizing number of tests for carpal tunnel syndrome. Muscle Nerve 2000;23:1880–2.
41. Robinson LR, Micklesen PJ, Wang L. Strategies for analyzing nerve conduction data: superiority of a summary index over single tests. Muscle Nerve 1998;21:1166–71.
42. Lew H, Wang L, Robinson LR. Test-retest reliability of combined sensory index: implications for diagnosing carpal tunnel syndrome. Muscle Nerve 2000;23:1261–4.
43. Celiker R. Corticosteroid injection vs. nonsteroidal antiinflammatory drug and splinting in carpal tunnel syndrome. Am J Phys Med Rehabil 2002;81:182–6.
44. Girlanda P, Venuto C, Mangiapane R, et al. Local steroid treatment in idiopathic carpal tunnel syndrome: short and long–term efficacy. J Neurol 1993;240:187–90.
45. Dammers JW, Vermeulen M. Injections with methylprednisolone proximal to the carpal tunnel: randomized double blind trial. BMJ 1999;319:884–6.
46. Malladi N, Micklesen PJ, Hou J, et al. Correlation between the combined sensory index and clinical outcome after carpal tunnel decompression: a retrospective review. Muscle Nerve 2010;41:453–7.
47. Spector J, Turner JA, Fulton-Kehoe D, et al. Pre-surgery disability compensation predicts long-term disability among workers with carpal tunnel syndrome. Am J Ind Med 2012;55(9):816–32.
48. Jarvik JG, Yuen E, Haynor DR, et al. MR nerve imaging in a prospective cohort of patients with suspected carpal tunnel syndrome. Neurology 2002;58:1597–602.
49. Jarvik JG, Yuen E, Kliot M. Diagnosis of carpal tunnel syndrome: electrodiagnostic and MR imaging evaluation. Neuroimaging Clin N Am 2004;14:93–102.
50. Descatha A. Huard Meta-analysison the performance of sonography for the diagnosis of carpal tunnel syndrome. Semin Arthritis Rheum 2012;41:914–22.

Electrodiagnosis of Lumbar Radiculopathy

Karen Barr, MD

KEYWORDS

- Electrodiagnosis • EMG • Lumbar radiculopathy

KEY POINTS

- It can often be clinically challenging to diagnose lumbar radiculopathy. Electrodiagnostic studies are helpful in this diagnosis because the test is very specific and is therefore a good complement to lumbar magnetic resonance imaging, which is a very sensitive, but not specific, test for lumbar spine disease. In addition, it is the only test that gives information about the physiologic function of the nerve root, or if damage to a nerve root has occurred.
- A thoughtfully planned study can also help rule out competing diagnoses that cause pain or neurologic changes in the lower extremity as well as rule in the diagnosis of radiculopathy.
- The utility of electrodiagnostic studies in the diagnosis of radiculopathy depends on the expertise of the examining physician to plan, perform, and interpret the study appropriately.

INTRODUCTION

Lumbosacral radiculopathies were first described by Mixter and Barr in 1934, and electrodiagnosis has been part of the clinical evaluation of this condition for over 50 years.[1] The question of whether a lumbar radiculopathy is present is one of the most common referrals to the electrodiagnostic laboratory.[2] This review describes the value and limitations of electrodiagnostic studies in evaluating for this condition, as well as the technical aspects of planning the optimal electrodiagnostic study to evaluate for the presence of radiculopathy and to rule out competing diagnoses. There is also a discussion regarding the use of electromyography (EMG) to help determine the prognosis and treatment of radiculopathy.

It is not always easy to diagnose lumbar radiculopathy. There are many different medical conditions that cause low back and lower extremity pain, or patients may have more than one disorder. Some patients are vague historians, without a clear recall of their symptoms; sometimes the clinical picture is confounded by issues regarding compensation or blame. The physical examination relies on the patient's

Rehabilitation Medicine, University of Washington, Box 356490, Seattle, WA 98195-6490, USA
E-mail address: barrk@u.washington.edu

Phys Med Rehabil Clin N Am 24 (2013) 79–91
http://dx.doi.org/10.1016/j.pmr.2012.08.011
1047-9651/13/$ – see front matter © 2013 Elsevier Inc. All rights reserved.

cooperation and may be difficult to interpret. Because of this, it is common for patients to undergo further testing to confirm or rule out this diagnosis. From an evidence-based medicine perspective, it can be difficult to assess the value of these tests, because there is no one gold standard for the diagnosis of lumbar radiculopathy. Therefore, in both research and the clinic, a combination of history, physical examination, imaging, and electrodiagnostic testing is used to come to a diagnosis.

MAGNETIC RESONANCE IMAGING VERSUS ELECTRODIAGNOSTIC STUDIES IN DIAGNOSING LUMBAR RADICULOPATHY

Most radiculopathies are caused by root compression, most commonly from intervertebral disk disease or other degenerative changes of the spinal column, such as ligamentous hypertrophy or the bony changes that accompany osteoarthritis. Other compressive lesions can less commonly cause radiculopathy, such as tumors and cysts. Magnetic resonance imaging (MRI) is exquisitely sensitive in detecting these anatomic changes. However, MRI often shows disk disease and other degeneration in asymptomatic people. Lumbar disk protrusions can be seen in as high as 67% of asymptomatic patients older than age 60, and more than 20% have lumbar central stenosis.[3] Therefore, MRI is very sensitive in detecting anatomic changes that could cause a radiculopathy but does not give any information about nerve function or whether these anatomic changes could be a source of symptoms.

There are other causes of radiculopathy besides nerve root compression, and MRI would not be helpful in the diagnosis of these types of radiculopathy. Motor radiculopathy can be seen in patients from varicella zoster virus, even in the absence of skin lesions.[4] Inflammatory mediator cytokines, perhaps from regional disk disease or other factors, can be a source of neuropathic pain and a "chemical radiculitis" without evidence of nerve root compression.[5,6]

STRENGTHS OF ELECTRODIAGNOSTIC TESTING FOR RADICULOPATHY

Studies have found that needle EMG is very specific in the diagnosis of lumbar radiculopathy when the appropriate electrodiagnostic criteria are used. For that reason clinically EMGs are commonly performed to rule in a radiculopathy, particularly in the following situations:

1. To determine if the structural changes seen on MRI are the common finding of an asymptomatic abnormality or are actually causing physiologic abnormalities in the nerve root
2. To determine the most likely affected level if clinical symptoms and imaging levels do not match
3. To look for physiologic evidence if noncompressive radiculopathies are suspected
4. To determine prognosis related to axonal loss
5. To search for other causes of neurologic symptoms
6. Electrodiagnostic studies for radiculopathy are rarely false positive: if an EMG shows evidence of a radiculopathy, the patient almost certainly has one. When the criteria used for diagnosis are the presence of positive sharp waves and fibrillation in 1-limb muscle plus lumbar paraspinal muscles at the corresponding level, or in 2-limb muscles innervated by the same nerve root, it is 100% specific, both in asymptomatic patients and in those patients with low back pain and sciatica. If evidence of either acute changes or chronic denervation (as demonstrated by more than 30% of motor units are polyphasic, have large amplitude, and have increased duration in a study that uses monopolar needles) is used as the

electrodiagnostic criteria, then specificity decreases, but still remains in the range of 81- nearly 100%, depending on the level tested.[7]

LIMITATIONS OF ELECTRODIAGNOSTIC STUDIES BECAUSE OF THE NATURE OF RADICULOPATHY

In contrast to the strength of very high specificity, one of the biggest limitations of electrodiagnostic testing for radiculopathy is that sensitivity is not that high. The exact sensitivity cannot be calculated, because of the lack of a gold standard, but it is often noted that a patient may clinically seem to have a radiculopathy that electrodiagnostic testing is unable to diagnose. It is also possible that an electrodiagnostician could determine that a radiculopathy is present, but be unable to ascertain the exact root level involved. Some reasons for this relative insensitivity follow.

WHY A PATIENT COULD HAVE A RADICULOPATHY AND STILL HAVE A NORMAL ELECTRODIAGNOSTIC STUDY

1. Inability to detect pure sensory radiculopathies: Clinically, most patients present with either purely sensory complaints (such as pain, parasthesias, or numbness) or primarily sensory complaints with some minimal complaints of weakness. However, because the site of nerve injury is proximal to the dorsal root ganglion in radiculopathies, sensory nerve conduction studies will be normal.[2] Therefore, there is no way for electrodiagnostic studies to evaluate these purely sensory nerve problems. Because there is no gold standard for the diagnosis of radiculopathy, it is unknown what percentage of radiculopathies is purely sensory.
2. Subtotal root involvement is the norm in lumbar radiculopathies: This root involvement may include demyelination, which would not cause most of the characteristic changes evaluated for on needle EMG, or limited axonal loss that goes undetected because only a few axons are involved. Therefore even in the presence of a motor radiculopathy, nerve fibers supplying much of the muscle are spared.[2]
3. If denervation is balanced with reinnervation, or the denervation is old, no fibrillations will be seen, and the denervation will be missed.[5]

WHY A PATIENT COULD HAVE A RADICULOPATHY, BUT THE LEVEL OF NERVE INJURY CANNOT BE DETERMINED
Imprecision of Myotomal Maps

Many myotomal maps have been published, but the primary root innervation of many muscles remains unclear. Besides a lack of consensus in this area, there is considerable individual variation in the innervation of individual muscles.[8] Because of this, if needle EMG changes are found in a muscle, the examining physician cannot say with 100% certainty what root level innervates that muscle; the examiner can only state what is thought to be the usual level for a typical patient.

Difficulty with Precise Localization of the Lesion in Patients with High Lumbar Radiculopathy

There are 2 issues that make this a difficult condition to diagnose precisely with electrodiagnostic testing. One issue is that lesions of L2, L3, and L4 radiculopathy have very extensive myotomal overlap, so it is often not possible to separate out which of these specific roots is the cause of the electrodiagnostic findings. The second issue is that it is often difficult to separate out plexopathy from radiculopathy at these levels. There are 2 main reasons for this. One is that, unlike brachial plexopathies, there are no good, reliable sensory nerve conduction studies for the nerves that arise for the upper lumbar plexus. If there were, this would give evidence to the electrodiagnostician that the problem is the plexus rather than the nerve root. The second reason is the limitation of paraspinal muscles in separating plexopathy from radiculopathy. In theory, abnormal paraspinal muscles would be expected in radiculopathy and would not be present with plexopathy. However, in reality, sometimes the paraspinal muscles are normal, and a radiculopathy is present; sometimes the paraspinal muscles are abnormal for reasons unrelated to radiculopathy.

Difficulty with Precise Localization of the Lesion in Patients with Lower Lumbar and Sacral Radiculopathies

Because of the anatomy of this region, there are many locations where the nerve root may be injured by a ruptured disk or other compressive force. For example, a disk herniation between the L4 and L5 vertebral bodies (which is the most common level) can affect the L4 root if it is a far lateral herniation, the L5 root if it is a posterior lateral herniation, and the S1–S4 roots if it is a central herniation. Within the cauda equina, roots are packed closely together so it is common for bilateral, multiroot lesions to be found in lumbar central stenosis.[2]

ANOTHER STUDY LIMITATION: EXAMINER EXPERTISE

Although these studies may seem to be objective; in reality, just as in other diagnostic tests, the skill of the physician performing and interpreting the study is the biggest factor in obtaining accurate results. This issue was studied by Kendall and Werner by comparing the diagnostic impressions of 6 cases of lumbar radiculopathy of an unblinded electromyographer with the impressions of the recorded study by a blinded resident or faculty electromyographer.[9] They found that the overall diagnostic agreement was only 46.9%. Faculty was twice as likely to agree on the final diagnosis as residents, demonstrating that extensive training is necessary to perform these studies accurately. Another study that looked at interrater reliability of needle EMG findings in lumbar radiculopathy used only expert examiners and compared the results of unblinded with blinded electrodiagnosticians. This study found an outstanding overall diagnostic impression agreement of greater than 90% between the unblinded and blinded examiners.[10]

PLANNING THE ELECTRODIAGNOSTIC STUDY

As mentioned earlier, the usefulness of electrodiagnostic testing for radiculopathy depends directly on the skills of the physician performing the study, and this applies to study planning as well as study interpretation. In general, there are 2 purposes of the electrodiagnostic study: to determine whether there is electrodiagnostic evidence of a radiculopathy, and to rule in or out competing diagnoses for the patient's symptoms.

The first part of this section addresses study planning in general. The second part addresses using electrodiagnostic studies to help in sorting out competing clinical diagnoses.

NEEDLE ELECTRODE EXAMINATION

The most important part of the electrodiagnostic testing to diagnose a radiculopathy is needle EMG. Other components may be helpful, but they are used primarily to rule in or out competing diagnoses that could explain all or part of the patient's symptoms. The presence of positive sharp waves and fibrillations in a myotomal distribution is the most reliable evidence of radiculopathy. Many electrodiagnosticians think there is a window of time when these acute changes are seen: They most likely first appear in the paraspinal muscles by about 7 days, but may not be seen in distal muscles for 5 or 6 weeks. Total myotomal involvement is rare—often many muscles within a myotome never show damage. If no further nerve damage occurs, these spontaneous changes generally disappear by about 9 months.[2] This limited duration of findings has also been shown in animal studies.[6] Other spontaneous activity, such as fasciculation potentials and complex repetitive discharges, are sometimes present and may help make the diagnosis. Abnormal motor unit action potential recruitment in a neurogenic pattern may be seen. Chronic neurogenic motor unit action potential changes are frequent in chronic radiculopathies, but if this alone is used for making the diagnosis, there is a significantly higher incidence of false positives, and many electrodiagnostic physicians think that this makes it unacceptable sole diagnostic criteria (**Fig. 1**).

WHAT MUSCLES TO CHOOSE TO STUDY FOR NEEDLE EMG

The best designed needle study is able to identify the level of radiculopathy, without causing unnecessary discomfort to the patient by testing unnecessary muscles. It also rules out another cause for an abnormal needle examination other than radiculopathy.

Principles of muscle selection include the following:

1. Several muscles with the same root innervations, but different peripheral nerves, should be tested.
2. Other muscles in the region and other muscles with the same peripheral nerve but different root levels should be tested, to rule out other causes of abnormal

MUSCLE	L2	L3	L4	L5	S1	S2
Proximal Nerves						
ILIOPSOAS (psoas from lumbar plexus and iliacus from femoral nerve)						
ADDUCTOR LONGUS (obturator nerve)						
VASTUS MEDIALIS/LATERALIS (femoral nerve)						
RECTUS FEMORIS (femoral nerve)						
TENSOR FASCIA LATA (superior gluteal nerve)						
GLUTEUS MEDIUS (superior gluteal nerve)						
GLUTEUS MAXIMUS (inferior gluteal nerve)						
Sciatic Nerve						
SEMITENDINOSUS/MEMBRANOSUS (tibial nerve)						
LONG HEAD BICEPS FEMORIS (tibial nerve)						
SHORT HEAD BICEPS FEMORIS (fibular nerve)						
Fibular nerve						
TIBIALIS ANTERIOR (deep fibular)						
EXTENSOR HALLUCIS LONGUS (deep fibular)						
PERONEUS LONGUS (superficial fibular)						
EXTENSOR DIGITORUM BREVIS (deep fibular)						
Tibial Nerve						
TIBIALIS POSTERIOR						
FLEXOR DIGITORUM LONGUS						
GASTROC LATERAL						
GASTROC MEDIAL						
SOLEUS						
ABDUCTOR HALLICUS (medial plantar nerve)						

Fig. 1. Lower extremity myotomal chart shows major and significant nerve root innervation of lower extremity muscles. Boxes shaded in green represent a dominant contribution, whereas boxes shaded in yellow represent a significant contribution. Minor contributions are not shown.

needle study, such as myopathy length-dependent peripheral neuropathy, or a mononeuropathy.

This framework for muscle selection still raises many questions: are some muscles more likely to be abnormal than others within a given root? Are there certain muscles that have less intersubject variation in root innervations, or more dominant root innervations, so that the examiner would be more confident that an abnormal muscle corresponded to a specific root?

One way of attempting to answer this question is to compare electrodiagnostic findings of patients with MRI evidence and surgically verified single-level spinal nerve root lesions as wasperformed by Tsao and colleagues.[11] In this study, 45 patients had positive electrodiagnostic studies, positive preoperative MRI, and surgically confirmed root lesions. Their findings are summarized below.

L2 and L3 Radiculopathy

There were very few patients in the study with L2 and L3 radiculopathies, and no particular pattern of muscle involvement was found that could distinguish one of these levels from another, most likely because of the marked overlap of muscle innervations in the anterior thigh. Both patients had abnormal iliacus, adductor longus, and paraspinal muscles as well as an abnormal quadriceps muscle.

L4 Radiculopathy

All patients had an abnormal adductor longus and, of those tested, an abnormal rectus femoris. They found no patients with L4 radiculopathies who had a positive anterior tibialis muscle, therefore concluding that this muscle is most likely highly L5 innervated. Most patients also had abnormal middle to upper paraspinal muscles.

L5 Radiculopathy

The muscles affected most commonly were the peroneus longus, tensor fascia lata, and posterior tibialis. Other commonly affected muscles were extensor digitorum brevis, anterior tibialis, and extensor hallucis longus. The biceps femoris short head was normal in all L5 patients in whom it was tested.

S1 Radiculopathy

The muscles affected most of the time included the long head of the biceps femoris, short head of the biceps femoris, the medial and lateral gastrocnemius, the abductor digiti quinti, and the gluteus maximus.

HOW MANY MUSCLES SHOULD BE INCLUDED IN A SCREENING EXAMINATION?

A second common question for the electromyographer to consider is how many muscles must be tested as an adequate screen before concluding that there is no electrodiagnostic evidence for a radiculopathy?

Dillingham and colleagues considered this question and performed a prospective study on patients referred for electrodiagnostic testing for suspected radiculopathy. For all patients, a standardized electrodiagnostic screen was performed that consisted of 11 muscles. Nonparaspinal muscles were considered abnormal if they had abnormal spontaneous activity, abnormal motor unit morphology consistent with nerve injury, or a neuropathic recruitment pattern (reduced recruitment). Paraspinals were considered abnormal if abnormal spontaneous activity was found. For the purpose of this study, they determined that if a patient had any abnormal muscle findings, they were considered to have an electrodiagnostically proven radiculopathy.

In this study, the paraspinal muscles were the most likely to be abnormal. The second most common muscle to show abnormalities was the medial gastrocnemius. They found that a 5-muscle screen that included parapinals identified 94% to 98% of radiculopathies that could be identified by needle EMG (which they defined as abnormality on an 11-muscle screen). A 6-muscle screen that included lumbar paraspinal muscles identified radiculopathy in 98% to 100% of the patients. Seven to 10 muscle screens that included parapinals did not identify a significant higher proportion of radiculopathies. If paraspinal muscles were not tested, a 5-muscle screen identified only 68% to 88% of radiculopathies, and to reach the level of 90% of radiculopathies identified, an 8-muscle screen was required.[5]

PARASPINAL MUSCLES AND THE ELECTRODIAGNOSIS OF RADICULOPATHY

Lumbar paraspinal muscles may be very helpful in the diagnosis of radiculopathy. It is thought that the lumbar paraspinal muscles are the first group of muscles to show spontaneous activity in acute radiculopathy, although this point has been disputed in the literature. Dillingham and colleagues performed a retrospective study of 139 patients with electrodiagnostically confirmed radiculopathy and found no evidence of correlation between abnormal paraspinal muscles and duration of symptoms.[12] They are also useful to prove that the lesion is located above the lumbar sacral plexus. One major drawback in their use in the diagnosis of radiculopathy is that, unlike most limb muscles, lumbar paraspinal muscles may show spontaneous activity in asymptomatic subjects. Date and colleagues found an overall prevalence of abnormal spontaneous activity in the lumbar paraspinal muscles of 14.5% of asymptomatic patients. This prevalence increased with age. They were very rare in patients under the age of 40 and were seen in 33% of those over the age of 60.[13] Another study found a prevalence of 42% had abnormal spontaneous activity in the paraspinal of asymptomatic patients. They characterized the activity as more commonly positive sharp waves than fibrillations, generally mild, and generally found in multiple locations.[14] This evidence has been disputed by others, who cite the close similarity in appearance of atypical-appearing endplate spikes with spontaneous activity. Dumitru and colleagues[15] reported a prevalence of 4% of true positive sharp waves or fibrillations in the paraspinal muscles of asymptomatic patients, but sited many examples of varied and atypical endplate spikes. At any rate, caution should be taken in making a diagnosis of radiculopathy in older patients when the only evidence is limited spontaneous changes in the paraspinal muscles.

NERVE CONDUCTION STUDIES AND RADICULOPATHY

Sensory nerve conduction studies are normal in radiculopathy, even if the physical examination reveals significant sensory loss, because the lesion occurs proximal to the dorsal root ganglion. Compound motor action potentials are usually normal unless severe damage has occurred, or if multiple root levels are involved, in which case there may be some diminished amplitude.

F WAVES

The evidence for the usefulness of F waves in the diagnosis of radiculopathy is limited. F waves are often normal in radiculopathy, most likely because the affected portion of the pathway is so small compared to the total pathway that the abnormality is not detected. If they are abnormal, the problem could be anywhere along the course of the nerve and cannot be localized to the root.[2] Some researchers have found that if multiple features of the F wave are taken into account (for example, considering the minimum latency, the maximum latency, and the number of repeaters), they can be helpful in making the diagnosis.[16,17] Overall, they appear less sensitive than the needle study. For example, Weber found that in patients with radiculopathy discovered on needle EMG, only 53% of L5 and 74% of S1 had abnormal F waves.[18] Aminoff and coworkers found similar results. Of 28 patients with unequivocal L5 or S1 radiculopathy, abnormal F waves were found in 14, and all of these patients also had abnormal needle EMG studies.[19]

H WAVES

H waves are helpful in the diagnosis of S1 radiculopathy. They have several strengths, including the ability to detect injury to sensory fibers, and they are not dependent on a window of opportunity to discover abnormalities as is the needle examination, because they become abnormal as soon as a compression occurs and the deficit can last indefinitely. Different waveform criteria are used to make the diagnosis by different examiners, such as side-to-side latency differences, side-to-side amplitude differences, or an absent response on one side and a present response on the other side. It is unclear which method is the best. Limitations of H waves include their inability to determine how acute or chronic the lesion is, and that they may be abnormal in other diseases, such as peripheral neuropathy. They also may be normal in radiculopathy if there is sparing of the fibers that relay the reflex.

SOMATOSENSORY-EVOKED POTENTIALS

Theoretically, somatosensory-evoked potentials (SEPs) should be helpful in the diagnosis of radiculopathy because they study the peripheral sensory pathway, including the sensory function of the proximal nerve root. Dermatomal SEPs should be particularly useful, because they assess the sensory fibers of a single root. However, the medical literature has not shown them to be useful in many cases.[2,20] Because of intersubject variations in SEP responses, only extreme changes can be interpreted as abnormal so more mild changes go unrecognized. Also, conduction in the normal fibers of the affected root may cause abnormalities to be missed. In addition, the small area of abnormality may be masked because of the long course of the pathway being tested.[19]

CONSIDERING A DIFFERENTIAL DIAGNOSIS FOR THOSE WITH BACK AND LOWER EXTREMITY PAIN

The differential of back pain with radiating leg pain is broad. Back pain affects most people at some point in their lifetime, and many structures in the back can cause referred pain into the thigh, such as facet joints, muscles, and the sacroiliac joint. Hip joint pain can cause buttock and thigh symptoms and therefore can be confused with radiculopathy. Other musculoskeletal conditions involving the hip can also cause symptoms in the thigh. A patient may have 2 conditions, such as back pain and plantar fasciitis, which could mimic radiculopathy. However, just because an examiner suspects the presence of a musculoskeletal disorder does not exclude the possibility of a radiculopathy being present. This theory was demonstrated in a study by Cannon and colleagues, in which 170 patients referred for electrodiagnostic testing were also examined for common musculoskeletal disorders.[21] They found a high prevalence of musculoskeletal disorders in this population, with an overall prevalence of 32%. Although there were a higher percentage of musculoskeletal disorders in those without electrodiagnostic evidence of radiculopathy (55%); musculoskeletal pain problems were a secondary diagnosis in 21% of those who did have electrodiagnostic evidence of a radiculopathy. The researchers concluded that the fairly high prevalence in all groups of musculoskeletal disorders makes it difficult to predict the outcome of electrodiagnostic testing based on their presence or absence.

CONSIDERING A DIFFERENTIAL DIAGNOSIS FOR THOSE WITH LOWER EXTREMITY WEAKNESS OR NUMBNESS

Electrodiagnostic studies are particularly useful if evidence for neurologic disease is discovered in the lower extremity to assist in determining their cause. Some conditions commonly confused with radiculopathy are described below and the electrodiagnostic study planning that will help differentiate these conditions is outlined.

Lumbosacral Plexopathy versus Radiculopathy

There are many causes of lumbosacral plexopathy, including trauma, compression during surgery or labor, compression from tumors, radiation damage from the treatment of tumors, vasculitic and idiopathic causes, among others.[22] Electrodiagnostically, key features that would separate this diagnosis from lumbar radiculopathy include the presence of abnormalities in the paraspinal muscles, which suggests radiculopathy, and diminished amplitude or absent sensory studies in the leg, which suggests plexopathy. In practice, however, changes in the paraspinal muscles can be seen in older patients and diabetic patients, and these same patients may have absent sensory studies in the leg, which can make differentiating these 2 diagnoses difficult. However, a combination of the history and the extent of changes found on the physical examination and electrodiagnostically can often assist the examiner in determining the most likely diagnosis.

Sciatic Nerve Lesions versus L5 or S1 Radiculopathy

Lesions isolated to the sciatic nerve are rarer than radiculopathy but may occur. Because of an overlap of electrodiagnostic findings, sciatic neuropathy is often confused with radiculopathy. Causes include trauma, local compression from positioning, a tumor, an abscess or other compressive lesion, and an idiopathic condition, among others.[23,24] Electrodiagnostically, needle changes should be sought in muscles that are innervated by the L5 and S1 nerve roots that do not arise from the sciatic nerve, such as gluteus medius, gluteus maximus, and paraspinal muscles, so that a clear diagnosis can be made.

Fibular Neuropathy versus L5 Radiculopathy

For patients with weak dorsiflexors, a differential to consider is a common fibular neuropathy at the fibular head versus L5 radiculopathy. Nerve conduction studies to the extensor digitorum brevis and anterior tibialis may show the presence of conduction block at the fibular head in fibular neuropathy if there is a significant demyelinating component. If the lesion is primarily axonal at the fibular head, the superficial fibular nerve should be absent or low amplitude, and this would be normal in radiculopathy. The needle study is also very helpful in differentiating these 2 diagnoses, in that L5 muscles not innervated by the fibular nerve are often abnormal in an L5 radiculopathy, but should be normal in a fibular neuropathy.

Tibial Neuropathy versus S1 Radiculopathy

Another peripheral mononeuropathy that could be confused with radiculopathy is tibial mononeuropathy (particularly tarsal tunnel syndrome) versus S1 radiculopathy. Again, specific nerve conduction studies to the tibial nerve, particularly sensory/mixed nerve studies, may be helpful, and the needle study of S1 innervated muscles above the ankle is helpful.

Lateral Femoral Cutaneous Neuropathy versus Radiculopathy

Lateral femoral cutaneous neuropathy (meralgia parasthetica) can cause numbness or parasthesias in the thigh that can be confused with radiculopathy. Specific testing of this nerve by either nerve conduction studies, or more sensitively by SEPs, can determine if this is the cause of thigh numbness.[25]

Polyperipheral Neuropathy versus Multilevel Radiculopathy

Often, a differential diagnosis of polyperipheral neuropathy versus multilevel radiculopathy is considered. Both of these conditions can cause bilateral numbness and weakness in the legs. The prevalence of both of these conditions increases with age, as does the prevalence of back pain from other causes, so it is not uncommon for a patient to have both back pain and peripheral neuropathy or both radiculopathy and peripheral neuropathy. Sometimes the history can be helpful in determining which of these is present: in general, the most common forms of polyperipheral neuropathy begin distally and symmetrically and progress slowly more proximally. In contrast, radiculopathy is often of a more acute onset with sensory and motor symptoms within a specific dermatome/myotome. However, with time, these dermatomes may overlap and appear to be distal and symmetric, and often the exact historical course of these changes is forgotten by the patient. Electrodiagnostic findings, particularly in patients older than 60 years of age, between the conditions may be similar. H waves are often unelicited in both conditions. Surals are commonly abnormal or absent in those with polyperipheral neuropathy but can be absent idiopathically in older patients, so their absence does not confirm one diagnosis as better than the other. What is helpful in differentiating these diagnoses is if proximal needle changes are seen, as this is unlikely to be due to a length-dependent peripheral neuropathy. Upper extremity nerve conduction studies, particularly sensory studies, may be abnormal in those with a typical length-dependent neuropathy severe enough to cause needle EMG changes in the leg, and this may help in the diagnosis of polyperipheral neuropathy rather than multilevel radiculopathy.

Early Motor Neuron Disease versus Radiculopathy

Sometimes motor neuron diseases, such as amyotrophic lateral sclerosis, may arise first in one or a few lumbosacral segments and therefore mimic radiculopathy. Features that suggest amyotrophic lateral sclerosis over radiculopathy include prominent, widespread fasciculation potentials, severe motor axonal loss in a patient without significant sensory complaints, and significant loss of axons in S1 distribution with an intact H reflex.[2] Additional needle EMG testing beyond one limb can be very helpful in determining this diagnosis.

EMG TO PREDICT PROGNOSIS

Several small studies have tried to determine if there is a clinical difference in patients who have EMG-positive radiculopathy, compared to those who have a presumed radiculopathy because of the history, physical examination, and imaging, but a normal EMG. One study compared 2 groups of patients who clinically met the diagnosis of radiculopathy, one group with positive EMG findings and the other group with normal EMGs. They found no difference between the groups in terms of pain scale ratings or Oswestry Disability Index scores.[26] Another study comparing the outcome of patients treated surgically compared to those treated conservatively for radiculopathy found that the initial EMG had no prognostic ability to predict outcome at 5 years. The overall outcome was influenced most by psychosocial factors.[27] In contrast to the findings of acute radiculopathy, one study found that, in long-term follow-up of patients diagnosed with radiculopathy, some treated surgically and some treated conservatively, those patients with a normal EMG at 1- and 5-year follow-up had better outcomes than those with signs of a remote radiculopathy, such as large motor units and reduced interference pattern at 1- and 5-year follow-up.

EMG to Predict Outcome of Lumbar Epidural Steroid Injection

A few studies have been performed to determine if those with EMG-positive radiculopathy have a different response to treatment than those with EMG-negative radiculopathy. One study found that the EMG-positive group who received the lumbar epidural steroid injections had a statistically better improvement on the Oswestry disability index after the injection, compared to the EMG-negative group, who had the injections. Improvement in both groups was so small, however, that there was only a minimally clinically significant difference. A similar but larger and more recent study by other researchers found those patients with EMG-positive radiculopathy had better pain improvement and functional improvement as measured by the pain disability questionnaire after lumbar epidural steroid injections than the group who was clinically diagnosed with radiculopathy, but who had normal EMGs.[28]

EMG to Predict Outcome of Lumbar Discectomy

Very little research has been done on the value of EMG to predict the outcome of surgery for radiculopathy. Spengler and colleagues included positive needle EMG findings in a scoring system of objective evaluations to assess who would improve with elective discectomy and found that EMG in combination with other objective measures, such as neurologic examination and imaging, correlated with operative findings of a disk, but psychological scores were the best predictor of clinical outcomes.[29] Falck and colleagues found similar results in their study of patients with positive EMG findings and lumbar disk herniation, some of whom were treated operatively, and some who were treated conservatively.[27] In contrast, in a small study of patients with cervical radiculopathy, patients with positive preoperative EMGs had a better outcome after discectomy and cervical fusion than patients who had normal preoperative EMGs.[30]

EMG and Persistent Neuropathic Pain in Radiculopathy

Whether an EMG is positive for radiculopathy does not appear to be a good indicator for the persistence of nerve related pain. In a study using a rat model of lumbar disk herniation, evidence of neuropathic pain improved with time, but the neuropathic pain persisted beyond the timeframe when positive needle EMG findings of fibrillations and positive sharp waves had already resolved.[6] Similar studies have not been conducted in humans.

SUMMARY

Electrodiagnosis still plays a major role in the diagnosis of lumbosacral radiculopathy. It has a complementary role to spine imaging. In the hands of a skilled examiner, the test is specific and can assist in ruling out competing diagnoses that may cause neurologic symptoms in the legs. Preliminary research is promising for the role of EMG in determining prognosis for some treatment outcomes. However, its power comes from the test's ability to determine physiologic function of the nerve root, not in detecting persistent neuropathic pain or predicting surgical outcomes.

REFERENCES

1. Shea PA, Woods WW, Werden DH. Electromyography in diagnosis of nerve root compression syndrome. Arch Neurol Psychiatry 1950;64(1):93–104.
2. Wilbourn AJ, Aminoff MJ. AAEM minimonograph 32: the electrodiagnostic examination in patients with radiculopathies. American Association of Electrodiagnostic Medicine. Muscle Nerve 1998;21(12):1612–31.
3. Weishaupt D, Zanetti M, Hodler J, et al. MR imaging of the lumbar spine: prevalence of intervertebral disk extrusion and sequestration, nerve root compression, end plate abnormalities, and osteoarthritis of the facet joints in asymptomatic volunteers. Radiology 1998;209(3):661–6.
4. Ter Meulen BC, Rath JJ. Motor radiculopathy caused by varicella zoster virus without skin lesions ('zoster sine herpete'). Clin Neurol Neurosurg 2010; 112(10):933.
5. Dillingham TR, Lauder TD, Andary M, et al. Identifying lumbosacral radiculopathies: an optimal electromyographic screen. Am J Phys Med Rehabil 2000; 79(6):496–503.
6. Kim SJ, Kim WR, Kim HS, et al. Abnormal spontaneous activities on needle electromyography and their relation with pain behavior and nerve fiber pathology in a rat model of lumbar disc herniation. Spine (Phila Pa 1976) 2011;36(24): E1562–7.
7. Tong HC. Specificity of needle electromyography for lumbar radiculopathy in 55- to 79-yr-old subjects with low back pain and sciatica without stenosis. Am J Phys Med Rehabil 2011;90(3):233–8 [quiz: 239–42].
8. Stewart JD. Electrophysiological mapping of the segmental anatomy of the muscles of the lower extremity. Muscle Nerve 1992;15(8):965–6.
9. Kendall R, Werner RA. Interrater reliability of the needle examination in lumbosacral radiculopathy. Muscle Nerve 2006;34(2):238–41.
10. Chouteau WL, Annaswamy TM, Bierner SM, et al. Interrater reliability of needle electromyographic findings in lumbar radiculopathy. Am J Phys Med Rehabil 2010;89(7):561–9.
11. Tsao BE, Levin KH, Bodner RA. Comparison of surgical and electrodiagnostic findings in single root lumbosacral radiculopathies. Muscle Nerve 2003;27(1): 60–4.
12. Dillingham TR, Pezzin LE, Lauder TD. Relationship between muscle abnormalities and symptom duration in lumbosacral radiculopathies. Am J Phys Med Rehabil 1998;77(2):103–7.
13. Date ES, Mar EY, Bugola MR, et al. The prevalence of lumbar paraspinal spontaneous activity in asymptomatic subjects. Muscle Nerve 1996;19(3):350–4.
14. Nardin RA, Raynor EM, Rutkove SB. Fibrillations in lumbosacral paraspinal muscles of normal subjects. Muscle Nerve 1998;21(10):1347–9.
15. Dumitru D, Diaz CA, King JC. Prevalence of denervation in paraspinal and foot intrinsic musculature. Am J Phys Med Rehabil 2001;80(7):482–90.
16. Pastore-Olmedo C, Gonzalez O, Geijo-Barrientos E. A study of F-waves in patients with unilateral lumbosacral radiculopathy. Eur J Neurol 2009;16(11):1233–9.
17. Toyokura M, Ishida A, Murakami K. Follow-up study on F-wave in patients with lumbosacral radiculopathy. Comparison between before and after surgery. Electromyogr Clin Neurophysiol 1996;36(4):207–14.

18. Weber F. The diagnostic sensitivity of different F wave parameters. J Neurol Neurosurg Psychiatry 1998;65(4):535–40.

19. Aminoff MJ, Goodin DS, Parry GJ, et al. Electrophysiologic evaluation of lumbosacral radiculopathies: electromyography, late responses, and somatosensory evoked potentials. Neurology 1985;35(10):1514–8.

20. Rodriquez AA, Kanis L, Lane D. Somatosensory evoked potentials from dermatomal stimulation as an indicator of L5 and S1 radiculopathy. Arch Phys Med Rehabil 1987;68(6):366–8.

21. Cannon DE, Dillingham TR, Miao H, et al. Musculoskeletal disorders in referrals for suspected lumbosacral radiculopathy. Am J Phys Med Rehabil 2007;86(12): 957–61.

22. Planner AC, Donaghy M, Moore NR. Causes of lumbosacral plexopathy. Clin Radiol 2006;61(12):987–95.

23. Srinivasan J, Ryan MM, Escolar DM, et al. Pediatric sciatic neuropathies: a 30-year prospective study. Neurology 2011;76(11):976–80.

24. Yuen EC, So YT, Olney RK. The electrophysiologic features of sciatic neuropathy in 100 patients. Muscle Nerve 1995;18(4):414–20.

25. el-Tantawi GA. Reliability of sensory nerve-conduction and somatosensory evoked potentials for diagnosis of meralgia paraesthetica. Clin Neurophysiol 2009;120(7):1346–51.

26. Fish DE, Shirazi EP, Pham Q. The use of electromyography to predict functional outcome following transforaminal epidural spinal injections for lumbar radiculopathy. J Pain 2008;9(1):64–70.

27. Falck B, Nykvist F, Hurme M, et al. Prognostic value of EMG in patients with lumbar disc herniation–a five year follow up. Electromyogr Clin Neurophysiol 1993;33(1):19–26.

28. Annaswamy TM, Bierner SM, Chouteau W, et al. Needle electromyography predicts outcome after lumbar epidural steroid injection. Muscle Nerve 2012; 45(3):346–55.

29. Spengler DM, Ouellette EA, Battie M, et al. Elective discectomy for herniation of a lumbar disc. Additional experience with an objective method. J Bone Joint Surg Am 1990;72(2):230–7.

30. Alrawi MF, Khalil NM, Mitchell P, et al. The value of neurophysiological and imaging studies in predicting outcome in the surgical treatment of cervical radiculopathy. Eur Spine J 2007;16(4):495–500.

Electrodiagnostic Testing in Lumbosacral Plexopathies

Ruple S. Laughlin, MD[a],*, P. James B. Dyck, MD[a,b]

KEYWORDS

- EMG • Lumbosacral plexopathy • Lumbosacral • Radiculoplexus neuropathy
- Lumbar plexopathy • Diabetic lumbosacral radiculoplexus neuropathy
- Diabetic amyotrophy

KEY POINTS

- Pure lumbosacral plexopathies are rare.
- Lumbosacral radiculoplexus neuropathies are more common than pure lumbosacral plexopathies.
- Inflammatory diabetic and nondiabetic lumbosacral radiculoplexus neuropathies are among the most common causes of lumbosacral plexopathies and are pathologically due to ischemic injury and microvasculitis.
- Lumbosacral plexopathies often do not occur alone but are found in association with thoracic and cervical radiculoplexus neuropathies.

INTRODUCTION

The lumbosacral roots and the lower extremity peripheral nerves are commonly involved in peripheral nervous system diseases (radiculopathies, length-dependent peripheral neuropathies). The lumbosacral plexus (composed of both the upper lumbar plexus and lower lumbosacral plexus) as a primary target for peripheral nervous system disease is less common. Despite this lesser frequency, the scope of processes that may be implicated in lumbosacral plexopathies is vast, ranging from compressive causes (ie, hematoma) and neoplastic diseases[1,2] to inflammatory conditions secondary to systemic disease (ie, diabetic radiculoplexus neuropathies [DRPN]).[1,2]

In all cases of lumbosacral plexopathy, electrodiagnostic studies incorporating nerve conduction studies and needle electromyography (EMG) can be helpful for localization and characterization of the underlying process. Localization to the lumbar

[a] Department of Neurology, Mayo Clinic Rochester, 200 First Street Southwest, Rochester, MN 55905, USA; [b] Peripheral Neuropathy Research Laboratory, Mayo Clinic Rochester, 200 First Street Southwest, Rochester, MN 55905, USA
* Corresponding author.
E-mail address: laughlin.ruple@mayo.edu

Phys Med Rehabil Clin N Am 24 (2013) 93–105
http://dx.doi.org/10.1016/j.pmr.2012.08.014
1047-9651/13/$ – see front matter © 2013 Elsevier Inc. All rights reserved.

plexus as opposed to nerve roots or individual roots is important, because diagnostic implications, evaluation, and treatment options may be different. Disorders that clinically present as a lumbosacral plexopathy often are not isolated to the lumbosacral plexus electrophysiologically and can extend into the roots (paraspinal involvement) as well as peripheral nerves. The concept of a radiculoplexus neuropathy (a process involving roots, plexus, and peripheral nerves) may therefore perhaps be more fitting when considering an electrodiagnostic approach to evaluating these patients.

This article focuses on nerve conduction studies and needle EMG in the diagnosis of lumbosacral plexopathies. In some clinical scenarios, there may be usefulness in other electrodiagnostic testing, including autonomic and quantitative sensation testing, to more firmly establish a diagnosis of lumbosacral plexopathy.

ANATOMY

Knowledge of the lumbosacral plexus anatomy is critical in assessment of the patient and planning a comprehensive electromyographic evaluation. Although often considered one entity, the lumbosacral plexus can be divided into 2 parts anatomically: the "upper" the lumbar plexus; and the "lower" the lumbosacral plexus.

Lumbar Plexus

The lumbar plexus lies within the psoas muscle and comprises the anterior rami of the T12 to L4 nerve roots (**Fig. 1**). Many of these muscles and nerves cannot be tested by standard EMG techniques because they are deep in the abdomen or are small cutaneous nerve branches. The 6 major branches of the lumbar plexus include[3]:

- Iliohypogastric nerve (T12/L1), which supplies the transverse and internal oblique muscles as well as sensation to the low abdomen.
- Ilioinguinal nerve (L1), a sensory branch to the inguinal region that also provides sensation to a small area of medial thigh and upper scrotum/labia sensation.
- Genitofemoral nerve (L1, L2) provides sensation to the skin of the femoral triangle. In men, this nerve provides muscular innervation to the cremasteric muscle and sensory innervation to the lower scrotum. In women, this nerve provides lower labial sensation.
- Lateral femoral cutaneous nerve (L2,L3) is a sensory branch to the lateral thigh. This sensory nerve, unlike those listed earlier, can be tested by nerve conduction techniques, although reliability of the results is questionable.
- Obturator nerve (L2, L3, L4 anterior rami) provides motor innervation to the thigh adductors and a small area of sensation to the medial thigh.
- Femoral nerve (L2, L3, L4 anterior rami, posterior divisions) is the largest branch of the lumbar plexus whose motor component can be tested by nerve conduction techniques. This branch supplies motor innervation to the iliopsoas, sartorius, and quadriceps muscles, and divides to form the saphenous nerve, which supplies sensation to the medial lower leg.

Unlike the brachial plexus, there are no subcomponents (trunks, cords) in the lumbar plexus (see **Fig. 1**).

Lumbosacral Plexus

The lumbosacral plexus primarily originates from the ventral rami L4 to S3 nerve roots (see **Fig. 1**).

- The lumbosacral trunk (also called the furcal nerve) has an L4 component that joins the L5 nerve root to form the lumbosacral trunk. This nerve then joins the

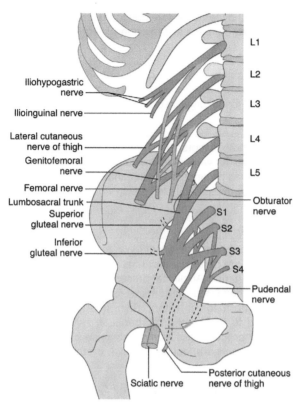

Fig. 1. Anatomy of the lumbosacral plexus. (Elsevier illustration from www.elsevierimages. com. © Elsevier Inc. All rights reserved.)

sacral plexus within the pelvic outlet. This structure is commonly affected in post-partum lumbosacral plexopathy, thought to be secondary to compression from the fetal head.[4]

- Superior gluteal nerve (L4, L5, S1) supplies motor innervation to the tensor fascia lata, gluteus medius, and gluteus minimus muscles.
- Inferior gluteal nerve (L5, S1, S2) provides motor innervation to the gluteus maximus muscle.
- Sciatic trunk/nerve (L5–S3) provides most motor innervation to the muscles of the posterior thigh and then into the leg via its 2 branches (common peroneal and tibial nerves).
- The pudendal nerve is formed from the anterior S2, S3, and S4 roots.

The tibial portion of the sciatic nerve innervates all the muscles of the posterior thigh except the short head of the biceps femoris, which is innervated by the peroneal division of the sciatic nerve or the common peroneal nerve branch of the sciatic nerve. This point is important when performing needle electromyogram studies for localization purposes.

HISTORY AND PHYSICAL EXAMINATION

When presented with a patient with lower limb symptoms, careful history and examination are imperative. Many different processes can cause lower extremity plexopathy,[2] and the responses to a few questions can be important in narrowing a differential diagnose and planning a subsequent electrodiagnostic study:

Onset

Did the process begin acutely (hours to days), subacutely (days to weeks), or is it chronic (months to years)? Most lumbosacral plexopathies have an acute to subacute onset, which is helpful in identifying the process.

Progression

Are the symptoms and findings worsening, stable, or improving? The disease course is a helpful feature to consider when thinking about the cause of a lumbosacral plexopathy as well as predicting prognosis. For instance, a slow, progressive course may point to a malignant cause, whereas a relapsing course may favor an inflammatory cause.

Extent

Is the process unilateral or bilateral at onset? We, and others, have described inflammatory plexopathies that are generally unilateral and focal in onset but become bilateral and widespread with time.[5] At clinical presentation, the disease may be bilateral but it should not be assumed that symptoms were bilateral at onset. This point should be clarified when taking a medical history. Also, it is important to confirm that the symptoms are confined to the lower limb, because involvement of the upper limb may make a structural process less likely, and raise concern for a more diffuse, possibly inflammatory, process affecting cervical, thoracic, as well as lumbosacral segments.

Pain, Sensation, and other Temporally Associated Symptoms

Associated pain and sensation changes are important clues in lumbosacral plexopathies. If the weakness seems to be confined to the plexus distribution, but the sensory loss seems to follow a more dermatomal distribution, this may increase the extent of needle examination and encourage imaging and further work-up, because concern for a primary root level process (ie, radiculopathy) may be heightened. Other clinical points to consider are associated systemic features that may support an inflammatory immune disorder such as sarcoidosis. Weight loss, in addition to constitutional symptoms such as fever and night sweats, may support the diagnosis of neoplastic infiltration or a paraneoplastic cause. A rash associated with the neuropathic symptoms may occur in the context of certain vasculitides.

ELECTROPHYSIOLOGIC EVALUATION
Nerve Conduction Studies

The electrophysiologic presence of lumbosacral plexopathy can be defined when there is evidence for electrophysiologic abnormalities in the distribution of at least 2 different peripheral nerves in at least 2 different nerve root distributions. Sparing of paraspinals on needle examination is also helpful in localizing a pure lumbosacral plexopathy.[6] However, most of these conditions are not pure and involve paraspinal denervation, hence our preferred term: radiculoplexus neuropathies.

Several sensory and motor nerve conduction studies are helpful in the diagnosis of a lumbosacral plexopathy (**Box 1**, **Table 1**). Several of these nerve conduction studies are not performed on routine lower limb studies and can be considered when evaluating for a lumbosacral plexopathy, especially if clinically involvement of the upper lumbar plexus is suspected. In many cases, if symptoms are unilateral, bilateral

---

Box 1
A nerve conduction study protocol for lumbosacral plexopathy

If the lumbar plexus is the most likely site of a lesion, then test:

1. Peroneal motor nerve conduction with F-wave study

2. If the peroneal compound muscle action potential (CMAP) amplitude is low or the conduction velocity is reduced then:

   Consider testing the opposite side

   Consider recording the peroneal motor nerve over the tibialis anterior muscle

3. Tibial motor nerve conduction with F-wave study

4. Femoral motor nerve conduction study with side-to-side comparisons (may require needle stimulation)

5. Sural sensory nerve conduction

6. Superficial peroneal sensory nerve conduction

7. Saphenous sensory nerve conduction

8. Lateral femoral cutaneous sensory nerve conduction

If the lumbosacral plexus is the most likely site of a lesion, then test:

1. Peroneal motor nerve conduction with F-wave study

2. If the peroneal CMAP amplitude is low or the conduction velocity is reduced then:

   Consider testing the opposite side

   Consider recording the peroneal motor nerve over the tibialis anterior muscle

3. Tibial motor nerve conduction with F-wave study

4. Sural sensory nerve conduction

   Superficial peroneal sensory nerve conduction

In both, it is likely necessary to compare abnormalities or borderline abnormalities with the contralateral limb.

If symptoms are bilateral, consider studying the upper limb to assess for a polyradiculoneuropathy or peripheral neuropathy.

---

studies can be helpful in determining a relative reduction in the size of the motor or sensory response (looking for axonal loss). Our laboratory uses a 50% difference from side to side as representing a significant and potentially pathologic difference.[7]

Sensory Nerve Conduction Studies

In cases of lumbosacral plexopathy, the sensory studies are likely to be most helpful for localization. Recall that, in most spinal segments, the dorsal root ganglion lies lateral to and outside the intervertebral foramen (**Fig. 2**). In electrodiagnostics, this feature is important because it helps assist in localization of a preganglionic process (ie, radiculopathy), versus a postganglionic process (ie, plexopathy or mononeuropathy). Therefore, a key point to remember is that, in most cases of lumbosacral plexopathy, reduced sensory nerve action potential amplitudes imply a postganglionic process and can help to exclude a radiculopathy as the main cause for clinical symptoms. The saphenous and lateral femoral cutaneous sensory nerve conductions in the upper lumbar plexus (see **Table 1**) are less technically reliable, whereas the sensory

Table 1
Useful nerve conduction studies in the evaluation of lumbar and lumbosacral plexopathies

	Stimulation Site	Recording Site	Pitfalls
Motor Nerves			
Lumbar Plexus			
Femoral (L2, L3, L4)	Femoral nerve in inguinal region	Quadriceps	Nerve is deep; often requires needle stimulation Proximity to femoral artery
Lumbosacral Plexus			
Peroneal (L4, L5)	Ankle and popliteal fossa	Extensor digitorum brevis (L5) Anterior tibialis (L4, L5)	Can be impaired in length-dependent neuropathies
Tibial (L5, S1, S2)	Ankle and popliteal fossa	Abductor hallucis (L5, S1)	Can be impaired in length-dependent neuropathies
Sensory Nerves			
Lumbar Plexus			
Saphenous (L3, L4)	Medial leg	Medial leg	Technically difficult
Lateral femoral cutaneous (L3, L4)	Lateral thigh	Lateral thigh	Technically difficult, deep, requires side-to-side comparison
Lumbosacral Plexus			
Superficial peroneal (L5)	Anterior shin	Distal anterior shin	Can be impaired in length-dependent neuropathies
Sural (S1, S2)	Ankle, midcalf and high calf	Ankle	Can be impaired in length-dependent neuropathies

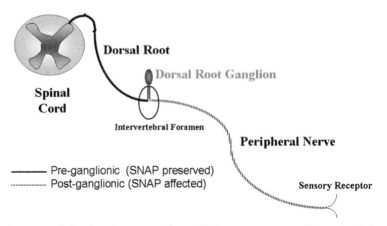

Fig. 2. Anatomy of the dorsal root ganglion. SNAP, sensory nerve action potential.

studies in the lumbosacral plexus (superficial peroneal, sural, and medial plantar) are more reliable and therefore more useful.

For example, the finding of the unilateral absence of superficial peroneal sensory and sural sensory nerve action potentials (SNAPs) suggests a lesion at or proximal to the sciatic nerve and lumbosacral plexus but distal to the dorsal root ganglion. When axonal loss is significant, a reduced or absent SNAP should be seen by 10 days after the inciting event. It is of note that although quite helpful, normal SNAPs do not completely exclude a plexopathy. This can be because the lesion may be proximal to the DRG (**Fig. 2**), there may be fascicular predilection for the motor fibers, or a conduction block. Additionally, in some lumbosacral plexopathies, the sensory responses are preserved because they primarily involve the upper lumbar plexus where the sensory studies are less reliable. An alternative explanation is the possible patchy involvement of nerves which spares sensory fascicles. It is dues to this latter situation that diabetic radiculoplexus neuropathy has also been called a "diabetic polyradiculopathy" (given the preservation of sensory responses in many cases).[8] As a result, if an electromyographer finds evidence for a polyradiculopathy on an electrodiagnostic study, an inflammatory plexopathy could still be considered in the differential diagnosis of that patient, depending on the clinical presentation.

Motor Nerve Conduction Studies

The femoral nerve is the only motor nerve conduction study likely to give meaningful information about the possibility of a pure lumbar plexopathy. As seen in **Table 1**, the most common method is to stimulate the nerve high in the inguinal region and record from a quadriceps muscle. Because of significant overlying connective tissue, needle stimulation is often necessary and may be contraindicated in some patients on anticoagulation given the proximity to the femoral artery, but the emphasis on this may be overstated.[9] In this case, side-to-side comparisons may not be as relevant as when using surface electrode recordings.

Peroneal and tibial motor studies are helpful in assessing axonal loss in the lumbosacral plexus; however, in elderly patients, these responses may be diminished or absent because of old age. Also, because the common recording sites are intrinsic foot muscles, patients with superimposed length-dependent peripheral neuropathies may have a reduction in CMAP amplitudes caused by their neuropathy and not by a lumbosacral plexopathy. In these cases, symmetric reductions are expected.

Needle Examination

The needle electromyographic examination may be the most important component of the electrodiagnostic evaluation of lumbosacral plexopathies, both for localization as well as determination of the severity of disease. The importance of a good examination and history cannot be overstated in deciding which muscles to test.

In suspected lumbosacral plexopathies, the planned needle EMG examination should be widespread and cover L2 to S1 innervated muscles as well as muscles innervated by the same root but different peripheral nerves to determine the extent of the abnormalities. Needle examination of the lumbosacral paraspinal muscles should also be performed (**Box 2**).[6,10] It is important that needle EMG evaluation of proximal L2/L3 muscles be conducted, because many providers do not routinely evaluate these muscles.

In lumbosacral plexopathies, one often sees a diffuse reduction of compound muscle and SNAP amplitudes, and needle examination shows neurogenic abnormalities in distal upper and lower limb muscles innervated by multiple lumbosacral roots.

Box 2
A needle examination protocol for lumbosacral plexopathy

To validate a diagnosis of lumbosacral plexopathy, involvement of at least 2 different muscles innervated by 2 different peripheral nerves must be shown:

1. Anterior tibialis (peroneal, L4/5)

2. Posterior tibialis/flexor digitorum longus (tibial, L5)

3. Medial gastrocnemius (tibial, S1/2)

4. Biceps femoris (sciatic, L5/S1)

5. Vastus medialis (femoral, L3/4)

6. Adductor longus (obturator, L2/3)

7. Tensor fascia latae/gluteus medius (inferior gluteal nerve, L5)

8. Gluteus maximus (superior gluteal nerve, S1/2)

9. Low lumbar paraspinals

If a sacral-predominant plexopathy is strongly suspected, consider also testing the anal sphincter and soleus muscles.

The needle examination abnormalities may be more severe in distal versus proximal muscles, with more fibrillation potentials. In these cases, it is tempting to interpret the findings as multiple lumbosacral radiculopathies superimposed on a length-dependent peripheral neuropathy. Although this interpretation at face value is not incorrect, it implies two pathophysiologically and temporally distinct processes. This pattern may be better characterized as a radiculoplexus neuropathy, in the appropriate clinical context.

Causes and Pathogenesis

As with other conditions of peripheral nerves, there are many potential causes of a lumbosacral plexopathy, including inflammatory, neoplastic, structural, and mechanical causes (**Box 3**).[11–15] Probably the most common cause of lumbosacral plexopathy that may mimic a lumbosacral radiculopathy electrophysiologically is diabetic lumbosacral radiculoplexus neuropathy (DLRPN). In these patients, careful history usually reveals an acute to subacute, asymmetrical, focal onset of lower limb pain followed by multifocal weakness, often associated with weight loss.[12] The natural history and underlying pathophysiologic mechanism of DLRPN has long been debated with many different names reflecting multiple views, including diabetic myelopathy,[16] diabetic amyotrophy,[17] Bruns-Garland syndrome,[18] diabetic mononeuritis multiplex,[19] proximal diabetic neuropathy,[20] diabetic lumbosacral plexopathy,[21] diabetic polyradiculopathy,[8] and multifocal diabetic neuropathy.[22] We use the term DLRPN because it emphasizes the frequent association of this syndrome with diabetes mellitus and its sites of involvement (roots, plexus, and nerves). We have studied these patients, as well as a cohort of patients with a similar syndrome without diabetes (lumbosacral radiculoplexus neuropathy [LRPN]) and found that clinically, electrophysiologically, and pathologically they are indistinguishable. Most of these patients have a monophasic course.

Electrophysiologic testing of these patients often shows axonal loss on routine lower limb motor nerve conduction studies, as shown by a reduction in CMAP amplitudes, as well as mild slowing of conduction velocity. This slowing is typically more in

---

Box 3
Causes of lumbosacral plexopathy

Inflammatory/immune

- Diabetic lumbosacral radiculoplexus neuropathy (microvasculitis)
- Nondiabetic lumbosacral radiculoplexus neuropathy (microvasculitis)
- Sarcoidosis
- Postsurgical inflammatory neuropathy

Neoplastic

- Metastatic diseases
  - Prostate
  - Cervix
  - Colorectum
  - Bladder
- Primary nerve sheath tumor
  - Benign schwannoma
  - Malignant nerve sheath tumor
- Perineurioma
- Lymphoma
- Paraneoplastic
- Amyloidosis

Compressive

- Retroperitoneal hematoma
- Retroperitoneal abscess

Stretch

- After hip or knee surgery

Trauma

Iatrogenic

- Injections
- Strict glucose in new diabetics

Pregnancy and parturition

Idiopathic

---

keeping with an axonal process as opposed to a demyelinating process, which typically translates to slowing that is greater than 70% of the upper limit of normal when the CMAP amplitude is greater than 50% of normal.[7] SNAP amplitudes are usually also reduced, supporting a postganglionic process.

As previously mentioned, needle EMG examination is often the most useful component of electrodiagnostic testing because of the lack of reliable nerve conduction study of the lumbar plexus. Needle EMG findings shows may be interpreted as multiple lumbosacral radiculopathies superimposed on a length-dependent peripheral neuropathy. This is because inflammatory cases of lumbosacral plexopathy such as

DLRPN (as opposed to a structural cause such as neoplastic infiltration), the pathologic process often involves the roots, plexus, and peripheral nerves simultaneously. Fibrillation potentials and long duration, high amplitude motor unit action potentials are commonly found extending from the lumbar paraspinals to distal leg muscles involving multiple myotomes. Extensive and often contralateral nerve conduction and needle EMG studies are often required to document the extent disease.

Additional testing in these patients can also be useful to help secure a diagnosis including quantitative sensation testing performed using CASE IV[23–25] and quantitative autonomic testing (a measure of postganglionic sudomotor, adrenergic, and cardiovagal function).[22] In a recent study of 17 DLRPN patients who underwent CASE IV testing, panmodality (small-fiber and large-fiber sensation) abnormalities were identified. Fourteen patients underwent autonomic testing (8 had clinical symptoms) all with abnormalities, 8 of which were severe.[5] Given these findings, additional testing of small and autonomic fibers is warranted when there is suspicion of a lumbosacral plexopathy, because these abnormalities would not be expected in radiculopathies, or other inflammatory polyradiculopathies.[26]

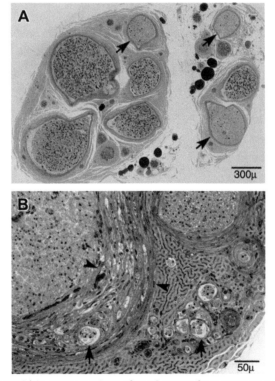

Fig. 3. Transverse semithin epoxy sections of sural nerves from patients with DLRPN stained with paraphenylenediamine (A) And methylene blue (B) Showing (1) multifocal fiber loss in which 3 fascicles (A, arrows) have almost no fibers, and the adjacent fibers are less affected; and (2) abortive repair with injury neuroma (B, arrows) and thickened perineurium (B, between arrowheads). These findings are typical for ischemic injury and repair and were commonly seen in both DLRPN an LRPN. (From Dyck PJB. Radiculoplexus neuropathies: diabetic and nondiabetic varieties. In: Dyck PJ, Thomas PK, eds. Peripheral Neuropathy. 4th ed. Vol. 2. Philadelphia: Elsevier; 2004; with permission.)

In the past, it has been suggested that the pathophysiologic basis of disease in diabetic patients who present with rapid asymmetrical plexopathies is caused by ischemic injury, which we and others have confirmed in DLRPN.[5,22,24] In our prospective series of 33 patients with DLRPN, distal cutaneous nerve biopsy samples in affected patients showed characteristic ischemic findings of multifocal fiber loss, perineurial degeneration or thickening, neovascularization, and abortive regeneration of nerve fibers forming microfasciculi (ie, an injury neuroma) (**Fig. 3**). We were able to compare these nerve samples with nerves of patients with diabetic peripheral neuropathy (DPN), and those with DLRPN showed significantly more ischemic changes. Axonal enlargements were also noted on transverse nerve sections; these were similar to enlargements described by others in experimental ischemia and were probably caused by accumulated organelles.[12,27,28] Teased nerve fiber evaluation showed increased rates of axonal degeneration and empty nerve strands compared with normal controls as well as DPN. In our recent prospective series, there were inflammatory infiltrates in all nerve biopsy samples. Inflammation involving the vessel walls suggesting microvasculitis was seen in half of the cases and, in several, diagnostic changes confirming microvasculitis were noted (**Fig. 4**).[15]

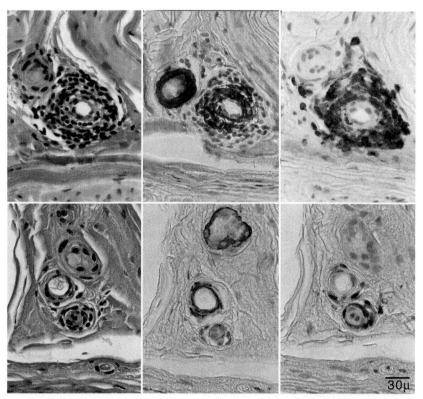

Fig. 4. Serial skip paraffin sections from a patient with painful DLRPN. Left panels are stained with hematoxylin and eosin, middle panels are stained with anti–smooth muscle actin, and the right panels reacted with leukocyte common antigen (CD45). The upper row shows fragmentation of the tunica media of the microvessel with mononuclear cells that show focal microvasculitis seen in DLRPN. (*From* Dyck PJB. Radiculoplexus neuropathies: diabetic and nondiabetic varieties. In: Dyck PJ, Thomas PK, eds. Peripheral Neuropathy. 4th ed. Vol. 2. Philadelphia: Elsevier; 2004; with permission.)

Symptomatic treatment in the form of narcotics in combination with neuropathic agents for pain as well as physical therapy should be considered at recognition of the condition. Patients need to be reassured that these inflammatory DRPN almost always seem to be monophasic in nature and, although complete resolution may not be seen, with time, meaningful improvement can usually be expected.

PITFALLS

Although electrodiagnostic testing is essential in the evaluation of a patient with a suspected lumbosacral plexopathy, it has limitations. For instance, in the case of a focal process such as a benign, slow-growing mass, the needle EMG findings may be limited to the distribution of only 1 nerve or 1 nerve root distribution, thereby failing to meet the definition of plexopathy (ie, the involvement of 2 different nerves and nerve roots in the lower extremity). However, if a high index of suspicion still exists, magnetic resonance imaging may be helpful to confirm a focal lesion. If the pathologic process is a lumbar radiculoplexus neuropathy, as discussed earlier, paraspinal denervation and long duration, high amplitude motor unit potentials on needle EMG are common.[5,13,29] The diagnosis of lumbosacral radiculoplexus neuropathy should also always be considered in patients presenting with what seems to be multiple radiculopathies superimposed on a length-dependent peripheral neuropathy, especially with a history of unilateral or asymmetrical onset of a painful, acute to subacute process associated with weight loss and autonomic derangements.

REFERENCES

1. Dyck PJB, Windebank AJ. Diabetic and nondiabetic lumbosacral radiculoplexus neuropathies: new insights into pathophysiology and treatment. Muscle Nerve 2002;25(4):477–91.
2. Planner AC, Donaghy M, Moore NR. Causes of lumbosacral plexopathy. Clin Radiol 2006;61:987–95.
3. Preston DC, Shapiro BE. Lumbosacral plexopathy. In: Preston DC, Shapiro BE, editors. Electromyography and neuromuscular disorders. 2nd edition. Philadelphia: Elsevier; 2005. p. 517–35.
4. Katirji B, Wilbourn AJ, Scarberry SL, et al. Intrapartum maternal lumbosacral plexopathy. Muscle Nerve 2002;26(3):340–7.
5. Dyck PJB, Norell JE, Dyck PJ. Microvasculitis and ischemia in diabetic lumbosacral radiculoplexus neuropathy. Neurology 1999;53(9):2113–21.
6. Dyck PJ. EMG approach to lumbosacral plexopathy. In: Course MCN, Lecture. Rochester (MN); 2010.
7. Daube JR, So ER. Application of clinical neurophysiology: assessing symptom complexes. In: Daube J, editor. Clinical neurophysiology. 2nd edition. New York: Oxford University Press; 2002. p. 597–8.
8. Bastron JA, Thomas JE. Diabetic polyradiculopathy: clinical and electromyographic findings in 105 patients. Mayo Clin Proc 1981;56(12):725–32.
9. Boon AJ, Gertken JT, Watson JC, et al. Hematoma risk after needle electromyography. Muscle Nerve 2012;45(1):9–12.
10. Tong HC, Haig AJ, Yamakawa KS, et al. Specificity of needle electromyography for lumbar radiculopathy and plexopathy in 55- to 79-year-old asymptomatic subjects. Am J Phys Med Rehabil 2006;85(11):908–12 [quiz: 913–5, 934].
11. Amato AA, Barohn RJ. Diabetic lumbosacral polyradiculoneuropathies. Curr Treat Options Neurol 2001;3(2):139–46.

12. Dyck PJ, Engelstad J, Norell J, et al. Microvasculitis in non-diabetic lumbosacral radiculoplexus neuropathy (LSRPN): similarity to the diabetic variety (DLSRPN). J Neuropathol Exp Neurol 2000;59(6):525–38.

13. Dyck PJB, Norell JE, Dyck PJ. Non-diabetic lumbosacral radiculoplexus neuropathy: natural history, outcome and comparison with the diabetic variety. Brain 2001;124(Pt 6):1197–207.

14. Mauermann ML, Amrami KK, Kuntz NL, et al. Longitudinal study of intraneural perineurioma–a benign, focal hypertrophic neuropathy of youth. Brain 2009; 132(Pt 8):2265–76.

15. Staff NP, Engelstad J, Klein CJ, et al. Post-surgical inflammatory neuropathy. Brain 2010;133(10):2866–80.

16. Garland H, Taverner D. Diabetic myelopathy. Br Med J 1953;1(4825):1405–8.

17. Garland H. Diabetic amyotrophy. Br Med J 1955;2(4951):1287–90.

18. Barohn RJ, Sahenk Z, Warmolts JR, et al. The Bruns-Garland syndrome (diabetic amyotrophy). Revisited 100 years later. Arch Neurol 1991;48(11):1130–5.

19. Raff MC, Asbury AK. Ischemic mononeuropathy and mononeuropathy multiplex in diabetes mellitus. N Engl J Med 1968;279(1):17–21.

20. Asbury AK. Proximal diabetic neuropathy. Ann Neurol 1977;2(3):179–80.

21. Bradley WG, Chad D, Verghese JP, et al. Painful lumbosacral plexopathy with elevated erythrocyte sedimentation rate: a treatable inflammatory syndrome. Ann Neurol 1984;15(5):457–64.

22. Low PA. Composite autonomic scoring scale for laboratory quantification of generalized autonomic failure. Mayo Clin Proc 1993;68(8):748–52.

23. Dyck PJ, Zimmerman I, Gillen DA, et al. Cool, warm, and heat-pain detection thresholds: testing methods and inferences about anatomic distribution of receptors. Neurology 1993;43(8):1500–8.

24. Dyck PJ, Zimmerman IR, Johnson DM, et al. A standard test of heat-pain responses using CASE IV. J Neurol Sci 1996;136(1–2):54–63.

25. Dyck PJ, Zimmerman IR, O'Brien PC, et al. Introduction of automated systems to evaluate touch-pressure, vibration, and thermal cutaneous sensation in man. Ann Neurol 1978;4(6):502–10.

26. Figueroa JJ, Dyck PJ, Laughlin RS, et al. Autonomic dysfunction in chronic inflammatory demyelinating polyradiculoneuropathy. Neurology 2012;78:702–8.

27. Korthals JK, Gieron MA, Wisniewski HM. Nerve regeneration patterns after acute ischemic injury. Neurology 1989;39(7):932–7.

28. Korthals JK, Wisniewski HM. Peripheral nerve ischemia. Part 1. Experimental model. J Neurol Sci 1975;24(1):65–76.

29. Garces-Sanchez M, Laughlin RS, Dyck PJ, et al. Painless diabetic motor neuropathy: a variant of diabetic lumbosacral radiculoplexus Neuropathy? Ann Neurol 2011;69(6):1043–54.

Clinical and Electrodiagnostic Features of Sciatic Neuropathies

B. Jane Distad, MD*, Michael D. Weiss, MD

KEYWORDS

- Sciatic neuropathy • Common fibular division • Tibial division
- Electrodiagnostic testing

KEY POINTS

- Sciatic neuropathy is the second most common neuropathy of the lower extremity.
- Sciatic neuropathy often presents with foot drop, mimicking common fibular neuropathy.
- The hip is the most common site of sciatic nerve injury.
- Trauma and masses account for most of the pathology leading to sciatic neuropathy.
- Electrophysiologic studies can help localize the lesion.
- Neuroimaging can sometimes identify an abnormality in more severe cases.

INTRODUCTION

Sciatic neuropathy is the one of the most common neuropathies of the lower extremities, second only to common fibular (peroneal) neuropathy. One of the most common presentations of sciatic neuropathy is foot drop. Because ankle dorsiflexion weakness, with or without lower extremity sensory impairment, may also be associated with several other clinical syndromes, a careful evaluation is necessary before confirming a diagnosis of sciatic neuropathy. Electrodiagnostic testing is of great value in confirming the diagnosis of suspected sciatic neuropathy and assessing the potential for recovery of nerve function.

ANATOMY

The sciatic nerve is the longest and widest single nerve in the body, originating just distal to the lumbosacral plexus and extending distal branches into the feet. It is responsible for most of the function of the lower extremity. It is derived from several

Division of Neuromuscular Diseases, Department of Neurology, University of Washington Medical Center, 1959 Northeast Pacific Street, Seattle, WA 98195, USA
* Corresponding author.
E-mail address: jdistad@uw.edu

Phys Med Rehabil Clin N Am 24 (2013) 107–120
http://dx.doi.org/10.1016/j.pmr.2012.08.023
1047-9651/13/$ – see front matter © 2013 Elsevier Inc. All rights reserved.

lumbosacral nerve roots and the lumbosacral plexus. A minor branch of L4 combines with the ventral ramus of L5 to form the lumbosacral cord or trunk. The lumbosacral trunk descends over the sacral ala and combines with the ventral rami of S1, S2, and S3 and a branch of S4 to form the sacral plexus.[1,2] The sciatic nerve forms the sacral plexus apex, located anteriorly to the sacroiliac joint and the piriformis muscle (**Fig. 1**).[3]

The sciatic nerve comprises the lateral division, which eventually forms the common fibular nerve, and the medial division, which forms the tibial nerve, each separately encased from the outset.[2] After arising at the exit of the superior and inferior gluteal nerves, the sciatic nerve leaves the pelvis via the sciatic notch, typically through the greater sciatic foramen, and is accompanied by the posterior femoral cutaneous nerve, inferior gluteal artery, pudendal vessels and nerves (**Fig. 2**). There is a close relationship to the piriformis muscle, which also exits the pelvis via the greater sciatic notch. The sciatic nerve usually travels under the piriformis muscle, except in 10%–30% of

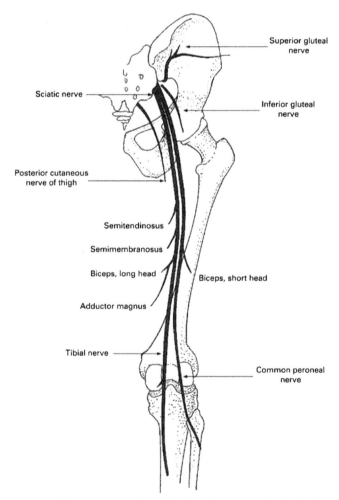

Fig. 1. The anatomy of the sciatic nerve from the gluteal region to the thigh. (*From* Stewart JD. Foot drop: where, why and what to do? Pract Neurol 2008;8:158–69; with permission.)

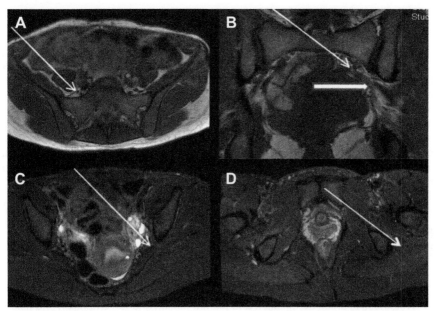

Fig. 2. The course of a normal sciatic nerve shown by MRI. (*A*) The lumbosacral trunk of the sciatic nerve (*arrow*) is shown lying posterior to the iliac vessels (axial T1). (*B*) The sacral plexus (*thin arrow*) and nerve at the notch sciatic notch (*thick arrow*) are denoted (coronal T1). (*C*) The sacral plexus (*arrow*) lies anterior to the piriformis muscle (axial T2). (*D*) The sciatic nerve (*arrow*) is situated between the ischial tuberosity and greater trochanter (axial T2).

cases, notably when the fibular division passes through or above the piriformis muscle.[4]

Distal to the piriformis muscle, the nerve is covered by the gluteus maximus muscle and soft tissue.[1] The nerve then travels halfway between the bony landmarks, greater trochanter laterally, and ischial tuberosity medially, and then descends into the sub-gluteal area. From there, it runs posteriorly in the midthigh, remaining dorsal to the adductor magnus and ventral to the long head of the biceps femoris. The tibial division of the sciatic nerve innervates the hamstring muscles (semimembranosus, semitendinosis, and long head of the biceps femoris) and the adductor magnus in the thigh. In the thigh, the common fibular division innervates the short head of the biceps femoris.

The nerve divides into the common fibular and tibial branches approximately 6 cm above the popliteal fossa crease.[5–7] The tibial nerve then continues posteriorly in the midline to the calf, innervating the muscles of the posterior compartment of the lower leg and supplying sensation to the posterior calf and lateral foot by the sural nerve (which also has a limited contribution from the common fibular nerve), the sole of the foot by the medial and lateral plantar nerves, and the heel by the medial calcaneal nerve. After passing through the upper popliteal fossa, the common fibular nerve travels laterally and around the fibular head, dividing into the deep fibular and superficial fibular branches, which supply the muscles of the anterior and lateral compartments of the lower leg, respectively. The superficial fibular nerve also forms a sensory branch that supplies sensation to the anterolateral lower leg and dorsum of the foot while the deep fibular nerve supplies sensation to the webspace between the first and second toes.[2]

PRESENTATION

Sciatic neuropathy often presents with foot drop. Patients often experience abrupt pain radiating down the posterolateral limb, with weakness and numbness evolving more gradually.[8–10] In sciatic neuropathy, the clinical findings are often more consistent with injury to the common fibular division rather than tibial division, sometimes mimicking a common fibular neuropathy at the knee. This finding is particularly true of more distal lesions, as they may not affect the flexors of the knee, or of less severe sciatic nerve injury. Because the common fibular division has fewer and larger fascicles and less supportive tissue compared with the tibial division, it is thought to be more vulnerable to compression. Also, the common fibular division is more taut, and secured at the sciatic notch and fibular neck, resulting in greater potential for stretch injury.[2]

In milder cases at the hip or thigh, the following features are typically noted:

- Foot drop that may mimic a common fibular neuropathy at the knee
- Weakness in knee flexion, ankle plantar flexion, ankle inversion
- Normal or decreased ankle jerk
- Pain and sensory loss in the foot and possibly the lateral shin

In severe lesions, these signs and symptoms are common:

- Weakness in ankle dorsiflexion and plantar flexion and toe extension and flexion
- Hamstring weakness
- Decreased ankle jerk
- Dysesthesic pain and numbness in the sole and dorsum of the foot and lateral lower leg

ELECTRODIAGNOSTIC STUDIES

Electrodiagnostic testing (EDx) is helpful in localizing the site of injury and the severity of the lesion. EDx studies are also useful for assessing both recovery and prognosis. Standard nerve conduction studies for evaluation of the sciatic nerve include testing the following:

- Ipsilateral common fibular and tibial motor nerve conduction and minimum F wave latencies
- Superficial fibular and sural sensory nerve conduction
- Comparison with the unaffected leg

Findings on motor nerve conduction studies most commonly include reduced fibular compound muscle action potential (CMAP) amplitudes often with a normal tibial CMAP amplitude. Given the depth and size of the sciatic nerve proximally, it is not possible to obtain reliable studies with more proximal stimulation using standard techniques. Tibial H reflex studies may be normal in fibular-predominant lesions, and therefore may not confirm the diagnosis or help localize the site of injury. In sensory nerve conduction studies, reduced superficial fibular and sural sensory nerve action potential amplitudes are seen in most cases (**Table 1**). Similar abnormalities are found in different age populations.[11–13] In one study of patients with sciatic neuropathy, nerve action potential amplitudes were reduced in the fibular motor nerve of 80% of adults and 83% of children; tibial motor nerve of 52% of adults and 67% of children; sural sensory of 71% of adults and 79% of children; and superficial fibular sensory of 83% of adults and 60% of children. Minimum F wave latencies in adult patients with sciatic neuropathy were abnormally prolonged in 85% of fibular and in 57% of tibial nerve studies.[11]

Table 1
Nerve conduction findings in sciatic neuropathy

Nerve	Latency	Amplitude	Velocity	F Wave
Common fibular motor				
Ankle	NL	Reduced		Abnl[a]
Below fibular head	NL	Reduced	NL	
Above fibular head	NL	Reduced	NL	
Tibial motor				
Ankle	NL	NL to reduced		NL/Abnl[a]
Knee	NL	NL to reduced	NL	
Sural sensory	NL	NL to reduced	NL	
Suprfl fibular sensory	NL	NL to reduced	NL	

Abbreviations: Abnl, abnormal; NL, normal; Suprfl, superficial.
[a] F wave abnormalities include prolonged latency or decreased persistence.

To maximize the yield for identifying signs of active denervation, needle electromyography should generally be performed 3 to 4 weeks after onset of symptoms. Positive sharp waves and fibrillation potentials can be identified reliably only after this period, initially in muscles closer to the lesion and then in those more distal, with reinnervation occurring in a similar pattern. In sciatic neuropathy, any muscle in the foot and lower leg is likely to show denervation. Commonly tested muscles include the extensor digitorum brevis, tibialis anterior, tibialis posterior and gastrocnemius. In general, however, needle EMG abnormalities in sciatic neuropathy are more commonly seen in fibular-innervated muscles (94%–100% of patients) than tibial-innervated muscles (74%–84% of patients).[11] Muscles innervated by the sciatic nerve in the thigh that often show denervation, depending on the site of the lesion, include both the short and long heads of the biceps femoris, semimembranosus, and semitendinosus.

In addition to studying muscles innervated by the sciatic nerve, the examiner should also study muscles that share the same root innervation but are supplied by a nerve other than the sciatic, such as the gluteus medius or tensor fascia latae (superior gluteal nerve) and the gluteus maximus (inferior gluteal nerve) to exclude L5 or S1 radiculopathy and lumbosacral plexopathy. To rule out a length-dependent process, such as a peripheral neuropathy, the electromyographer should also compare distal with proximal muscles of the leg, including those muscles in the proximal leg not supplied by the sciatic nerve. For example, the examiner could compare the extensor hallucis longus muscle (supplied by the sciatic nerve) with the vastus medialis muscle (supplied by the femoral nerve). Paraspinal muscle abnormalities of the lumbosacral spine on needle examination support a diagnosis of lumbosacral radiculopathy rather than sciatic neuropathy or a superimposed additional site of neuropathic injury.

Performed together, nerve conduction studies and needle electromyography can detect subclinical involvement of the tibial nerve and thereby exclude a common fibular mononeuropathy, for example, by showing involvement in the gastrocnemius or hamstring muscles. It is important to recognize that more distal tibial-innervated muscles, such as the gastrocnemius, tibialis posterior, and flexor digitorum longus, are more likely to show denervation than the hamstring muscles in chronic lesions, because the hamstring muscles may have had adequate time to reinnervate.[11]

IMAGING TECHNIQUES
Magnetic Resonance Imaging

Of all imaging techniques, magnetic resonance imaging (MRI) seems to be the best technique to identify sciatic nerve pathology. Depending on the severity of the injury, T2-weighted magnetic resonance images may show high signal intensity in the nerve fibers or increased nerve dimension, deformation of the nerve, or total loss of nerve integrity.[14] Short tau inversion recovery (STIR) sequences of the nerve help identify the extent of a lesion, with a more diffuse area of high signal indicating an inflammatory etiology (**Fig. 3**). Chhabra and colleagues[15] found higher nerve-to-vessel signal intensity ratios and higher incidences of T2 hyperintensity, nerve enlargement, and abnormal fascicular shape in affected nerves compared with normal nerves, with excellent interobserver and intraobserver reliability. Affected muscles showed more fatty infiltration, edema, and atrophy. However, findings on MRI may sometimes be difficult to interpret, because abnormal signal may occasionally be seen in normal individuals on both T2 and STIR imaging.

Other

Computerized axial tomography is helpful in finding lesions that impact the sciatic nerve involving bone (eg, sacrum fracture), vessel abnormalities (eg, aneurysm), or hematoma.[3] Ultrasonographic studies have limited utility in the diagnosis of sciatic neuropathy and have been used more frequently for sciatic nerve blocks rather than to identify sciatic nerve pathology. However, a few recent studies have tried to use ultrasound scan to foster a greater understanding of the causes of sciatic nerve injury. For instance, Moayeri and Groen[16] and Brull and colleagues,[17] with the use of specific ultrasonographic settings, found more neural than nonneural tissue in the hip region than in the thigh, which might contribute to the greater proximal vulnerability of the sciatic nerve.

ETIOLOGIES

Different conditions can lead to sciatic neuropathy (**Table 2**). In one retrospective study of individuals referred for electrodiagnostic evaluation of sciatic neuropathy, hip trauma and surgery were the most common etiologies. Sciatic neuropathy has

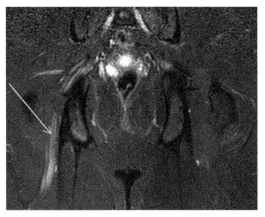

Fig. 3. Increased signal (*arrow*) is shown in an idiopathic right sciatic neuropathy in a proximal nerve segment. (coronal STIR).

Table 2
Etiologies of sciatic neuropathy

Infection	Abscess[3,20]: tubo-ovarian, pelvic, psoas
Inflammation	Sacroiliitis[40,53,54]
Trauma	Intramuscular injection,[8,9,55,56] abdominal surgery,[57] fracture,[58] hematoma,[59] open injury including gunshot or knife wound[21,60,61]
Tumor: intraneural	Schwannoma,[3] intraneural perineurioma,[24,26] neurofibroma,[25] neurilemoma,[25] neurolymphomatosis,[3,24,27] malignant neurofibrosarcoma[25,62,63]
Compressive	Leiomyosarcoma,[28] rhabdomyosacroma,[24] lipoma,[64] metastasis[3]
Vascular	Vasculitis,[23] iliac artery occlusion[21–23] venous varix,[65] arteriovenous malformation[20,66] ischemic,[67] deep venous thrombosis[68]
Gynecologic	Endometriosis,[46,51] fibroids[69]
Other	Piriformis syndrome,[41,42] radiotherapy,[70] hereditary neuropathy with liability to pressure palsy,[71] cryoglobulinemia[72]
Surgery, hip	Traction,[73] arthroplasty debris[74]
Surgery, other	Compartment syndrome,[75] anesthesia,[19] positioning[76]

Data from Ergun T, Lakadamyali H. CT and MRI in the evaluation of extraspinal sciatica. Br J Radiol 2010;83(993):791–803.

been reported in as many as 1%–3% of patients after total hip replacement surgery.[18,19] The neuropathy is usually discovered immediately postoperatively and is typically a consequence of stretch injury. The next most common causes include external compression and open injuries, such as gunshot wounds and knife injury, and ischemia, which may occur secondary to vasculitis or atherothrombosis or after bypass surgery. Endometriosis, iatrogenic nerve injection, and compartment syndrome are also less commonly reported causes. Not infrequently, a cause cannot be identified (ie, idiopathic sciatic neuropathy).[20] An etiology for sciatic neuropathy was uncertain in 16% in the series reported by Yuen and colleagues[21] of 73 patients. Vascular malformations may also uncommonly lead to sciatic neuropathy as a consequence of nerve compression.[22,23]

Tumors involving the sciatic nerve are uncommon in adults, but in the pediatric population, sciatic neuropathy is often associated with a neoplasm. In a series of 7 pediatric cases, etiologies included nerve infiltration by an adjacent neoplasm (neuroblastoma, rhabdomyosarcoma, and leukemic and lymphomatous infiltration) as well as an intrinsic neurogenic tumor (perineurioma).[24] Although tumors are more common presentations in childhood, occurring often in the first decade, neurilemmomas, neurofibromas, neurofibrosarcomas, perineuriomas, lymphoma, leiomyosarcoma, and malignant peripheral nerve sheath tumors have been reported rarely in adults.[25–29]

Certain etiologies for sciatic neuropathy often are associated with specific sites of injury to the sciatic nerve:

Hip

Given its proximal location to the hip joint and its long course, the sciatic nerve is predisposed to injury in the hip region. Partial entrapment of the sciatic nerve at the hip affects the lateral (fibular) division more commonly. Etiologies include hip arthroplasty, dislocation, and fracture in up to 30% of patients.[10,30] Acute external compression can occur in patients in coma, with or without compartment syndrome, or after prolonged sitting. Mass lesions are more common at this site than elsewhere, occurring in up to 14% of cases.[19,31–35]

Gluteal

Gluteal compartment hemorrhage, misplaced intramuscular gluteal injections, and repeated injections leading to fibrosis can lead to sciatic nerve injury at this location.[8,36–39] The sciatic nerve may also be at risk of compression based on its close association with the piriformis muscle at the level of the sciatic notch. Compression of the nerve by the piriformis muscle as a clinical syndrome was proposed by Freiberg and Vinke in 1934.[40] Robinson[41] is credited with coining the term *piriformis syndrome*.[41] Individuals with piriformis syndrome typically present with buttock tenderness and pain, which may radiate down the posterior thigh. Prolonged sitting, bending at the waist, and activities involving hip adduction and internal rotation exacerbate the pain. Paresthesias may occur in the buttocks and thigh, but weakness is not usually evident. The pain can be reproduced with palpation over the sciatic notch or with rectal or pelvic examination.[41] Additionally, several maneuvers have been described to assess for piriformis syndrome in eliciting buttocks pain by either (1) passive stretching of the piriformis muscle (the Freiberg or flexion adduction internal rotation/FAIR maneuver) or (2) active contraction against resistance to the piriformis muscle (the Pace and Beatty maneuver).[42] Although helpful, the Freiberg and Pace maneuvers only have a sensitivity of about 75% in confirmed cases.[41] Potential causes of piriformis syndrome include hypertrophy of the piriformis muscle, which can cause impingement of the sciatic nerve at the greater sciatic foramen; inflammation of the piriformis muscle secondary to adjacent infectious or inflammatory processes; hematoma or fibrous adhesions of the piriformis muscle; and local ischemia of the nerve at this site.[43]

Thigh

Causes of sciatic neuropathy at the thigh include external compression from coma and posterior thigh compartment syndrome. Prolonged positioning on a toilet seat, lotus position or craniotomy[32,33,44,45] have been described as causes of sciatic neuropathy. Transient symptoms of sciatic neuropathy may also occur in endometriosis associated with menses.[46] Sciatic nerve injury can also occur at this site as a consequence of a gunshot wound or penetrating injury.[21]

DIFFERENTIAL DIAGNOSIS

The differential diagnosis of sciatic neuropathy is largely limited to L5 or S1 radiculopathies, lumbosacral plexopathy, and common fibular neuropathy (**Table 3**). Additionally, distal lower extremity weakness mimicking sciatic neuropathy may be the presenting feature of motor neuron disease, distal myopathy or polyneuropathy. Some clinical findings may be helpful in distinguishing a sciatic nerve insult from these other nerve injuries. With L5 or S1 radiculopathies, patients typically describe low back pain radiating into the lateral (L5 distribution) or posterior (S1 distribution) leg. The pain in radiculopathy is better with standing and walking and worse with sitting. In contrast, sciatic nerve pain usually originates in the buttocks or more distally. Lumbosacral plexopathy often involves more weakness than sciatic neuropathy, including involvement of the gluteal muscles, and pain is usually more diffuse.[47] Unlike sciatic neuropathy, common fibular neuropathy should not affect knee flexion, and sensory symptoms in this neuropathy do not involve the posterior leg or plantar aspect of the foot.

Table 3
Differential diagnosis of sciatic neuropathy

	Sciatic Neuropathy	Common Fibular Neuropathy	LS Plexopathy	Radiculopathy	
				L5	S1
Pain	Foot + radiating posterolateral thigh	Rare	Posterolateral thigh	Low back to lateral thigh	Low back to posterior thigh
Weakness	Foot inversion, toe flexion, ± knee flexion	Ankle dorsiflexion/foot eversion	Ankle dorsiflexion and plantar flexion	Ankle dorsiflexion ± foot inversion	Ankle plantar flexion
Sensory	Upper 1/3 lateral leg/sole	Distal 2/3 lateral leg	± Antero- or posterolateral thigh and shin	± Lateral thigh across to medial foot	± Posterior thigh
Reflex	Depressed/absent - ankle	Normal	Norm/depressed at ankle	Normal	Depressed/absent - ankle
SLR	+	–	–	+	+
Common Fibular CMAP	Reduced	Reduced	± Reduced	± Reduced	Normal
Tibial CMAP	± Reduced	Normal	± Reduced	Normal	± Reduced
Sural SNAP	± Reduced	Normal	± Reduced	Normal	Normal
Sup. Fibular SNAP	Reduced	Reduced	Reduced	Normal	Normal

Abbreviations: SLR, straight leg raise sign; SNAP, sensory nerve action potential; Sup, superficial.

TREATMENT

Identification of the cause of sciatic neuropathy is vital in determining prognosis and therapy. For instance, in piriformis syndrome, conservative therapy is key, including stretching in flexion, adduction, and internal rotation of the hip joint, supine and standing.[47] Physical therapy and ankle foot orthotic for foot drop are commonly indicated. Steroid or botox injections have been used in cases of suspected piriformis syndrome.[48] Two randomized, controlled trials showed efficacy of botulinum toxin injection into the piriformis muscle compared with placebo.[49,50] Pharmacologic suppression of the ovarian cycle may reverse sciatic neuropathy in endometriosis.[51] Immunosuppressant therapy, such as prednisone, would be warranted as therapy for vasculitis affecting the sciatic nerve. Neuropathic pain is common in all causes of sciatic neuropathy and is generally treated with neuropathic pain medications such as tricyclic antidepressants like amitriptyline or nortriptyline; anticonvulsants, including gabapentin, pregabalin, or carbamazepine; and lidocaine patch. Surgery is indicated in compartment syndrome, hip fracture or dislocation, and tumors involving the sciatic nerve to prevent progressive symptoms.[52]

Nerve grafting may play a role in treatment of severe sciatic nerve injuries from trauma but is a challenge in a nerve of this size and length. In a large retrospective review of 353 patients by Kim and colleagues,[52] individuals with gluteal or thigh-level injury were examined to determine the degree of recovery after neurolysis if an intraoperative nerve action potential could be generated or after end-to-end suture repair or graft in severe sciatic neuropathy without an elicitable intraoperative nerve action potential. Outcomes varied depending on the mechanism of injury, with better responses to surgery noted in patients suffering from tibial division lesions than in those sustaining insults primarily to the common fibular division. Partial recovery ranged from 71%–96% of patients undergoing neurolysis, 30%–93% of those treated with end-to-end suture repair, and 24%–80% of those undergoing nerve grafts.

OUTCOME

In general, the prognosis for sciatic neuropathy is chiefly dependent on the severity of the lesion rather than the location. Yuen and colleagues[21] found that most individuals with sciatic neuropathy had a good outcome at 3 years, whereas only 30% had a good or better recovery at 1 year. Good but incomplete recovery occurred primarily in those who did not show severe motor axonal loss on EDx study. In patients with an acute or subacute onset, a moderate or better recovery occurred in most patients: 30% recovered within 1 year, 50% within 2 years, and 75% within 3 years.[21] Two factors predicted an earlier or better recovery: (1) presence of a common fibular compound muscle action potential recording from the extensor digitorum brevis, as all of these patients had moderate to excellent recovery by 3 years, and (2) an initial absence of paralysis of muscles controlling ankle plantar flexion and dorsiflexion.[11]

SUMMARY

Sciatic neuropathy is a common cause of foot drop and the second most common neuropathy of the lower extremity. Sciatic neuropathy must be distinguished from other causes of foot drop, including common fibular neuropathy, lumbosacral plexopathy, and L5 radiculopathy. Less commonly, distal lower extremity weakness mimicking sciatic neuropathy may be the presenting feature of motor neuron disease, distal myopathy, or polyneuropathy. There are multiple potential sites of injury along the sciatic nerve, determined in part by the mechanism of insult, such as trauma, compression, mass, inflammation, and vascular lesions. Diagnosis is augmented by careful EDx studies and imaging, which help to distinguish sciatic neuropathy from other neuropathic conditions. EDx may also help gauge recovery and aide in prognosis.

REFERENCES

1. Katirji B, editor. Compressive and entrapment neuropathies of the lower extremity in Neuromuscular Disorders in Clinical Practice. Boston: Butterworth Heinemann; 2002. p. 787–96.
2. Sunderland S. Nerve and nerve injuries. 2nd edition. Edinburgh (United Kingdom): Churchill Livingstone; 1978.
3. Ergun T, Lakadamyali H. CT and MRI in the evaluation of extraspinal sciatica. Br J Radiol 2010;83(993):791–803.
4. Pezina M. Contribution of the etiological explanation of the piriformis syndrome. Acta Anat 1979;105:181–4.
5. Schwemmer U, Markus CK, Greim CA, et al. Sonographic imaging of the sciatic nerve division in the popliteal fossa. Ultraschall Med 2005;26:496–500.
6. Vloka JD, Hadzic A, April E, et al. The division of the sciatic nerve in the popliteal fossa: anatomical implications for popliteal nerve blockade. Anesth Analg 2001; 92:215–7.
7. Moayeri N, van Geffen GJ, Bruhn J, et al. Correlation among ultrasound, cross-sectional anatomy, and histology of the sciatic nerve: a review. Reg Anesth Pain Med 2010;35(5):442–9.
8. Streib EW, Sun SE. Injection injury of the sciatic nerve: unusual anatomic distribution of nerve damage. Eur J Neurol 1981;20:481–4.
9. Mishra P, Stringer MD. Sciatic nerve injury from intramuscular injection: a persistent and global problem. Int J Clin Pract 2010;64(11):1573–9.
10. Yuen EC, So YT. Sciatic neuropathy. Neurol Clin 1999;17(3):617–31, viii.
11. Yuen EC, So YT, Olney RK. The electrophysiologic features of sciatic neuropathy in 100 patients. Muscle Nerve 1995;18:414–20.
12. Srinivasan J, Ryan MM, Escolar DM, et al. Pediatric sciatic neuropathies: a 30-year prospective study. Neurology 2011;76(11):976–80.
13. Katirji B, Wilbourn AJ. High sciatic lesion mimicking peroneal neuropathy at the fibular head. J Neurol Sci 1994;121(2):172–5.
14. Maravilla KR, Bowen BC. Imaging of the peripheral nervous system: evaluation of peripheral neuropathy and plexopathy. AJNR Am J Neuroradiol 1998;19: 1011–23.
15. Chhabra A, Chalian M, Soldatos T, et al. 3-T high-resolution MR neurography of sciatic neuropathy. AJR Am J Roentgenol 2012;198(4):W357–64.
16. Moayeri N, Groen GJ. Differences in quantitative architecture of sciatic nerve may explain differences in potential vulnerability to nerve injury. Anesthesiology 2009; 111(5):1128–34.
17. Brull R, McCartney CJ, Chan VW, et al. Neurological complications after regional anesthesia: contemporary estimates of risk. Anesth Analg 2007;104:965–74.
18. Schmalzried TP, Amstutz HC, Dorey FJ. Nerve palsy associated with total hip replacement: risk factors and prognosis. J Bone Joint Surg Am 1991;73A: 1074–80.
19. Brown GD, Swanson EA, Nercessian OA. Neurologic injuries after total hip arthroplasty. Am J Orthop (Belle Mead NJ) 2008;37(4):191–7.
20. Goh KJ, Tan CB, Tjia HT. Sciatic neuropathies: a retrospective review of electrodiagnostic features in 29 patients. Ann Acad Med Singapore 1996;25:566–9.

21. Yuen EC, Olney R, So YT. Sciatic neuropathy: clinical and prognostic features in 73 patients. Neurology 1994;4:1669–74.
22. Van Gompel JJ, Griessenauer CJ, Scheithauer BW, et al. Vascular malformations, rare causes of sciatic neuropathy: a case series. Neurosurgery 2010;67(4):1133–42.
23. Srinivasan J, Escolar D, Ryan M, et al. Pediatric sciatic neuropathies due to unusual vascular causes. J Child Neurol 2008;23(7):738–41.
24. McMillan HJ, Srinivasan J, Darras BT, et al. Pediatric sciatic neuropathy associated with neoplasms. Muscle Nerve 2011;43(2):183–8.
25. Thomas JE, Piepgras DG, Scheithauer B, et al. Neurogenic tumors of the sciatic nerve. A clinicopathologic study of 35 cases. Mayo Clin Proc 1983;58(10):640–7.
26. Emory TS, Scheithauer BW, Hirose T, et al. Intraneural perineurioma. A clonal neoplasm associated with abnormalities of chromosome 22. Am J Clin Pathol 1995;103(6):696–704.
27. Misdraji J, Ino Y, Louis DN, et al. Primary lymphoma of peripheral nerve: report of four cases. Am J Surg Pathol 2000;24(9):1257–65.
28. Borvorn S, Praditphol N, Nakornchai V. Leiomyosarcoma in peripheral nerve: the first case report. J Med Assoc Thai 2003;86(11):1080–5.
29. Sharma RR, Pawar SJ, Mahapatra AK, et al. Sciatica due to malignant nerve sheath tumour of sciatic nerve in the thigh. Neurol India 2001;49(2):188–90.
30. Stewart JD, Angus E, Gendron J. Sciatic neuropathies. BMJ 1983;287:1108–9.
31. Shields RW Jr, Root KE Jr, Wilbourn AJ. Compartment syndromes and compression neuropathies in coma. Neurology 1986;36:1370–4.
32. Holland NR, Schwartz-Williams L, Blotzer JW. "Toilet seat" sciatic neuropathy. Arch Neurol 1999;56:116.
33. Vogel CM, Albin R, Alberts JW. Lotus foot-drop: sciatic neuropathy in the thigh. Neurology 1991;41:605–6.
34. Gozal Y, Pomeranz S. Sciatic nerve palsy as a complication after acoustic neurinoma resection in the sitting position. J Neurosurg Anesthesiol 1994;6:40–2.
35. Wilbourn AJ, Mitsumoto H. Proximal sciatic neuropathies caused by prolonged sitting. Neurology 1988;38:400.
36. Chan VO, Colville J, Persaud T, et al. Intramuscular injections into the buttocks: are they truly intramuscular? Eur J Radiol 2006;58:480–4.
37. Ahuja B. Post injection sciatic nerve injury. Indian Pediatr 2003;40:368–9.
38. Pandian JD, Bose S, Daniel V, et al. Nerve injuries following intramuscular injections: a clinical and neurophysiological study from Northwest India. J Peripher Nerv Syst 2006;11:165–71.
39. Tak SR, Dar GN, Halwai MA, et al. Post-injection nerve injuries in Kashmir: a menace overlooked. J Res Med Sci 2008;13:244–7.
40. Freiberg AH, Vinke TH. Sciatica and the sacro-iliac joint. J Bone Joint Surg Am 1934;16:126–36.
41. Robinson DR. Pyriformis syndrome in relation to sciatic pain. Am J Surg 1947;73: 355–8.
42. Beatty RA. The piriformis muscle syndrome: a simple diagnostic maneuver. Neurosurgery 1994;34(3):512–4.
43. Hopayian K, Song F, Riera R, et al. The clinical features of the piriformis syndrome: a systematic review. Eur Spine J 2010;19(12):2095–109.
44. Beltran LS, Bencardino J, Ghazikhanian V, et al. Entrapment neuropathies III: lower limb. Semin Musculoskelet Radiol 2010;14(5):501–11.
45. Wang JC, Wong TT, Chen HH, et al. Bilateral sciatic neuropathy as a complication of craniotomy performed in the sitting position: localization of nerve injury by using magnetic resonance imaging. Childs Nerv Syst 2012;28(1):159–63.

46. Vilos GA, Vilos AW, Haebe JJ. Laparoscopic findings, management, histopathology, and outcome of 25 women with cyclic leg pain. J Am Assoc Gynecol Laparosc 2002;9:145–51.

47. Katirji B. Electromyography in clinical practice. St. Louis (MO): Mosby; 1998.

48. Barton PM. Piriformis syndrome: a rational approach to management. Pain 1991; 47:345–51.

49. Fishman LM, Anderson C, Rosner B. BOTOX and physical therapy in the treatment of piriformis syndrome. Am J Phys Med Rehabil 2002;81(12):936–42.

50. Childers MK, Wilson DJ, Gnatz SM, et al. Botulinum toxin type A use in piriformis muscle syndrome: a pilot study. Am J Phys Med Rehabil 2002;81(10):751–9.

51. Salazar-Grueso E, Roos R. Sciatic endometriosis: a treatable sensorimotor mononeuropathy. Neurology 1986;36:1360–3.

52. Kim DH, Murovic JA, Tiel R, et al. Management and outcomes in 353 surgically treated sciatic nerve lesions. J Neurosurg 2004;101:8–17.

53. Wong M, Vijayanathan S, Kirkham B. Sacroiliitis presenting as sciatica. Rheumatology 2005;44:1323–4.

54. Liu XQ, Li FC, Wang JW, et al. Postpartum septic sacroiliitis misdiagnosed as sciatic neuropathy. Am J Med Sci 2010;339(3):292–5.

55. Senes FM, Campus MD, Becchetti F, et al. Sciatic nerve injection palsy in the child: early microsurgical treatment and long-term results. Microsurgery 2009;29:443–8.

56. Akyüz M, Turhan N. Post injection sciatic neuropathy in adults. Clin Neurophysiol 2006;117(7):1633–5.

57. Yasin A, Patel AG. Bilateral sciatic nerve palsy following a bariatic operation. Obes Surg 2007;17(7):983–5.

58. Al-Atassi T, Phillips JR, Eid AS, et al. Late recovery of sciatic nerve palsy at twelve years following pelvis fracture. Injury 2011;42(10):1188–9.

59. Weir Y, Mattan Y, Goldman V, et al. Sciatic nerve palsy due to hematoma after thrombolysis therapy for acute pulmonary embolism after total hip arthroplasty. J Arthroplasty 2006;21(3):456–9.

60. Saroyan JM, Winfree CJ, Schechter WS, et al. Sciatic neuropathy after lower-extremity trauma: successful treatment of an uncommon pain and disability syndrome in an adolescent. Am J Phys Med Rehabil 2007;86(7):597–600.

61. Plewnia C, Wallace C, Zochodne D. Traumatic sciatic neuropathy: a novel cause, local experience, and a review of the literature. J Trauma 1999;47(5):986–91.

62. Feinberg J, Sethi S. Sciatic neuropathy: case report and discussion of the literature on postoperative sciatic neuropathy and sciatic nerve tumors. HSS J 2006; 2(2):181–7.

63. Rao SB, Dinakar I, Rao KS. Neurofibrosarcoma of sciatic nerve. Indian J Cancer 1970;7(3):226–9.

64. Botwin KP, Shah CP, Zak PJ. Sciatic neuropathy secondary to infiltrating intermuscular lipoma of the thigh. Am J Phys Med Rehabil 2001;80(10):754–8.

65. Maniker A, Thurmond J, Padberg FT Jr, et al. Traumatic venous varix causing sciatic neuropathy: case report. Neurosurgery 2004;55(5):1224.

66. Ney JP, Shih W, Landau ME. Sciatic neuropathy following endovascular treatment of a limb vascular malformation. J Brachial Plex Peripher Nerve Inj 2006;1:8.

67. Forester ND, Parry D, Kessel D, et al. Ischaemic sciatic neuropathy: an important complication of embolisation of a type II endoleak. Eur J Vasc Endovasc Surg 2002;24(5):462–3.

68. Kara M, Ozçakar L, Eken G, et al. Deep venous thrombosis and inferior vena cava agenesis causing double crush sciatic neuropathy in Behçet's disease. Joint Bone Spine 2008;75(6):734–6.

69. Bodack MP, Cole JC, Nagler W. Sciatic neuropathy secondary to a uterine fibroid: a case report. Am J Phys Med Rehabil 1999;78(2):157–9.
70. Gikas PD, Hanna SA, Aston W, et al. Post-radiation sciatic neuropathy: a case report and review of the literature. World J Surg Oncol 2008;6:130.
71. Lynch JM, Hennessy M. HNPP presenting as sciatic neuropathy. J Peripher Nerv Syst 2005;10(1):1–2.
72. Pérez D, de la Torre RG, Carrio I, et al. Cryoglobulinaemic neuropathy: a further cause of bilateral sciatic neuropathy. Int Arch Med 2008;1(1):18.
73. Kemler MA, de Vries M, van der Tol A. Duration of preoperative traction associated with sciatic neuropathy after hip fracture surgery. Clin Orthop Relat Res 2006;445:230–2.
74. Fischer SR, Christ DJ, Roehr BA. Sciatic neuropathy secondary to total hip arthroplasty wear debris. J Arthroplasty 1999;14(6):771–4.
75. Rodríguez Uranga JJ, Uclès Sánchez AJ, Pérez Díaz JM. Neuropathy of common sciatic nerve secondary to compartment syndrome as a complication after bariatric surgery. Neurologia 2005;20(2):94–7 [in Spanish].
76. Roy S, Levine AB, Herbison GJ, et al. Intraoperative positioning during cesarean as a cause of sciatic neuropathy. Obstet Gynecol 2002;99(4):652–3.

Fibular (Peroneal) Neuropathy
Electrodiagnostic Features and Clinical Correlates

Christina Marciniak, MD

KEYWORDS

• Fibular • Peroneal • Neuropathy • Electrodiagnostic

KEY POINTS

- Fibular (peroneal) neuropathy is the most common mononeuropathy encountered in the lower limbs.
- Clinically, sciatic mononeuropathies, radiculopathies of the 5th lumbar root, and lumbosacral plexopathies may present with similar findings of ankle dorsiflexor weakness, thus evaluation is needed to distinguish these disorders.
- The most common site of injury to the fibular nerve is at the fibular head.
- The deep fibular branch is more frequently abnormal than the superficial branch.
- Electrodiagnostic studies are useful to determine the level and type (axonal, demyelinating) of injury.
- The presence of any compound muscle action potential response on motor nerve conduction studies, recorded from either the tibialis anterior or extensor digitorum brevis, is associated with good long-term outcome.

INTRODUCTION

Fibular or peroneal neuropathy is the most frequent mononeuropathy encountered in the lower limb and the third most common focal neuropathy encountered overall, after median and ulnar neuropathies.[1,2] Following revised anatomic terminology published in 1998, the peroneal nerve is also now known as the fibular nerve, to prevent confusion of this nerve with those regions with similar names.[3] Perone is another term for the fibula and, thus, this revised terminology for this nerve, its branches, and related musculature is based on language describing the location.[3] While both fibular and peroneal are considered acceptable terms, "fibular" and it related terminology is preferred and therefore will be used throughout this article.

Weakness of ankle dorsiflexion and the resultant foot drop are common presentations of fibular neuropathy, but may also be seen in a wide variety of other clinical conditions, including sciatic mononeuropathy, lumbosacral plexopathy, or a lumbar (L) 5

Disclosures: No relevant disclosures.
Department of Physical Medicine and Rehabilitation, Northwestern University, Feinberg School of Medicine, The Rehabilitation Institute of Chicago, 345 East Superior, Chicago, IL 60611, USA
E-mail address: cmarciniak@ric.org

Phys Med Rehabil Clin N Am 24 (2013) 121–137
http://dx.doi.org/10.1016/j.pmr.2012.08.016
1047-9651/13/$ – see front matter © 2013 Elsevier Inc. All rights reserved.

radiculopathy. Additionally, ankle dorsiflexion weakness may be the initial presentation of generalized disorders, such as amyotrophic lateral sclerosis, or a hereditary neuropathy.[1] In a retrospective series of 217 patients presenting with paresis or paralysis of foot dorsiflexors, of whom 68% had peripheral nerve abnormalities as the cause of their weakness, 31% had weakness related to a common fibular nerve lesion, 30% an L5 radiculopathy, and 18% due to a polyneuropathy.[4] Fibular neuropathies may also present with predominantly sensory symptoms limited to the distribution of the deep or superficial fibular nerve or its branches.[5] In addition to documenting fibular nerve abnormalities and the level of the injury, electrodiagnostic techniques have also been used to assess the potential for recovery of nerve function.[6,7]

ANATOMY
Common Fibular (Peroneal) Nerve

The common fibular (peroneal) nerve is derived from the lateral division of the sciatic nerve. Fibers from the dorsal fourth and fifth lumbar, as well as the first and second sacral nerve roots, join with tibial axons to form the sciatic nerve (**Fig. 1**). Though bound in the nerve sheath with the tibial nerve in the thigh, the fibular and tibial axons are separate even within the sciatic nerve at this level.[8] In the thigh, a branch arises from the fibular division of the sciatic nerve to innervate the short head of the biceps femoris. Following bifurcation of the sciatic nerve in the distal thigh at the superior popliteal fossa, the common fibular nerve travels along the lateral side of the fossa at the border of the biceps femoris muscle to the lateral knee. At this level, the nerve gives off a branch, the lateral cutaneous nerve of the calf, which supplies sensation to the upper third of the anterolateral leg. The sural communicating branch of the lateral sural cutaneous nerve joins with the medial sural cutaneous nerve to form the sural nerve. The common fibular nerve then travels superficially at the lateral fibula and is located about 1 to 2 cm distal to the fibular head before entering the anterior compartment of the leg where it divides into deep and superficial branches at the fibular head (**Fig. 2**).

Deep Fibular (Peroneal) Nerve

The deep fibular (peroneal) nerve supplies motor innervation to all anterior compartment muscles (the tibialis anterior, the extensor digitorum longus, and extensor hallucis longus) and the fibularis tertius, also known as the peroneus tertius. The anterior tibialis is the strongest foot dorsiflexor, although the extensor digitorum longus and the fibularis tertius assist with this movement. The deep fibular nerve travels distally in the calf and at the level of the ankle joint, fascia overlying the talus and the navicular bind the deep fibular nerve dorsally. Ventrally, the extensor hallucis longus muscle fibers and tendon and the inferior extensor retinaculum overlay the nerve. The inferior extensor retinaculum is a Y-shaped band anterior to the ankle; the anterior tarsal tunnel is considered the space located between the inferior extensor retinaculum and the fascia overlying the talus and navicular. Just rostral or under the inferior extensor retinaculum, the deep fibular nerve branches into medial and lateral branches. The lateral branch of the deep fibular nerve travels under the extensor retinaculum, as well as the extensor digitorum and hallucis brevis muscles to innervate these muscles and nearby joints. The medial branch travels under the extensor hallucis brevis tendon to supply sensation to the skin between the first and second toes.

Superficial Fibular (Peroneal) Nerve

The superficial fibular (or peroneal) nerve arises from the common fibular nerve in the proximal leg and travels distally in the leg through the lateral compartment. After

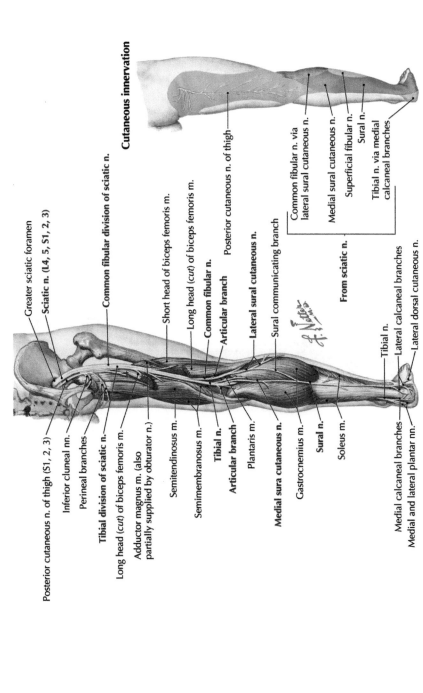

Cutaneous innervation

Greater sciatic foramen

Sciatic n. (L4, 5, S1, 2, 3)

Common fibular division of sciatic n.

Short head of biceps femoris m.

Long head (cut) of biceps femoris m.

Common fibular n.

Articular branch   Posterior cutaneous n. of thigh

Lateral sural cutaneous n.

Sural communicating branch

Common fibular n. via lateral sural cutaneous n.

Medial sural cutaneous n.

Superficial fibular n.

Sural n.

Tibial n. via medial calcaneal branches

From sciatic n.

Tibial n.

Lateral calcaneal branches

Lateral dorsal cutaneous n.

Tibial division of sciatic n.

Posterior cutaneous n. of thigh (S1, 2, 3)

Inferior cluneal nn.

Perineal branches

Tibial division of sciatic n.

Long head (cut) of biceps femoris m.

Adductor magnus m. (also partially supplied by obturator n.)

Semitendinosus m.

Semimembranosus m.

Tibial n.

Articular branch

Plantaris m.

Medial sura cutaneous n.

Gastrocnemius m.

Sural n.

Soleus m.

Medial calcaneal branches

Medial and lateral plantar nn.

Fig. 1. Sciatic nerve: anatomy. Netter illustration from www.netterimages.com. © Elsevier Inc. All rights reserved.

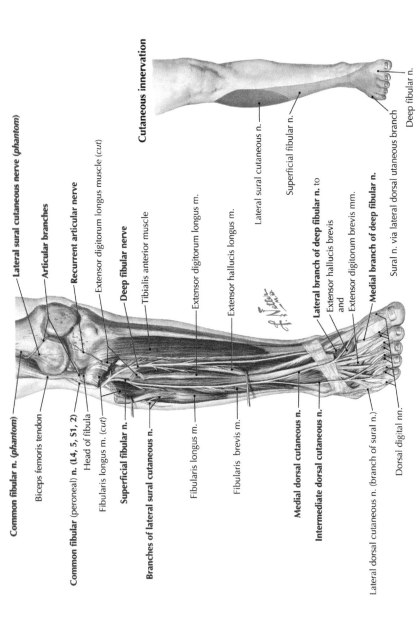

Cutaneous innervation

Common fibular n. (*phantom*)

Biceps femoris tendon

Lateral sural cutaneous nerve (*phantom*)

Articular branches

Common fibular (peroneal) n. (L4, 5, S1, 2)

Head of fibula

Fibularis longus m. (*cut*)

Recurrent articular nerve

Extensor digitorum longus muscle (*cut*)

Superficial fibular n.

Deep fibular nerve

Tibialis anterior muscle

Branches of lateral sural cutaneous n.

Extensor digitorum longus m.

Extensor hallucis longus m.

Lateral sural cutaneous n.

Superficial fibular n.

Fibularis longus m.

Fibularis brevis m.

Lateral branch of deep fibular n. to
Extensor hallucis brevis
and
Extensor digitorum brevis mm.

Medial dorsal cutaneous n.

Intermediate dorsal cutaneous n.

Medial branch of deep fibular n.

Sural n. via lateral dorsal utaneous branch

Lateral dorsal cutaneous n. (branch of sural n.)

Dorsal digital nn.

Deep fibular n.

Fig. 2. Common peroneal nerve and branches: anatomy. Netter illustration from www.netterimages.com. © Elsevier Inc. All rights reserved.

providing muscular innervation to the fibularis (peroneus) longus and brevis muscles in the lateral compartment of the leg, the terminal sensory branch supplies sensation to the lower two-thirds of the anterolateral leg and the dorsum of the foot, except for the first web space. It becomes superficial within the muscular compartment about 5 cm above the ankle joint where it pierces the fascia to become subcutaneous. It divides into its two terminal sensory branches, the intermediate and medial dorsal cutaneous nerves. The intermediate dorsal cutaneous nerve travels to the third metatarsal space and then divides into the dorsal digital branches to supply sensation to the lateral two digits. The medial dorsal cutaneous branch passes over the anterior aspect of the ankle overlying the common extensor tendons, runs parallel to the extensor hallucis longus tendon, and divides distal to the inferior retinaculum into three dorsal digital branches.

Accessory Fibular (Peroneal) Nerve

A common anatomic variant, the accessory fibular (peroneal) nerve, may be identified in the performance of studies to the extensor digitorum brevis.[9] It generally arises from the superficial fibular nerve as it courses under the fibularis brevis muscle, traveling distally to the foot posterior to the lateral malleolus.[10] It subsequently branches to innervate ligaments, joints, and the extensor digitorum brevis muscle. Prevalence as a normal anatomic variant has been reported to be 17% to 28% in anatomic studies and 12% and 22% electrophysiologically.[9,11–13]

CAUSES

Fibular neuropathies are most often traumatic in origin; stretch or compression is a common feature in the history (**Box 1**).[14,15] Recurring external pressure at the fibular head may result in this complication, such as that seen in patients at bed rest or in individuals who habitually cross their legs.[16] Intrinsic compression of the superficial and/or deep fibular nerves has also been described, such as that occurring from fascial bands or intraneural ganglia.[17]

Acute fibular neuropathies located at the fibular head may be found in the setting of recent weight loss, frequently in conjunction with a history of leg crossing.[1,18–20] Fibular nerve palsies were reported in prisoners of war during World War II who lost from 5 to 11 kg.[21] In another case series, it was noted that 20% of 150 cases of fibular mononeuropathy were associated with dieting and weight loss.[1] The mean weight decrease in these patients was 10.9 kg, with most patients having moderate to severe weakness of foot dorsiflexion and eversion.[1] It has been theorized that loss of subcutaneous fat leads to increased susceptibility of the nerve to compression at this level.[2] Fibular neuropathy associated with weight loss most often demonstrates conduction block on electrodiagnostic testing, with the severity correlating with clinical weakness.[1] More recently fibular neuropathy has been described following bariatric surgery.[22]

Significant trauma around the knee or ankle may result in fibular nerve injuries due to the nerve's proximate and superficial locations at the level of these joints. Lacerations from saws, boat propellers, or lawn mowers have all been described.[23] Not surprisingly, those with nerve in continuity have better recovery of function. Knee dislocations, particularly open, rotatory, or posterolateral corner injuries can results in proximal fibular nerve involvement.[24] Deep fibular nerve abnormalities may be localized following spiral fibular fractures.[25] Fractures requiring external fixation of the ankle may result in more distal injury.[26] However, in the case of fractures, it has been noted that fibular neuropathy may be localized to the fibular head electrodiagnostically, though the fracture is an alternative location.

Box 1
Fibular (Peroneal) neuropathy: reported causes

Knee or fibular head
- Anaphylactoid purpura
- Arthroplasty (knee)
- Arthroscopy (Knee)
- Baker cyst
- Bed rest
- Birth trauma
- Boney exostoses
- Casts
- Crossed-leg sitting
- Cryotherapy
- Fractures (femur, tibia, fibular)
- Fibrous arch
- Foot boards
- Ganglion
- Gun shot wounds
- Heterotopic ossification
- Hematoma
- Hemangiomas
- Intravenous infiltration or injections
- Knee dislocation
- Knee stabilization by helicopter pilots
- Kneepads
- Kneeling
- Lacerations
- Lipoma
- Knee surgery
- Schwannoma
- Sequential compression devices
- Sesamoid bone of the lateral head of gastrocnemius
- Severe valgus or varus deformity at the knee
- Splints
- Squatting (childbirth, strawberry picking, farm workers)
- Synovial cysts
- Traction
- Varicose vein surgery
- Venous thrombosis
- Water ski kneeboards

- Weight loss

Ankle or distal leg

- Ankle sprain
- Arthroscopy
- Boots
- Burn scar
- Edema
- Exertional compartment syndrome
- External fixator
- Fasciotomy for compartment syndrome
- Fascia
- Fracture
- Ganglion cyst
- Inferior extensor retinaculum
- Kneeling in prayer position
- Tightly fitting shoes

Although the most common site of injury following surgical procedures is at the fibular head, focal fibular neuropathies have also been reported at the level of the calf, ankle, and foot. Following total knee replacements, fibular nerve abnormalities may present with sensory symptoms or decreased range of motion.[27] Following high tibial osteotomies, done in association with fibular osteotomies, fibular nerve abnormalities have been noted in 2% to 27% of cases.[28–32] The abnormalities of ankle and toe extension and the sensory loss described following these procedures are thought to result from hardware placement, tourniquet effects, or the fibular osteotomy.[28] Nerve abnormalities as the result of surgeries may be subclinical. In 11 cases studied prospectively with electrophysiologic testing, pre- and post-osteotomy surgery, abnormalities were present postoperatively in 27%, though only one patient was clinically symptomatic.[28]

Fibular neuropathy is the most common lower limb mononeuropathy encountered in athletes.[33,34] Common or proximal deep fibular nerve injuries at or near the level of the fibular head are most often found, particularly in football or soccer players, and may be seen in isolation or in association with severe ligamentous knee injuries or fractures.[33,34] Some athletes reporting pain and weakness in a fibular nerve distribution have been found to have constriction of the nerve by the fibularis longus muscle.[35] Acute or chronic exertional compartment syndrome may also result in foot drop and should be considered, particularly in athletes with intermittent complaints.[36] Superficial fibular nerve injuries at the ankle have been described in soccer players.[34] Due to excursion of superficial nerve with inversion, injury may be seen in association with ankle inversion sprains.[37,38] Nerve abnormalities may also occur at the fibular head in the setting of ankle sprains due to traction of the nerve at the posterolateral knee because the patient's foot is forced into plantar flexion and inversion.[39]

Fibular neuropathies, though more frequently reported in adults, can also be seen in childhood. In a case series of 17 children, findings were similar to those of adults in that the common fibular nerve was most often injured (59%), as opposed to the deep (12%), superficial (5%), or a nonlocalizable level of injury (24%).[40] Compression, trauma, or entrapment were the most common causes encountered.[40]

CLINICAL FEATURES

Patients with fibular neuropathy often present with complaints of "foot drop" or catching their toe with ambulation, which may develop acutely or subacutely depending on the precipitating cause. There may also be complaints of sensory loss over the foot dorsum.

Clinical motor examination demonstrates weakness in ankle dorsiflexion and great toe extension with deep fibular and eversion weakness with superficial fibular involvement. Superficial peroneal nerve abnormalities are rarely present in isolation.[16,41] Toe flexion and ankle plantar flexion strength should be normal. In the setting of a deep fibular neuropathy in conjunction with an accessory deep fibular nerve supplying complete innervation of the extensor digitorum brevis muscle, foot drop with preserved toe extension can be seen.[42]

Sensory loss may be found over the foot dorsum (superficial branch) and/or in the first web space (deep branch). However, sensory symptoms may also be absent.[41] More proximally, neuropraxia of the poster lateral cutaneous nerve of the calf has been reported with sensory deficits in the posterolateral upper calf. When symptoms are limited to the superficial sensory branches, generally patients complain of tingling, numbness, and/or pain in the distribution of the involved sensory fibers.[43] In patients with entrapment of the superficial fibular nerve in the calf, these symptoms extend proximally or distally from the anterolateral leg. The distribution depends on whether one or both terminal branches of the superficial fibular nerve are involved.[44] Those patients with entrapment in the calf fascia may note aggravation of symptoms with exercise.[45] In these cases, a soft tissue bulge with resisted dorsiflexion of the ankle, and a Tinel sign or tenderness at the bulge has been described.[44] In the case of more distal nerve involvement at the ankle, findings may be limited to the involved branches and isolated sensory loss involving specific superficial fibular nerve branches to digits 2 to 5 has also been documented.[5]

The term anterior tarsal tunnel syndrome refers to compression of the deep fibular nerve under the inferior extensor retinaculum.[43,46] Although the fibular nerve is a mixed sensorimotor nerve at the ankle, patients with anterior tarsal tunnel syndrome have been reported to describe more sensory symptoms. Primary complaints include numbness and paresthesias in the first dorsal web space that may awaken the patient from sleep.

ASSESSMENT
Electrodiagnostic Evaluation

Electrodiagnostic studies should include an evaluation of motor and sensory axons of the fibular nerve and its branches using nerve conduction studies and electromyographic examination of relevant muscles (**Table 1**). Appropriate testing to rule out other disorders that may mimic fibular neuropathy (radiculopathy, plexopathy, or generalized disorders) should also be included.

Motor conduction studies
Motor conduction studies have been used for localization of the site of the nerve injury, assessing the severity of the injury and following the recovery process. Motor nerve conduction studies are most often performed to the extensor digitorum brevis. Stimulation sites should include the ankle, fibular neck, and popliteal fossa using an 8 to 10 cm

Table 1
Standard electrophysiologic testing used in the evaluation of a fibular or peroneal mononeuropathy

Electrophysiologic Study	Nerve or Muscle	Recording Site	Stimulation Site	Findings in Fibular Neuropathy and the Fibular Head
Motor Nerve Conduction Study				
	Fibular (Peroneal)	Extensor digitorum brevis	Ankle / Below fibular head / Above fibular head	Low amplitude, or drop in amplitude across fibular head, or both. Slowed conduction velocity across fibular head
	Fibular (Peroneal)	Anterior tibialis	Below fibular head / Above fibular head	Low amplitude or drop in amplitude across the fibular head. Slowed conduction velocity.
	Tibial	Abductor hallucis	Ankle / Popliteal fossa	Normal
Sensory Nerve Conduction Study				
	Superficial fibular (peroneal)	Ankle	Calf	Low amplitude or absent
	Sural	—	—	Usually normal
Electromyography				
	Anterior tibialis	NA	NA	Abnormal (may be normal if purely demyelinating lesion)
	Fibularis (peroneus) longus	NA	NA	Abnormal (may be normal if purely demyelinating lesion)
	Biceps femoris, Short head	NA	NA	Normal
	Tibial-innervated L5 (posterior tibialis, flexor digitorum longus)	NA	NA	Normal
	Gluteus medius or tensor fascia lata	NA	NA	Normal
	Paraspinal muscles	NA	NA	Normal

Abbreviation: NA, not applicable.

segment across the fibular head.[47] In severe or chronic cases, no response may be recorded. Because the goal is to assess for conduction slowing, conduction block and axon loss, an absent response does not give information about the underlying pathophysiology. Thus, motor nerve conduction studies should be performed recording over the tibialis anterior muscle, with stimulation sites at the fibular neck and in the popliteal fossa, if there is no response on studies to the extensor digitorum brevis muscle.[48] Focal conduction slowing or block may be evident on such studies. If motor or sensory fibular studies are abnormal, then further nerve conduction studies should be performed to exclude a more diffuse process.

In case series, muscles supplied by the deep compared with the superficial fibular nerve are most frequently reported as abnormal and more severely involved in fibular neuropathy at the fibular head. The intraneural topography of the common fibular nerve at this level may explain the particular pattern of involvement, in the same way it has been used to explain the differential involvement of fascicles within the ulnar nerve at the elbow. At the level of the fibular head, the fascicles of the deep fibular nerve are located anteriorly and, thus, are more sensitive to pressure or stretch.[8,49] It is also possible that this branch is preferentially affected due to tethering in the fibular tunnel.[50]

Electrophysiologically, the accessory fibular nerve may result in unexpected changes on motor nerve conduction studies recording at the extensor digitorum brevis muscle. In such cases, maximal stimulation of the deep fibular nerve at the ankle produces a smaller response with recording at the extensor digitorum brevis muscle, compared with responses with maximal stimulation at the knee. A response may be recorded from the extensor digitorum brevis if stimulation is applied posterior to the lateral malleolus.[9]

Nerve conduction study parameters should be compared between the below fibular head and the across fibular head segment. The following suggest a focal lesion at the fibular head: a significant drop in conduction velocity between the ankle to the below fibular head segment compared with the across fibular segment and/or a significant decrease in the compound muscle action potential negative peak amplitude from the below fibular head stimulation site to the above fibular head site, which suggests conduction block or focal demyelination. A greater than 20% drop in fibular motor amplitude across the knee segment had a specificity of 99% in localizing fibular nerve lesions at the knee.[51] Short segment stimulation of the fibular nerve across the knee segment has also been described.[52] Though motor conduction is most often recorded proximally from the anterior tibialis, it may also be recorded over the fibularis brevis muscle.[53] Comparison of side-to-side amplitudes distally can be used to assess relative amounts of axonal loss.[14]

Katirji and Wilbourn[2] reported electrophysiological findings in 116 nerves of 103 patients with fibular neuropathies. In this study, motor nerve conduction studies to the extensor digitorum brevis and tibialis anterior muscles were performed bilaterally. No response was recorded in 45 nerve lesions to the extensor digitorum brevis, but the fibular motor response to the tibialis anterior was unobtainable in only 13% (15 limbs). Axonal loss was uniformly present. In 52 of the 116 limbs, a conduction block was localized to the region of the fibular head. The motor nerve conduction study to the tibialis anterior muscle was helpful in localizing lesions to conduction block at the fibular head. In a study assessing the relative contributions of motor axonal loss versus focal conduction block, axonal degeneration was found to be greater in motor fibers to the extensor digitorum brevis, whereas, conversely, conduction block was more often found in anterolateral compartment recordings.[14] Interestingly, it has been found that, despite extensive axonal loss, conduction velocity distal to the fibular head may not be slowed. This suggests that larger myelinated fibers are less involved. Major conduction abnormalities were most often found between the midfibular head and the popliteal fossa.[14]

Sensory Nerve Conduction Studies

Antidromic evaluation of the two sensory branches of the superficial fibular nerve at the ankle can be done with surface stimulation applied 14 cm proximal to the recording electrodes at the anterior edge of the fibula, with the recording electrodes at the level of the malleoli, placed over the intermediate and medial dorsal cutaneous nerves (as located with palpation with the ankle inverted and plantarflexed)[54] or 3 cm proximal to the bimalleolar line.[54,55] Jabre[56] reported a similar technique using the intermediate dorsal cutaneous branch, but stimulating 12 cm proximal to the recording site. The superficial fibular nerve conduction studies may be normal in a common fibular neuropathy despite severe abnormalities in the deep fibular distribution.[57] There seems to be selective vulnerability of the deep fibular fibers to compression or stretch. Sural conduction studies may be normal in fibular neuropathies at the fibular head, despite contributions from the fibular nerve to the sural, and should be normal with more distal lesions.[16,58] Sensory studies may be normal in some cases despite abnormalities documented in motor nerve conduction studies.[59]

If focal involvement of a distal sensory branch is suspected, nerve conduction studies to each of the digital branches of the superficial fibular nerve may be performed.[60] Patients with clinical findings limited to sensory distribution of the deep fibular sensory nerve (first web space of the foot) may be evaluated with nerve conduction studies to evaluate this specific branch.[61] Finally, if focal sensory abnormalities are reported in the upper posterolateral calf, nerve conduction studies to evaluate the posterolateral cutaneous nerve of the calf can also be performed.[62]

Needle Electromyography

Needle electromyographic examination should include the tibialis anterior muscle. This muscle is the most likely muscle to demonstrate abnormalities on the needle examination.[16] The examination should also include at least one muscle innervated by the superficial fibular nerve, the short head of the biceps femoris, and at least one tibial innervated muscle distal to the knee. The short head of the biceps femoris, the only fibular-innervated muscle above the knee, is abnormal with a more proximal mononeuropathy involving the fibular division of the sciatic. Sciatic nerve lesions may mimic fibular neuropathies because of the fascicular arrangement of the nerve in the thigh.[63,64] The fibular nerve fibers in the thigh seem to be more susceptible to injury compared with those of the tibia, and clinically only fibular nerve involvement may be suspected. This susceptibility is thought to arise from several factors, including the fibular nerve's more lateral location, the larger funiculi, or its tethering and course around the fibular head. Electrophysiologically, a sciatic neuropathy can be distinguished by assessing tibial motor and sensory conduction, as well as evaluating for axonal loss in tibial nerve innervated muscles, including those in the thigh. If a distal tibial innervated muscle is abnormal or if the short head of the biceps femoris is abnormal, then the examination should be extended to include more proximal sciatic innervated muscles to exclude a sciatic neuropathy as well as an evaluation of gluteal muscles (abnormal in a lumbosacral plexopathy), and a lumbosacral paraspinal examination to exclude a radiculopathy or polyradiculopathy. Deep fibular abnormalities may be severe with common fibular neuropathy, with normal superficial sensory responses.

Evidence for the use of electrodiagnostic studies

An evidence-based review conducted by the American Association of Neuromuscular and Electrodiagnostic Medicine concluded that there was class III evidence supporting the use of nerve conduction studies for the diagnosis of fibular neuropathy, specifically motor nerve conductions of the fibular nerve recording from the tibialis anterior and extensor digitorum brevis muscles (including conduction through the leg and across the fibular head), and orthodromic and antidromic superficial fibular sensory nerve conduction studies.[65] In addition, class III and IV evidence was found for its usefulness in providing information with regard to recovery of function, whereas evidence was limited to class IV for the role of needle electromyography.[65]

Complementary Assessment Techniques

Ultrasonography has been used to assess the fibular nerve across the fibular head, as well as the superficial fibular nerve as it exits in the calf. The superficial fibular nerve became subcutaneous at about one-fourth of the fibular length.[66] High-resolution ultrasonography may easily evaluate the nerve in its more superficial locations, such as around the fibular head. Body mass index has been found to be positively correlated with fibular nerve and fibular tunnel cross-sectional area and, thus, these parameters should be considered in evaluation with ultrasonography.[67]

Magnetic resonance (MR) neurography is increasingly being used to define the site and extent of peripheral nerve disorders.[68,69] High-field MR scanners allow high resolution and soft tissue contrast imaging of peripheral nerves. Secondary muscle denervation changes may also be seen.[68,69] As with the results of MRI, it may be used to detect space-occupying lesions.[70] Use of these imaging modalities is more important in nontraumatic fibular neuropathies because they may detect intraneural ganglia.[70]

ASSESSMENT OF RECOVERY

Electrodiagnostics have been used to identify the potential for recovery of functional movement. Smith and Trojaborg[7] followed a group of 14 subjects with fibular palsy at the head of the fibula, related either to compression at the time of surgery, crossed legs, or occurring spontaneously. At the time of follow-up, which spanned 5 months to 3 years, less than half of the subjects demonstrated complete recovery. All subjects with full clinical recovery had normal sensory conduction distal to the fibular head at the time of the initial study and only one had reduced amplitude SNAP. Similarly, all patients who recovered clinically had normal initial conduction velocities distal to the fibular head.[7]

Derr and colleagues[6] evaluated electrodiagnostic features associated with good recovery of function at follow-up in persons with fibular neuropathy diagnosed electrophysiologically. Good recovery in this study was defined by Medical Research Council Scale muscle strength grade 4 or 5 for ankle dorsiflexion. Any compound muscle action potential response recorded from the tibialis anterior or extensor digitorum brevis at baseline was associated with a good response (81% and 94%, respectively) compared with absent responses.[6] However, it has been found that good outcome was still possible with an absent compound muscle action potential response.[6,71] Recruitment in the tibialis anterior has also found to be predictive in cases of traumatic injury. Subjects with discrete or absent recruitment in the tibialis anterior tend to have a poorer outcome.[6] Individuals with nontraumatic compression are more likely to have a good outcome.[6]

Treatment Options

Treatment of fibular nerve injuries depends on the cause and the degree of weakness or sensory symptoms. In cases of compression, relief from external compressive sources should be in the initial intervention or in the case of intraneural ganglia, surgical referral. Open lacerations should undergo exploration and surgical repair as appropriate. If weakness is incomplete, strengthening exercises can be used to improve function. With complete loss of dorsiflexion, stretching to maintain ankle range of motion should be performed to prevent equinovarus deformity. Orthotic interventions include a lateral wedge shoe insert in the case of isolated superficial fibular neuropathies to decrease supination of the foot or an ankle foot orthosis with common or deep fibular neuropathy and significant ankle dorsiflexor weakness.

Options for intervention with persistent nerve injury include neurolysis, nerve repair, and nerve and tendon transfers.[24,72] Electrophysiologic studies may identify reinnervation along with clinical examinations and the need for surgical intervention. Posterior tibialis tendon transfers have been used to restore ankle dorsiflexion with absent recovery.[73]

Surgical outcomes for fibular neuropathy have been reported in large case series. Follow-up outcomes of 318 operatively-managed common fibular nerve lesions associated with a variety of mechanisms (stretch or contusions, lacerations, tumors, entrapments, stretch dislocations with fractures or dislocations, compression, iatrogenic injures and gun shot wounds) found that of the 19 subjects who underwent end-to-end suture repair, 84% achieved good recovery by 24 months. In subjects requiring graft repair, graft length correlated with recovery; of those with grafts less than 6 cm long, 75% had good recovery of function.[23] Longer grafts generally correlated with more severe injuries and poorer outcomes.[23] Decompression surgery when symptoms were limited to sensory findings has associated with recovery of function at follow-up in other studies.[74] Posterior tibial tendon transfers through the interosseous membrane followed by fixation to the anterior tibial and long fibular tendons have been reported to allow gait without an orthosis and improved quality of life in most patients.[73]

SUMMARY

Fibular (peroneal) neuropathy is the most common mononeuropathy found in the lower limb and may be encountered as the result of acute traumatic injuries, surgical intervention, or with chronic stretch or compression. Clinically, sciatic mononeuropathies, L5 radiculopathies, and lumbosacral plexopathies may present with similar findings of ankle dorsiflexor weakness. More generalized disorders may also present with this symptom and, thus, evaluation is needed to distinguish these various disorders. The most common site of injury to the fibular nerve is at the fibular head. Electrodiagnostic studies have shown that the deep fibular branch is more frequently abnormal than the superficial branch; however, findings may be limited to specific motor or sensory branches, depending on the mechanism of injury. Electrodiagnostic studies are useful to determine the level and type (axonal, demyelinating) of injury. Studies should include motor nerve conduction studies to the extensor digitorum brevis and anterior tibialis muscles, superficial fibular sensory nerve conduction studies, and other motor nerve conduction studies outside the fibular distribution to distinguish a disorder localized to the fibular nerve from more extensive nerve abnormalities. The presence of any compound muscle action potential response on motor nerve conduction studies, recorded from either the tibialis anterior or extensor digitorum brevis, is associated with good long-term outcome. However, recovery is still possible despite an initial absent response.

REFERENCES

1. Cruz-Martinez A, Arpa J, Palau F. Peroneal neuropathy after weight loss. J Peripher Nerv Syst 2000;5:101–5.
2. Katirji MB, Wilbourn AJ. Common peroneal mononeuropathy: a clinical and electrophysiologic study of 116 lesions. Neurology 1988;38:1723–8.
3. Federative Committee on Anatomical Terminology. Terminologia anatomica. Stuttgart (Germany): Thieme; 1998. p. 140.
4. Van Langenhove M, Pollefliet A, Vanderstraeten G. A retrospective electrodiagnostic evaluation of footdrop in 303 patients. Electromyogr Clin Neurophysiol 1989;29:145–52.
5. Collins MP, Mendell JR, Periquet MI, et al. Superficial peroneal nerve/peroneus brevis muscle biopsy in vasculitic neuropathy. Neurology 2000;55:636–43.
6. Derr JJ, Micklesen PJ, Robinson LR. Predicting recovery after fibular nerve injury: which electrodiagnostic features are most useful? Am J Phys Med Rehabil 2009; 88:547–53.
7. Smith T, Trojaborg W. Clinical and electrophysiological recovery from peroneal palsy. Acta Neurol Scand 1986;74:328–35.
8. Sunderland S. Nerves and nerve injuries. Baltimore, (MD): Williams and Wilkins; 1968. p. 1012.
9. Lambert EH. The accessory deep peroneal nerve. A common variation in innervation of extensor digitorum brevis. Neurology 1969;19:1169–76.
10. Prakash, Bhardwaj AK, Singh DK, et al. Anatomic variations of superficial peroneal nerve: clinical implications of a cadaver study. Ital J Anat Embryol 2010; 115:223–8.
11. Infante E, Kennedy WR. Anomalous branch of the peroneal nerve detected by electromyography. Arch Neurol 1970;22:162–5.
12. Mapelli G, Pavoni M, Di Bari M, et al. The accessory deep peroneal nerve. Acta Neurol (Napoli) 1978;33:349–54.
13. Neundorfer B, Seiberth R. The accessory deep peroneal nerve. J Neurol 1975; 209:125–9.
14. Brown WF, Watson BV. Quantitation of axon loss and conduction block in peroneal nerve palsies. Muscle Nerve 1991;14:237–44.
15. Wilbourn AJ. AAEE case report #12: common peroneal mononeuropathy at the fibular head. Muscle Nerve 1986;9:825–36.
16. Sourkes M, Stewart JD. Common peroneal neuropathy: a study of selective motor and sensory involvement. Neurology 1991;41:1029–33.
17. Dubuisson AS, Stevenaert A. Recurrent ganglion cyst of the peroneal nerve: radiological and operative observations. Case report. J Neurosurg 1996;84:280–3.
18. Marwah V. Compression of the lateral popliteal (common peroneal) nerve. Lancet 1964;2:1367–9.
19. Sherman DG, Easton JD. Dieting and peroneal nerve palsy. JAMA 1977;238:230–1.
20. Sotaniemi KA. Slimmer's paralysis—peroneal neuropathy during weight reduction. J Neurol Neurosurg Psychiatry 1984;47:564–6.
21. Kaminsky F. Peroneal palsy by crossing the legs. JAMA 1947;134:206.
22. Elias WJ, Pouratian N, Oskouian RJ, et al. Peroneal neuropathy following successful bariatric surgery. Case report and review of the literature. J Neurosurg 2006; 105:631–5.
23. Kim DH, Murovic JA, Tiel RL, et al. Management and outcomes in 318 operative common peroneal nerve lesions at the Louisiana State University Health Sciences Center. Neurosurgery 2004;54:1421–8 [discussion: 8–9].

24. Cush G, Irgit K. Drop foot after knee dislocation: evaluation and treatment. Sports Med Arthrosc 2011;19:139–46.
25. Hey HW, Tan TC, Lahiri A, et al. Deep peroneal nerve entrapment by a spiral fibular fracture: a case report. J Bone Joint Surg Am 2011;93(1–5):e113.
26. Lui TH, Chan LK. Deep peroneal nerve injury following external fixation of the ankle: case report and anatomic study. Foot Ankle Int 2011;32:S550–5.
27. Zywiel MG, Mont MA, McGrath MS, et al. Peroneal nerve dysfunction after total knee arthroplasty: characterization and treatment. J Arthroplasty 2011;26:379–85.
28. Aydogdu S, Cullu E, Arac N, et al. Prolonged peroneal nerve dysfunction after high tibial osteotomy: pre- and postoperative electrophysiological study. Knee Surg Sports Traumatol Arthrosc 2000;8:305–8.
29. Ferkel RD, Heath DD, Guhl JF. Neurological complications of ankle arthroscopy. Arthroscopy 1996;12:200–8.
30. Gibson MJ, Barnes MR, Allen MJ, et al. Weakness of foot dorsiflexion and changes in compartment pressures after tibial osteotomy. J Bone Joint Surg Br 1986;68:471–5.
31. Jackson JP, Waugh W. The technique and complications of upper tibial osteotomy. A review of 226 operations. J Bone Joint Surg Br 1974;56:236–45.
32. Wootton JR, Ashworth MJ, MacLaren CA. Neurological complications of high tibial osteotomy—the fibular osteotomy as a causative factor: a clinical and anatomical study. Ann R Coll Surg Engl 1995;77:31–4.
33. Kouyoumdjian JA. Peripheral nerve injuries: a retrospective survey of 456 cases. Muscle Nerve 2006;34:785–8.
34. Krivickas LS, Wilbourn AJ. Peripheral nerve injuries in athletes: a case series of over 200 injuries. Semin Neurol 2000;20:225–32.
35. Mitra A, Stern JD, Perrotta VJ, et al. Peroneal nerve entrapment in athletes. Ann Plast Surg 1995;35:366–8.
36. Popovic N, Bottoni C, Cassidy C. Unrecognized acute exertional compartment syndrome of the leg and treatment. Acta Orthop Belg 2011;77:265–9.
37. Nitz AJ, Dobner JJ, Kersey D. Nerve injury and grades II and III ankle sprains. Am J Sports Med 1985;13:177–82.
38. O'Neill PJ, Parks BG, Walsh R, et al. Excursion and strain of the superficial peroneal nerve during inversion ankle sprain. J Bone Joint Surg Am 2007;89:979–86.
39. Hyslop GH. Injuries to the deep and. superficial peroneal nerves complicating ankle sprain. Am J Surg 1941;51:436.
40. Jones HR Jr, Felice KJ, Gross PT. Pediatric peroneal mononeuropathy: a clinical and electromyographic study. Muscle Nerve 1993;16:1167–73.
41. Garland H, Moorhouse D. Compressive lesions of the external popliteal (common peroneal) nerve. Br Med J 1952;2:1373–8.
42. Kayal R, Katirji B. Atypical deep peroneal neuropathy in the setting of an accessory deep peroneal nerve. Muscle Nerve 2009;40:313–5.
43. Krause KH, Witt T, Ross A. The anterior tarsal tunnel syndrome. J Neurol 1977;217:67–74.
44. Sridhara CR, Izzo KL. Terminal sensory branches of the superficial peroneal nerve: an entrapment syndrome. Arch Phys Med Rehabil 1985;66:789–91.
45. Styf J, Morberg P. The superficial peroneal tunnel syndrome. Results of treatment by decompression. J Bone Joint Surg Br 1997;79:801–3.
46. Marinacci AA. Medial and anterior tarsal tunnel syndrome. Electromyography 1968;8:123–34.
47. Buschbacher RM. Peroneal nerve motor conduction to the extensor digitorum brevis. Am J Phys Med Rehabil 1999;78:S26–31.

48. Buschbacher RM. Reference values for peroneal nerve motor conduction to the tibialis anterior and for peroneal vs. tibial latencies. Am J Phys Med Rehabil 2003;82:296–301.
49. Urushidani H. The funicular pattern of the sciatic nerve in Japanese adults (author's transl). Nihon Geka Hokan 1974;43:254–75 [in Japanese].
50. Mackinnon SE, Dellon AL. Surgery of the peripheral nerve. New York: Thieme Medical Publishers; 1988. p. 320.
51. Pickett JB. Localizing peroneal nerve lesions to the knee by motor conduction studies. Arch Neurol 1984;41:192–5.
52. Kanakamedala RV, Hong CZ. Peroneal nerve entrapment at the knee localized by short segment stimulation. Am J Phys Med Rehabil 1989;68:116–22.
53. Devi S, Lovelace RE, Duarte N. Proxial peroneal nerve conduction velocity: recording from the anterior tibial and peroneaus brevis muscles. Ann Neurol 1977;2:116–9.
54. Izzo KL, Sridhara CR, Rosenholtz H, et al. Sensory conduction studies of the branches of the superficial peroneal nerve. Arch Phys Med Rehabil 1981;62: 24–7.
55. Levin KH, Stevens JC, Daube JR. Superficial peroneal nerve conduction studies for electromyographic diagnosis. Muscle Nerve 1986;9:322–6.
56. Jabre JF. The superficial peroneal sensory nerve revisited. Arch Neurol 1981;38: 666–7.
57. Kang PB, Preston DC, Raynor EM. Involvement of superficial peroneal sensory nerve in common peroneal neuropathy. Muscle Nerve 2005;31:725–9.
58. Kwon HK, Kim L, Park YK. Compound nerve action potential of common peroneal nerve and sural nerve action potential in common peroneal neuropathy. J Korean Med Sci 2008;23:117–21.
59. de Carvalho M, Miguel S, Bentes C. Sensory potential can be preserved in severe common peroneal neuropathy. Electromyogr Clin Neurophysiol 2000;40:61–3.
60. Oh SJ, Demirci M, Dajani B, et al. Distal sensory nerve conduction of the superficial peroneal nerve: new method and its clinical application. Muscle Nerve 2001; 24:689–94.
61. Lee HJ, Bach JR, DeLisa JA. Deep peroneal sensory nerve. Standardization in nerve conduction study. Am J Phys Med Rehabil 1990;69:202–4.
62. Campagnolo DI, Romello MA, Park YI, et al. Technique for studying conduction in the lateral cutaneous nerve of calf. Muscle Nerve 2000;23:1277–9.
63. Berry H, Richardson PM. Common peroneal nerve palsy: a clinical and electrophysiological review. J Neurol Neurosurg Psychiatry 1976;39:1162–71.
64. Katirji B, Wilbourn AJ. High sciatic lesion mimicking peroneal neuropathy at the fibular head. J Neurol Sci 1994;121:172–5.
65. Marciniak C, Armon C, Wilson J, et al. Practice parameter: utility of electrodiagnostic techniques in evaluating patients with suspected peroneal neuropathy: an evidence-based review. Muscle Nerve 2005;31:520–7.
66. Park GY, Im S, Lee JI, et al. Effect of superficial peroneal nerve fascial penetration site on nerve conduction studies. Muscle Nerve 2010;41:227–33.
67. Meylaerts L, Cardinaels E, Vandevenne J, et al. Peroneal neuropathy after weight loss: a high-resolution ultrasonographic characterization of the common peroneal nerve. Skeletal Radiol 2011;40:1557–62.
68. Chhabra A, Faridian-Aragh N, Chalian M, et al. High-resolution 3-T MR neurography of peroneal neuropathy. Skeletal Radiol 2012;41:257–71.
69. Wadhwa V, Thakkar RS, Maragakis N, et al. Sciatic nerve tumor and tumor-like lesions-uncommon pathologies. Skeletal Radiol 2012;41(7):763–74.

70. Kim S, Choi JY, Huh YM, et al. Role of magnetic resonance imaging in entrapment and compressive neuropathy - what, where, and how to see the peripheral nerves on the musculoskeletal magnetic resonance image: part 1. Overview and lower extremity. Eur Radiol 2007;17:139–49.
71. Sorell DA, Hinterbuchner C, Green RF, et al. Traumatic common peroneal nerve palsy: a retrospective study. Arch Phys Med Rehabil 1976;57:361–5.
72. Strazar R, White CP, Bain J. Foot reanimation via nerve transfer to the peroneal nerve using the nerve branch to the lateral gastrocnemius: case report. J Plast Reconstr Aesthet Surg 2011;64:1380–2.
73. Steinau HU, Tofaute A, Huellmann K, et al. Tendon transfers for drop foot correction: long-term results including quality of life assessment, and dynamometric and pedobarographic measurements. Arch Orthop Trauma Surg 2011;131: 903–10.
74. Fabre T, Piton C, Andre D, et al. Peroneal nerve entrapment. J Bone Joint Surg Am 1998;80:47–53.

Electrodiagnosis of Motor Neuron Disease

Anuradha Duleep, MD*, Jeremy Shefner, MD, PhD

KEYWORDS

- Motor neuron disease • Amyotrophic lateral sclerosis • Awaji criteria
- Electrodiagnosis

KEY POINTS

- ALS, a relentlessly progressive disorder of upper and lower motor neurons and the most common form of motor neuron disease, is examined here as a model for the electrodiagnosis of all motor neuron disease.
- Electrodiagnostic testing in ALS should be guided by the clinical manifestations noted on physical examination.
- The most sensitive and specific criteria for the diagnosis of ALS are the principles of the revised El Escorial criteria combined with the Awaji modifications to the diagnostic categories of the revised El Escorial criteria.
- Nerve conduction study and needle electromyography remain the most important diagnostic testing for ALS. The former is used primarily to help rule out other disorders, and the latter to establish evidence for widespread active denervation and chronic reinnervation.

CLINICAL FEATURES OF AMYOTROPHIC LATERAL SCLEROSIS

Amyotrophic lateral sclerosis (ALS) is a progressive neurodegenerative disorder of upper motor neurons (UMN) and lower motor neurons (LMN). It has a worldwide incidence of approximately 1.5 per 100,000, with a male/female ratio of approximately 1.5.[1] Although occasional patients present before the age of 25, the incidence increases after age 40 and does not clearly decline in the elderly population.[2] Approximately 10% of cases are familial and include autosomal recessive, X-linked, and

Dr Shefner receives research funding from NIH, ALSA, MDA, ALS Therapy Alliance, Biogen-Idec, Sanofi Aventis, Neuraltus. He receives personal compensation as an Editor for UpToDate, and as a consultant for Trophos, ISIS, Glaxo SmithKline, Biogen-Idec, Cytokinetics.
No disclosures (Anuradha Duleep).
Department of Neurology, SUNY Upstate Medical University, 750 East Adams Street, Syracuse, NY 13210, USA
* Corresponding author.
E-mail address: duleepa@upstate.edu

autosomal-dominant patterns, with autosomal-dominant being most common.[3] The first causative mutation reported was a point mutation in the gene that encodes SOD1; since this discovery in 1993, more than 75 other mutations have been described.[4,5] Most recently, a hexanucleotide repeat expansion of the chromosome 9 open reading frame 72 (C9orf72) gene has been described, and is likely to be the most common mutation in familial cases with or without frontotemporal dementia.[6] A total of 90% of cases of ALS remain sporadic or idiopathic.

The only clear risk factor is increasing age, but this is too nonspecific to be clinically useful. Sporadic ALS has been linked to cigarette smoking, military service, agricultural or factory work, and periods of heavy muscle use, but a definite causal relationship with any one factor has not been established.[7,8] Multiple genetic risk factors have been identified in sporadic ALS, including duplication of the survival motor neuron 1 gene and trinucleotide repeat expansion of the ataxin 2 gene.[9–12] Hexanucleotide repeat expansions of the C9orf72 gene are not only associated with familial ALS, but may be found in approximately 5% to 7% of apparently sporadic cases.[13,14]

The cause of sporadic ALS is unknown, and many of the multiple genetic defects that cause ALS do so in a manner that is still obscure. The finding that mutations in SOD1 cause ALS has raised the question of the role of oxidative stress in ALS, because SOD1 is a ubiquitous free radical scavenger in neural and nonneural tissue. However, it is clear that SOD1 mutations cause disease as a result of a toxic gain of function, rather than reduction of activity of the SOD1 protein.[15,16] Mitochondrial dysfunction has been noted early in genetic models, and likely plays a role in the disease pathway.[17] Excitotoxicity by excessive activation of glutamate receptors has been shown in a variety of models, caused at least in part by reduction in glutamate uptake in areas of the brain damaged by ALS.[18] This leads to increased intracellular calcium, which triggers damage to mitochondria and nucleic acids, and ultimately neuronal death. Protein misaggregation has been noted pathologically, and several recently discovered causative mutations in the genes for fused in sarcoma (FUS), TAR DNA binding protein-43 (TDP-43), and potentially C9orf72 result in abnormal protein being deposited in the cytoplasm of motor neurons.[19,20] Because these genes have a major role in RNA trafficking, impairment of this function has been suggested as a potential cause of ALS.[21]

Riluzole (Rilutek), which reduces glutamate-induced excitotoxicity, is the only drug that has been shown to affect the course of ALS.[22,23] Death usually occurs through respiratory muscle insufficiency or complications from dysphagia, with a median survival from time of diagnosis of 3 to 5 years. Approximately 10% of patients with ALS may live beyond 10 years, but the relentlessly progressive nature of this disease, the significant morbidity, and impact on family and society is common to all.

The clinical presentation of ALS is varied, given the number of body segments and predominance of UMN versus LMN symptoms and signs that are possible. We speak of ALS affecting four body segments, referring to motor neurons involved in a craniobulbar, cervical, thoracic, or lumbosacral distribution. A fundamental quality of ALS is the presence of UMN and LMN findings that spread without remission to ultimately involve multiple body segments, often in a predictable pattern. UMN findings include muscle spasticity, defined as increased tone in the muscle that renders it resistant to stretch and causes stiff and slow movement with little weakness, and heightened deep tendon reflexes. An interesting feature of UMN dysfunction is pseudobulbar affect. This manifests with sudden outbursts of involuntary laughter or crying that is often excessive or incongruent to mood, caused by loss of voluntary cortical inhibition to brainstem centers that produce the facial and respiratory functions associated with those behaviors, through bilateral corticobulbar lesions, or through interruption of corticocerebellar control of affective displays.[24]

Clinical features resulting from loss of LMNs are flaccid weakness, muscle atrophy, hyporeflexia, muscle cramps, and fasciculations, which may be visible as brief twitching under the skin or in the tongue. LMN loss in axial muscles may result in abdominal protuberance or impaired ability to hold the body or head upright against gravity. LMN loss to the diaphragm results in dyspnea or orthopnea that usually disturbs sleep. Flaccid weakness affecting bulbar muscles may present as slurred, nasal, or hoarse speech; dysphagia; or drooling. The initial clinical presentation of ALS may start in any body segment, and may manifest as UMN, LMN, or both, with a pattern of spread from one body segment to others that is often predictable. In time, UMN and LMN findings develop in the same body segment, if they did not start concurrently. Asymmetric limb weakness, often distal with hand weakness or foot drop, is the initial presentation in 80% of patients, with bulbar symptoms, such as dysarthria or dysphagia, in most of the rest.

Extraocular motor neurons are spared until very late in the disease. Autonomic symptoms are not typical, but multifactorial constipation and urinary urgency from a spastic bladder may occur late in the course. Sensory symptoms, such as distal limb paresthesias, may occur in 20% of patients, but usually with a normal clinical sensory examination. Cognitive symptoms in the form of frontotemporal dementia or dysfunction may be present in anywhere from 15% to 50% of patients.[25] This may manifest as subtle impairment of language, judgment, or personality.[26] Mutations involving certain genes, including TDP-43, FUS, and C9orf72, are associated with a higher likelihood of cognitive impairment.[27–29]

ELECTRODIAGNOSIS

ALS is a clinical diagnosis, but is supported by electrophysiologic study, which can either help to rule out other possible diagnoses or show characteristic abnormalities in body areas not yet clinically affected. The electrophysiologic studies that are in common practice, such as needle electromyography (EMG) and nerve conduction studies (NCS), directly identify LMN pathology, and at best may suggest UMN pathology by the observation of decreased activation on EMG. How do needle EMG and nerve conduction testing, together referred to as electrodiagnostic testing (EDX), support the diagnosis of ALS? EDX primarily helps rule out other causes of similar symptoms (**Table 1**) and uncovers subclinical LMN loss, which can speed time to diagnosis and increase diagnostic sensitivity.

Review of the diagnostic criteria for ALS illustrates the importance of uncovering subclinical LMN loss with EDX, particularly with EMG. The El Escorial World Federation of Neurology criteria, first proposed in 1994 and revised in 2000 (**Tables 2** and **3**), is still in effect, with two key modifications proposed in December 2006 during a consensus conference in Awaji-shima, Japan, sponsored by the International Federation of Clinical Neurophysiology.[30]

Using EMG to uncover subclinical LMN dysfunction in the form of active denervation with compensatory chronic reinnervation in the same muscle can change the diagnosis of ALS from "Clinically Possible ALS" to "Laboratory Supported Clinically Probable ALS." A limitation of the revised El Escorial criteria is that it is not sufficient to demonstrate LMN dysfunction by EMG alone in a limb, but that the category of "Laboratory Supported Clinically Probable ALS" requires a demonstration of LMN by physical examination in one limb. Another limitation is that the revised El Escorial criteria restricts EMG evidence of acute denervation to fibrillations or positive sharp waves, which may not be as demonstrable in bulbar muscles and those muscles of normal bulk and strength. These limitations have contributed to the fact that 22% of patients

Table 1
Mimics of motor neuron disease

Disease	Presentation	Distinguishing Features	Role of Electrodiagnostic Testing
Cervical radiculomyelopathy	LMN dysfunction at the level of stenosis with UMN findings below	Neck pain and radicular sensory symptoms in arms	No EMG findings in bulbar or thoracic paraspinal muscles
Concomitant cervical and lumbar stenosis	Like cervical radiculomyelopathy, but with LMN findings also in lumbosacral myotomes	Neck and back pain, radicular sensory symptoms in the arms and legs	No EMG findings in bulbar or thoracic paraspinal muscles
Benign fasciculation syndrome	Frequent fasciculations, diffuse or focal; cramps	Normal neurologic examination	No EMG findings other than fasciculation potentials
Multifocal motor neuropathy with conduction block	LMN limb weakness, often upper extremities	Not myotomal, often in patients younger than 45 yr old	Conduction block in motor nerve NCS nonentrapment sites
Inflammatory myopathies	LMN limb weakness, dysphagia	IBM: finger flexor, quadriceps weakness Polymyositis or dermatomyositis: proximal muscle weakness	Fibrillation potentials/ positive sharp waves; small amplitude and short duration motor unit potentials and occasionally neuropathic MUPs (IBM only) with normal or early recruitment

Abbreviations: IBM, inclusion body myositis; MUPs, motor unit potentials.

die from ALS without being assigned a level of certainty about the disease higher than the "Clinically Possible ALS" category.[31]

To increase the sensitivity for detection of a probable or definite diagnosis of ALS, the Awaji criteria were recently proposed (**Table 4**). Using these criteria, EMG findings of LMN dysfunction, specifically active denervation with chronic reinnervation in a muscle, are assigned equal diagnostic significance to the findings of LMN dysfunction on physical examination. This eliminates the need for the category of "Laboratory Supported Clinically Probable ALS" and is based on the observation that EMG is an extension of the physical examination in detecting features of denervation and reinnervation.

Although no change was suggested to the general principles of the revised El Escorial criteria (see **Table 2**), the Awaji criteria stipulates that the diagnostic categories of ALS should be defined by clinical or electrophysiologic evidence of LMN dysfunction, and UMN dysfunction, in specified numbers of body segments. Specifically, this means that in using the Awaji criteria, individual muscles that show active and chronic denervation with reinnervation electrophysiologically may be used to help diagnose

Table 2
The diagnostic principles of the revised El Escorial criteria

Presence	Absence
Evidence of LMN degeneration by clinical, electrophysiologic, or neuropathologic examination	Electrophysiologic or pathologic evidence of another disease process that might explain the signs of LMN or UMN degeneration
Evidence of UMN dysfunction by clinical examination	Evidence of another disease process by neuroimaging that might explain the observed clinical and electrophysiologic signs
Progressive spread of symptoms or signs within a region or to other regions, as determined by history, physical examination, or electrophysiologic tests	

ALS in conjunction with the clinical examination, obviating the need to demonstrate needle EMG changes in an entire limb. One other change from revised El Escorial criteria is that using Awaji criteria, in the presence of chronic neurogenic findings on EMG in a patient with a clinical history suggestive of ALS, fasciculation potentials are equivalent to fibrillation potentials and positive sharp waves in denoting acute denervation, especially if the fasciculation potentials have unstable or complex morphology. Studies evaluating the utility of the Awaji modifications compared with the revised El Escorial criteria for the diagnosis of ALS suggest improved sensitivity from 28% to 61% with no change in specificity, which remains at 96%.[32–35]

Electrodiagnosis of ALS begins with the recognition of a clinically suggestive history and examination. The role of NCS is to help rule out other causes of similar symptoms, as required by the general principles outlined in the revised El Escorial criteria for the diagnosis of ALS and endorsed by the Awaji consensus group (see **Table 2**). The role

Table 3
Diagnostic categories in the revised El Escorial criteria

Category of ALS	UMN Findings Body Segments[a] on Physical Examination		LMN Findings Body Segments on Physical Examination		Additional Tests
Clinically definite	3	+	3		
Clinically probable	2 Some UMN signs rostral to the LMN signs	+	2		
Clinically probable Laboratory supported	1 At least 1 +	+ OR +	1 0	+ +	Acute and chronic denervation in at least two limbs by EMG
Clinically possible	1 At least 2	+ OR	1 0		
Definite familial Laboratory supported	1	+	1	+	Documented genetic mutation

[a] Body segments are craniobulbar, cervical, thoracic, and lumbosacral.

Table 4
Awaji modifications to the diagnostic categories of the revised El Escorial criteria

Category of ALS	UMN Findings Body Segments[a] on Physical Examination		LMN Findings Body Segments[a] on Physical Examination Or Electrophysiologic Testing[b]		Additional Tests
Clinically definite	3	+	3		
Clinically probable	2 Some UMN signs rostral to the LMN	+	2		
Clinically possible	1	+	1		
	At least 2	+	0		
Definite familial Laboratory supported	1	+	1	+	Documented genetic mutation

[a] Body segments are craniobulbar, cervical, thoracic, and lumbosacral.
[b] Electrophysiologic examination:
- Evidence of acute denervation in the form of fibrillation potentials and positive sharp waves
AND
- Evidence of chronic reinnervation in the form of voluntary motor unit potentials of increased amplitude, increased duration, or polyphasia, that may exhibit decreased recruitment (if there is concomitant UMN dysfunction, a decreased recruitment pattern may not be clear)
OR
- Evidence of chronic reinnervation as above, with evidence of acute denervation in the form of fasciculation potentials, preferably of complex morphology, or instability when studied with a high band pass filter and trigger delay line, which suggests their origin from reinnervated motor units.

of needle EMG is to establish concomitant acute denervation and compensatory chronic reinnervation in specific body segments, according to the specifications set out by the Awaji modifications to the revised El Escorial criteria (see **Table 4**). The following is a summary of features of NCS and EMG that are most relevant to ALS.

NERVE CONDUCTION STUDIES

Because the fundamental pathology in the disease is motor neuron loss resulting in retrograde axonal degeneration followed by reinnervation, features that are not seen on NCS in ALS include the following:

- *Evidence of demyelination or conduction block on motor nerve conduction.* Evidence for demyelination suggests pathology at the level of the myelinated axon rather than the motor neuron. Demyelination is characterized by prolonged distal latencies or slowing of conduction velocity, with the caveat that loss of larger and faster motor axons may cause a mild prolongation of distal latency (but not more than 130% the upper limit of normal) or mild slowing of conduction velocity (but not less than 75% the lower limit of normal). Conduction block of motor nerves in areas not associated with entrapment, with sparing of sensory nerves, suggests multifocal motor neuropathy with conduction block, an immune-mediated demyelinating neuropathy that is responsive to intravenous immunoglobulin.[36] Conduction block, as distinguished from normal temporal dispersion, is defined as a drop in the compound muscle action potential (CMAP) area of greater than 50% between proximal and distal stimulation sites.[37]

- *Abnormalities of sensory nerve conduction.* Sensory nerves are not typically affected in ALS. Sensory nerve conduction abnormalities in a patient with motor neuron disease suggests a diagnosis of X-linked bulbospinal muscular atrophy, also known as Kennedy disease. Kennedy disease is a slowly progressive form of spinal muscular atrophy, found in men in their third to fifth decade with LMN degeneration in proximal limb and bulbar muscles. Unlike other motor neuron diseases, Kennedy disease is associated with low amplitude or absent sensory nerve action potentials (SNAPs) caused by degeneration of dorsal root ganglia. SNAP abnormalities should also prompt consideration of other diagnoses, including plexopathies and peripheral and multiple entrapment neuropathies. It is also possible for a patient with ALS to have an unrelated peripheral neuropathy or entrapment neuropathy.

Features on NCS that are consistent with the diagnosis of ALS include the following:

- *Normal or reduced CMAP amplitudes.* Reduced CMAP amplitude reflects axonal loss, but does not distinguish between lesions at the motor neuron, nerve root, plexus, or peripheral nerve. Loss of larger, faster motor neurons may cause prolongation of distal latency up to but not beyond 130% of the upper limit of normal, or decrease in conduction velocity but not less than 75% of the lower limit of normal.
- *Normal SNAP amplitudes.* Although expected in ALS, this may be seen in cervical or lumbar radiculopathies, and because these lesions are proximal to the dorsal root ganglia.
- *Normal F wave latencies.* F waves, representing antidromic stimulation of 1% to 5% of the motor neurons in the anterior horn of the spinal cord, are often normal early in the course of ALS. As the disease progresses and motor neurons are lost from the anterior horn, F response abnormalities begin to be seen. Impersistence, defined by less than 50% of F waves obtained per number of stimulations, and repetition of similar F wave morphologies from stimulation of the same motor units, reflect the decreased pool of motor units overall from motor neuron loss. If the largest and fastest motor units are lost, F wave latency may be slightly prolonged. F wave abnormalities are actually more likely to occur in radiculopathy rather than motor neuron disease, but cannot be used reliably to distinguish between the two.

RECOMMENDATION FOR NCS

At a minimum, NCS of a patient with suspected ALS should include testing of at least one motor nerve with F wave study and one sensory nerve in an upper and lower extremity on the most symptomatic side. If suspicion is high for multifocal motor neuropathy with conduction block, multiple upper and lower extremity nerves should be studied, with stimulation as proximal as is feasible.

NEEDLE EMG

The hallmark of ALS on needle EMG is chronic and active loss of LMNs innervating muscles with multiple nerve root innervation and spread within an initial body segment and to other body segments. Although NCS is used primarily to help rule out other causes of the same clinical symptoms, such as neuropathy and radiculopathy, needle

EMG is primarily used to establish evidence of ongoing denervation and chronic compensatory reinnervation. EDX is particularly helpful in uncovering subclinical evidence of this process, so needle EMG should not be limited to the testing of muscles or body segments where LMN dysfunction is clinically apparent.

Evidence for acute denervation in ALS on needle EMG includes the following:

- *Fibrillations and positive sharp waves.* In ALS, these waveforms reflect the spontaneous depolarization of a denervated muscle fiber at rest. Although they are pathologic, they are also seen in other denervating conditions, such as radiculopathy and axonal neuropathies, and myopathies in which muscle necrosis occurs, such as polymyositis.
- *Fasciculation potentials.* These potentials reflect the spontaneous and involuntary discharge of a single motor unit, and as such may arise from the motor neuron or its axon, and are considered the hallmark of ALS. However, they may be a benign finding in normal muscles, in the setting of a serially normal neurologic examination and no other findings suggestive of acute or chronic denervation on EMG, as in the case of benign fasciculation syndrome (see **Table 1**). Unfortunately, there is no definitive way to distinguish between pathologic and benign fasciculation potentials. However, pathologic fasciculation potentials usually have a more regular activation frequency and a morphology of motor unit potentials (MUPs) characterized by increased amplitude, polyphasia, and duration. Pathologic fasciculation potentials are also commonly complex or unstable, with peaks appearing or disappearing with sustained observation. Yoked discharges appearing more than 10 milliseconds after the initial discharge are also suspicious for a pathologic process. As such, these complex and unstable fasciculation potentials are given equal weight as a sign of denervation as fibrillations and positive sharp waves when seen in the context of chronic neurogenic changes on EMG, in the Awaji modified criteria for the diagnosis of ALS (see **Table 4**).

Evidence for chronic denervation in ALS on needle EMG includes the following morphologic changes of MUPs:

- *Increased duration.* Increased duration results from the reinnervation process of collateral axonal sprouting, because duration reflects the number of muscle fibers within the motor unit, which increases as motor units with intact axons reinnervate adjacent muscle fibers from a denervated motor unit.
- *Increased polyphasicity.* MUPs are commonly polyphasic in ALS, although in very slowly progressive disease, polyphasic motor units may be rare. Polyphasia is defined by greater than four phases in a MUP and may occur normally up to 10% of the MUPs in any given muscle, and up to 25% in the deltoid. Polyphasia beyond this normal range is a sign of dyssynchrony of the muscle fibers firing within the motor unit, reflecting the process of reinnervation through collateral sprouting from adjacent normal axons after denervation within a motor unit.
- *Increased amplitude.* Amplitude increases in a chronically reinnervated muscle because of an expansion of the territory of the motor unit. Depending on the rate of progression of the disease process, abnormally small MUPS can also be seen, which reflect the inability of individual axons to support the normal number of nerve sprouts. This is often a reflection of a diseased axon just before death of the associated neuron.
- *Decreased recruitment.* Decreased recruitment of motor units reflects the loss of MUPs and manifests as increased firing of an inappropriately low number of

MUPs when the muscle is called on to generate a greater force of contraction. With motor neuron dropout, a common observation is that a reduced number of rapidly firing motor units is noted when subjects exert maximum or near maximum strength. This is a subjective finding, but often a sensitive and early indicator of neurogenic change. Decreased recruitment of motor units is often an early and sensitive indicator of LMN abnormality.

- *MUP instability.* This is often reflective of rapid loss of motor units and is not always seen. It may reflect more aggressive disease. MUP instability is noted subjectively when a voluntarily activated unit changes with respect to number of peaks or amplitude of individual peaks from potential to potential. This can be characterized more objectively by measuring jitter and blocking of MUPs with a trigger delay line. MUP instability, while common, is not specific to the diagnosis of ALS.[38]

RECOMMENDATIONS FOR NEEDLE EMG TESTING

At a minimum, needle EMG study of a patient with suspected ALS should include testing of at least three limbs, sampling muscles innervated by at least two different nerve roots, and peripheral nerves and proximal and distal muscles. Additionally, testing should be performed on at least one bulbar muscle, such as a facial muscle, the masseter muscle, or tongue. Finally, needle EMG should be done on at least two thoracic paraspinal muscles.

OTHER ELECTRODIAGNOSTIC TOOLS

Motor unit number estimation (MUNE), a sensitive technique for identifying lower motor unit loss, particularly before the onset of clinical weakness, is not yet widely performed and is used primarily in the research setting. MUNE can be used as marker for disease progression in ALS, because it can be linked to important outcomes, such as survival.[39–41] A recently described standardized technique for multipoint incremental MUNE generates highly reproducible data, and can be rapidly performed on basic EDX equipment with minimal discomfort to the patient through use of low stimulus intensities.[42] When studied as percent change from baseline, this measurement of decline in ALS compares favorably with the more commonly used Amyotrophic Lateral Sclerosis Functional Rating Scale-Revised.

Transcranial magnetic stimulation (TMS) physiologically evaluates UMN function. A brief magnetic pulse is directed to the motor cortex, which induces an electric current that is capable of exciting corticomotor neurons or interneurons. The activation of these cells creates a motor volley recordable in the extremities as a motor evoked potential. Central motor conduction time is derived by subtracting peripheral conduction time from the total response latency. Prolongation may reflect loss of corticospinal axons.[43,44] Peripheral conduction time can be estimated using F waves, or directly measured by stimulating ventral roots at their origin using a magnetic stimulator. Similar studies can be performed using routine electrical stimulation, but needle-stimulating electrodes must be used to approach the ventral root and this procedure is usually perceived as uncomfortable by patients. Another parameter of TMS that is associated with ALS is shortening of the cortical silent period recorded from muscle during voluntary contraction.[45,46] The cortical silent period duration is evoked by asking a subject to tonically contract the muscle from which recordings are being made. Stimulation of motor cortex induces a period of suppression of the tonic contraction known as the cortical silent period. This is a function of cortical inhibitory interneurons activated during voluntary contraction. Reduced cortical inhibition has also been reported in ALS, measured by pairing two magnetic stimuli at varying laten-cies and looking at inhibition of the second response by the first as a function of time between the two stimuli.[47–49]

TMS can be used to measure short interval intracortical inhibition (SICI) and shows a reduction in inhibition in ALS, suggesting cortical hyperexcitability from ion channel dysfunction. SICI is the increase in TMS stimulus required to generate a constant motor evoked potential, when a conditioning stimulus representing a selected percentage of the resting motor threshold is first applied. Reduction in SICI across a variety of subthreshold stimuli correlates with reductions in resting motor threshold and increase in motor evoked potential/CMAP ratio, suggesting that the decreased net central inhibition that results in cortical hyperexcitability is mediated through reduced inhibitory cortical interneurons and excessive intracortical excitation.[50,51]

Threshold tracking techniques are applicable to the study of LMNs in ALS.[52] A criterion response from a mixed nerve is selected, such as percentage of the maximal motor response. Then the stimulus intensity required to maintain that crite-rion response is measured while varying stimuli duration (strength-duration relation-ship) or before or after administering a hyperpolarizing or depolarizing conditioning stimulus below the threshold for activation (latent addition if the conditioning stimulus is brief, and threshold electrotonus if it is prolonged). The differences in axonal membrane excitability observed with threshold tracking reflect nodal and internodal processes across ion channels. Prolonged strength-duration time constants and latent addition reflect persistent sodium channel conductance, whereas threshold electrotonus provides information on internodal processes, such as reduction of fast potassium conduction.[53,54] LMN hyperexcitability may be appreciated with threshold tracking techniques before clinical manifestations of spontaneous axonal activity, such as fasciculation potentials, are seen. At present time, threshold tracking is primarily a research tool to investigate the basic mechanisms of hyperexcitability in ALS, and thus target therapies. It is not specific enough to contribute to diagnosis, and has not been studied in relation to rate of progression, but prolonged strength-duration time constant and latent addition have been linked to decreased survival in ALS.[55]

SUMMARY

ALS is a disease diagnosed primarily on clinical grounds, because specific imaging abnormalities or other biomarkers have not been clearly identified. Clinical neurophys-iology, as an extension of the neurologic examination, has proved useful in helping to establish a diagnosis, by eliminating possible disease mimics and providing evidence of abnormalities in body areas that may yet be clinically unaffected. Electrodiagnosis begins with an understanding of the clinical features of the disease, because clinical correlation is important to an accurate interpretation of the electrophysiologic findings. To improve the sensitivity of the electrophysiologic evaluation, the Awaji criteria has been proposed as a modification to the revised El Escorial criteria, which is currently accepted as the gold standard for the diagnosis of ALS. The Awaji criteria incorporate needle EMG findings of ongoing denervation and reinnervation in LMNs in a fashion similar to that of the El Escorial criteria but assigns increased importance to the pres-ence of fasciculation potentials. NCS are primarily used to help rule out other diseases that could mimic ALS, such as multifocal motor neuropathy. Although techniques have been developed to evaluate abnormalities of corticomotor neurons and to quantify loss of LMNs, they remain primarily research tools and have not yet influenced clinical practice.

REFERENCES

1. Ragonese P, Cellura E, Aridon P, et al. Incidence of amyotrophic lateral sclerosis in Sicily: a population based study. Amyotroph Lateral Scler 2012;13(3):284–7.
2. Belzil VV, Langlais JS, Daoud H, et al. Novel FUS deletion in a patient with juvenile amyotrophic lateral sclerosis. Arch Neurol 2012;69(5):653–6.
3. Byrne S, Walsh C, Lynch C, et al. Rate of familial amyotrophic lateral sclerosis: a systematic review and meta-analysis. J Neurol Neurosurg Psychiatry 2011; 82(6):623.
4. Rosen DR, Siddique T, Patterson D, et al. Mutations in Cu/Zn superoxide dismutase gene are associated with familial amyotrophic lateral sclerosis. Nature 1993; 362(6415):59–62.
5. Siddique N, Siddique T. Genetics of amyotrophic lateral sclerosis. Phys Med Rehabil Clin N Am 2008;19(3):429.
6. Renton AE, Majounie E, Waite A, et al. A hexanucleotide repeat expansion in C9ORF72p21 is the cause of chromosome 9p21-linked ALS-FTD. Neuron 2011; 72(2):257.
7. Armon C. Smoking may be considered an established risk factor for sporadic ALS. Neurology 2009;73(20):1693.
8. Weisskopf MG, O'Reilly EJ, McCullough ML, et al. Prospective study of military service and mortality from ALS. Neurology 2005;64(1):32.
9. Corcia P, Camu W, Halimi JM, et al. SMN1 gene, but not SMN2, is a risk factor for sporadic ALS. Neurology 2006;67(7):1147.
10. Lee T, Li YR, Chesi A, et al. Evaluating the prevalence of polyglutamine repeat expansions in amyotrophic lateral sclerosis. Neurology 2011;76(24):2062.
11. Elden AC, Kim HJ, Hart MP, et al. Ataxin-2 intermediate length polyglutamine expansions are associated with increased risk for ALS. Nature 2010;466(7310): 1069.
12. Bonini NM, Gitler AD. Model organisms reveal insight into human neurodegenerative disease: ataxin-2 intermediate-length polyglutamine expansions are a risk factor for ALS. J Mol Neurosci 2011;45(3):676–83.
13. DeJesus-Hernandez M, Mackenzie IR, Boeve BF, et al. Expanded GGGGCC hexanucleotide repeat in noncoding region of C9orf72 causes chromosome 9p-linked FTD and ALS. Neuron 2011;72(2):245.
14. Gijselinck I, Van Langenhove T, van der Zee J, et al. A C9orf72 promoter repeat expansion in a Flanders-Belgium cohort with disorders of the frontotemporal lobar degeneration-amyotrophic lateral sclerosis spectrum: a gene identification study. Lancet Neurol 2012;11(1):54–65.
15. Gurney ME. Transgenic animal models of familial amyotrophic sclerosis. J Neurol 1997;244(Suppl 2):S15.
16. Harraz MM, Marden JJ, Zhou W, et al. SOD1 mutations disrupt redox-sensitive Rac regulation of NADPH oxidase in a familial ALS model. J Clin Invest 2008; 118(2):659.
17. Beal MF. Mitochondria take center stage in aging and neurodegeneration. Ann Neurol 2005;58(4):495.
18. Lin CL, Bristol LA, Jin L, et al. Aberrant RNA processing in a neurodegenerative disease: the cause for absent EAAT2, a glutamate transporter, in amyotrophic lateral sclerosis. Neuron 1998;20(3):589.
19. Ince PG, Highley JR, Kirby J, et al. Molecular pathology and genetic advances in amyotrophic lateral sclerosis: an emerging molecular pathway and the significance of glial pathology. Acta Neuropathol 2011;1122(6):657–71.

20. Ling SC, Albuquerque CP, Han JS, et al. ALS-associated mutations in TDP-43 increase its stability and promote TDP-43 complexes with FUS/TLS. Proc Natl Acad Sci U S A 2010;107(30):13318.
21. Ito D, Suzuki N. Conjoint pathologic cascades mediated by ALS/FTLD-U linked RNA binding proteins TDP-43 and FUS. Neurology 2011;77(17):1636–43.
22. Miller RG, Mitchell JD, Lyon M, et al. Riluzole for amyotrophic lateral sclerosis (ALS)/ motor neuron disease (MND). Cochrane Database Syst Rev 2007;24(1): CD001447.
23. Morren JA, Galvez-Jimenez N. Current and prospective disease-modifying therapies for amyotrophic lateral sclerosis. Expert Opin Investig Drugs 2012;21(3): 297–320.
24. Parvizi J, Andersen SW, Martin CO, et al. Pathological laughter and crying: a link to the cerebellum. Brain 2001;124:1708–19.
25. Ringholz GM, Appel SH, Bradshaw M, et al. Prevalence and patterns of cognitive impairment in sporadic ALS. Neurology 2005;65(4):586.
26. Phukan J, Pender NP, Hardiman O. Cognitive impairment in amyotrophic lateral sclerosis. Lancet Neurol 2007;6(11):994.
27. Byrne S, Elamin M, Bede P, et al. Cognitive and clinical characteristics of patients with amyotrophic lateral sclerosis carrying a C9orf72 repeat expansion: a population-based cohort study. Lancet Neurol 2012;11(3):232–40.
28. Geser F, Lee VM, Trojanowski JQ. Amyotrophic lateral sclerosis and frontotemporal lobar degeneration: a spectrum of TDP-43 proteinopathies. Neuropathology 2010;30(2):103–12.
29. Huang C, Zhou H, Tong J, et al. FUS transgenic rats develop the phenotypes of amyotrophic lateral sclerosis and frontotemporal lobar degeneration. PLoS Genet 2011;7(3):e1002011.
30. De Carvalho M, Dengler R, Eisen A, et al. Electrodiagnostic criteria for diagnosis of ALS. Clin Neurophysiol 2007;119:497–503.
31. Traynor BJ, Codd MB, Corr B, et al. Clinical features of amyotrophic lateral sclerosis according to the El Escorial criteria and airlie house diagnostic criteria. Arch Neurol 2000;57:1171–6.
32. Douglass CP, Kandler RH, Shaw PJ, et al. An evaluation of neurophysiologic criteria used in the diagnosis of motor neuron disease. J Neurol Neurosurg Psychiatry 2010;81(6):646.
33. Chen A, Weimer L, Brannagan T III, et al. Experience with the Awaji Island modifications to the ALS diagnostic criteria. Muscle Nerve 2010;42(5):831–2.
34. Noto Y, Misawa S, Kanai K, et al. Awaji ALS criteria increase the diagnostic sensitivity in patients with bulbar onset. Clin Neurophysiol 2012;123(2):382–5.
35. De Carvalho M, Swash M. Awaji diagnostic algorithm increases sensitivity of El Escorial criteria for ALS diagnosis. Amyotroph Lateral Scler 2009;10(1):53.
36. Kimura J, Kaji R, editors. Multifocal motor neuropathy and conduction block. In: Physiology of ALS and related diseases. Amsterdam: Elsevier Science; 1997. p. 57–72.
37. Preston D, Shapiro B. Electromyography and neuromuscular disorders. Philadelphia (Pennsylvania): Elsevier; 2005. p. 40–3.
38. Erminio F, Buchthal F, Rosenfalck P. Motor unit territory and muscle fiber concentration in paresis due to peripheral nerve injury and anterior horn cell involvement. Neurology 1959;9:657–71.
39. Shefner JM, Cudkowicz M, Brown RH Jr. Motor unit number estimation predicts disease onset and survival in a transgenic mouse model of amyotrophic lateral sclerosis. Muscle Nerve 2006;34:603–7.

40. Armon C, Brandstater ME. Motor unit number estimate-based rates of progression of ALS predict patient survival. Muscle Nerve 1999;22:1571–5.
41. Olney RK, Yuen EC, Engstrom JW, et al. Statistical motor unit number estimation: reproducibility and sources of error in patients with amyotrophic lateral sclerosis. Muscle Nerve 2000;23:193–7.
42. Shefner JM, Watson ML, Simionescu L, et al. Multipoint incremental motor unit number estimation as an outcome measure in ALS. Neurology 2011;77(3): 235–41.
43. Berardelli A, Inghilleri M, Formisano R, et al. Stimulation of motor tracts in motor neuron disease. J Neurol Neurosurg Psychiatry 1987;50:732–7.
44. Daube JR, editor. Motor unit estimates in ALS. In: Physiology of ALS and related diseases. Amsterdam: Elsevier Science; 1997. p. 203–16.
45. Attarian S, Azulay JP, Lardillier D, et al. Transcranial magnetic stimulation in lower motor neuron diseases. Clin Neurophysiol 2005;116:35–42.
46. Triggs WJ, Menkes D, Onorato J, et al. Transcranial magnetic stimulation identifies upper motor neuron involvement in motor neuron disease. Neurology 1999;53:605–11.
47. Kobayashi M, Pascual Leone A. Transcranial magnetic stimulation in neurology. Lancet Neurol 2003;2:145–56.
48. Rossini PM, Rossi S. Transcranial magnetic stimulation: diagnostic, therapeutic and research potential. Neurology 2007;68:484–8.
49. Ziemann U, Winter M, Reimers CD, et al. Impaired motor cortex inhibition in patients with amyotrophic lateral sclerosis: evidence from paired transcranial magnetic stimulation. Neurology 1997;49:1292–8.
50. Vucic S, Cheah BC, Yiannikas C, et al. Cortical excitability distinguishes ALS form mimic disorders. Clin Neurophysiol 2011;122(9):1860–6.
51. Vucic S, Cheah B, Kiernan M. Defining the mechanisms that underlie cortical hyperexcitability in amyotrophic lateral sclerosis. Exp Neurol 2009;220:177–82.
52. Shefner J. Excitability testing in clinical neurophysiology: what, why and when? Muscle Nerve 2001;24(7):845–7.
53. Bostock H, Sharief MK, Reid G. Brain 1995;119(Pt 1):217–25.
54. Vucic S, Kiernan MC. Axonal excitability properties in amyotrophic lateral sclerosis. Clin Neurophysiol 2006;117(7):1458–66.
55. Kanai K, Shibuya K, Sato Y, et al. Motor axonal excitability properties are strong predictors for survival in amyotrophic lateral sclerosis. J Neurol Neurosurg Psychiatry 2012;83:734–8.

An Electrodiagnostic Approach to the Evaluation of Peripheral Neuropathies

Mark B. Bromberg, MD, PhD

KEYWORDS

- Peripheral neuropathy • Diagnosis of peripheral neuropathies
- Nerve conduction studies • EMG studies

KEY POINTS

- A planned approach to electrodiagnostic testing provides the most information.
- Electrodiagnostic testing is highly sensitive for defining the pattern and degree of nerve involvement.
- Electrodiagnosis can provide information on the chronicity of a neuropathy.
- Electrodiagnostic testing can provide insight into the underlying pathophysiology, defining the neuropathy as either primary axonal or primary demyelinating.

INTRODUCTION

In the clinical setting of a suspected peripheral neuropathy, the history and neurologic examination provide information about general features but cannot define the nature of the pathologic changes and the clinical features may underrepresent the distribution of nerve involvement or time course. Electrodiagnostic tests allow for a more detailed characterization of a neuropathy.[1] Electrodiagnostic tests include nerve conduction and needle electromyographic (EMG) studies. Reliable interpretation of the data assumes recognition of potential technical issues and overall must be within the context of the clinical information.[2,3] A systematic electrodiagnostic approach is based on an understanding of basic nerve anatomy and physiology and how pathologic changes affect electrodiagnostic data, and this foundation will be reviewed. Electrodiagnostic findings in prototypic axonal and demyelinating neuropathies are presented. These principles are put together as a diagnostic strategy to aid in planning informative tests and interpreting outside studies.

Disclosure: The author has no financial interest in any company or product that is related to the content of this article.
Department of Neurology, University of Utah, 175 North Medical Drive, Salt Lake City, UT 84132, USA
E-mail address: mbromberg@hsc.utah.edu

Phys Med Rehabil Clin N Am 24 (2013) 153–168
http://dx.doi.org/10.1016/j.pmr.2012.08.020
1047-9651/13/$ – see front matter © 2013 Published by Elsevier Inc.

PERIPHERAL NERVE ANATOMY

A nerve consists of individual nerve fibers of different types bundled together and can be divided along several lines: somatic and autonomic fibers, motor and sensory fibers, large and small fibers. Each fiber consists of an axon insulated by segments of myelin, which is thick and tightly wrapped for large myelinated fibers and thin and loosely wrapped for small unmyelinated fibers. The functional and electrodiagnostic implications of different nerve fiber diameters and their degree of myelination is varied in nerve fiber conduction velocities. Myelinated fibers have faster velocities as a result of saltatory conduction (30–60 m/s), whereas unmyelinated fibers conduct relatively slowly (<1 m/s). Routine nerve conduction studies assess exclusively larger myelinated nerve fibers, as the contributions from smaller myelinated and unmyelinated fibers to the recorded signal are by comparison minimal. Special tests can assess these fibers but are not commonly performed and rarely help with characterization of common neuropathies.

Named (large) peripheral nerves contain all fiber types (large and small fiber somatic, autonomic, and motor and sensory nerves) before branching in the end organs, where somatic motor and sensory nerves separate and are accessible for study. Sensory nerves contain 3000 to 6000 fibers. Motor nerves frequently innervate a group of muscles, such as the thenar or hypothenar groups, and 100 to 300 motor nerve fibers innervate muscle(s) in the groups. However, each motor axon branches into 500 to 800 terminal branches within a muscle and each branch innervates a muscle fiber.

Another anatomic feature of motor nerves is the motor unit, which is the axon and its terminal branches. Terminal branches and the muscle fibers they innervate are distributed over a circular area within a muscle with a diameter of 5 to 10 mm. With more than 100 motor units innervating a muscle, the territories of approximately 20 motor units overlap at any given site in the muscle.

PRINCIPLES OF NERVE CONDUCTION PHYSIOLOGY

During nerve conduction studies, the entire nerve is electrically activated. Sensory and motor responses are recorded separately by the position of electrodes over sensory nerves or over muscles. The sensory response is recorded as the sensory nerve action potential (SNAP) and the motor response as the compound muscle action potential (CMAP). The SNAP represents the sum of single nerve fiber action potentials. The SNAP waveform shape is determined by the arrival times of nerve fiber action potentials, the duration of the action potentials, and the degree of phase cancellation.[4] Nerve fiber action potential waveforms are biphasic (negative-positive) with a duration of approximately 1 millisecond. Sensory nerves conduct over a range of approximately 25 m/s. The arrival of slower conducting nerve action potentials positions their negative peaks at the time of the positive portions of the faster conducting action potentials, resulting in significant phase cancellation and a lower SNAP amplitude than might be expected from the simple algebraic addition of the nerve fiber action potentials (**Fig. 1**). With greater conduction distances, the effect of phase cancellation is marked and the SNAP amplitude decreases greatly with longer conduction distances. The shape of the CMAP is affected by the same elements. However, motor nerves activate muscle fibers whose action potentials are approximately 6 milliseconds in duration. Further, motor nerves conduct over a smaller range of conduction velocities, approximately 15 m/s, and the slower arriving muscle fiber potentials are minimally affected by phase cancellation (see **Fig. 1**).[4] Accordingly, the CMAP amplitude is higher and decreases little with longer conduction distances.

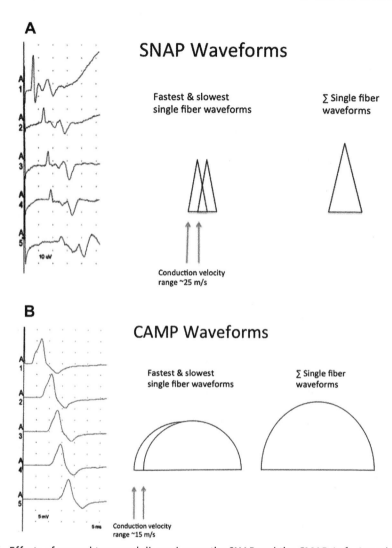

Fig. 1. Effects of normal temporal dispersion on the SNAP and the CMAP. *Left,* Actual wave-forms from ulnar nerve study (stimulating at the wrist, A1, and up the arm to Erb point, A5) are shown for sensory (*A*) and motor (*B*) nerve conduction. *Right,* Model of summation of action potentials. Sensory nerve action potentials have an approximately 1-millisecond-duration waveform and conduct over an approximately 25 m/s range, leading to marked phase cancellation and relative low amplitude when nerve fiber waveforms are summed in the SNAP. Muscle fiber action potentials have an approximately 6-millisecond-duration waveform and conduct over an approximately 15 m/s range, leading to much less phase cancellation and a relative high amplitude when muscle fiber waveforms are summed in the CMAP.

Another difference between sensory nerve fibers and muscle fibers is their diame-ters: sensory nerve fibers that contribute to the SNAP have diameters of 8 to 12 μm, whereas muscle fibers that contribute to the CMAP have diameters of 30 to 70 μm. The amplitudes of individual action potentials are proportional to the diameter of the fiber; SNAP amplitude (normal range) is 6 to 90 μV, whereas CMAP amplitude (normal range) is 2000 to 15,000 μV, or 2 to 15 mV.

Nerve stimulation is accomplished by passing current between anode and cathode electrodes (which are 3–4 cm apart) on the skin over the nerve. Current flows from the anode to the cathode with hyperpolarized beneath the anode and depolarization under the cathode (the site of impulse initiation). With sufficient current, all axons are activated to produce a maximal SNAP or CMAP response. The cathode must be placed closest to the recording site, for if the anode is placed closest, 2 situations occur. Because the distance between the electrodes is 3 to 4 cm, the intended measured distance between recording and stimulating electrodes will be approximately 3 to 4 cm greater, leading to artificially longer distal latencies or slowed conduction velocities. The other is the phenomenon of anodal block that can cause partial conduction block along the nerve caused by hyperpolarization of some axons under the anode, leading to artificially lower SNAP and CMAP amplitudes.

Nerve conduction studies yield 2 types of metrics: the amplitude of the evoked response and a set of timing measures (**Fig. 2**). SNAP and CMAP amplitudes are roughly proportional to the number of axons conducting between the stimulating and recording electrodes. With progressive axonal loss, both responses lose amplitude but the CMAP amplitude drops less than the SNAP amplitude because of the effects of collateral reinnervation of motor nerves (to be discussed later). Timing measures generally reflect activity of the fastest myelinated fibers and include distal latency (conduction over set distances), F-wave latency (conduction over twice the whole length of motor nerves), and conduction velocity (over segments of nerve). The duration of the CMAP waveform (negative peak duration) provides an estimate of the spectrum of more slowly conducting myelinated fibers.

Nerve fiber conduction velocity is slowed at lower temperatures in a linear manner. However, the effects of temperature are more apparent with sensory than with motor nerves. With lower nerve temperatures, sensory nerve action potentials are longer in duration, resulting in less phase cancellation and larger SNAP amplitudes. Although muscle fiber action potentials also lengthen in duration, the effect on CMAP amplitude is negligible. For both, the lower nerve temperature slows conduction, approximately 2 m/s/°C.[5] Correction factors can be applied when limb temperature is low, but the factors are approximate and diagnostic interpretation uncertainties can be avoided by warming limbs to approximately 31°C.

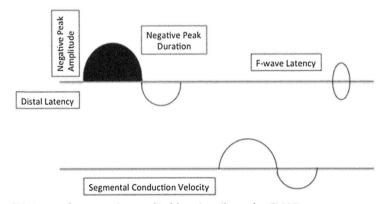

Fig. 2. CMAP waveform metrics, applicable primarily to the CMAP.

PRINCIPLES OF NEEDLE EMG

Needle EMG records electrical activity from muscle fibers to assess the integrity and architecture or arrangement within the muscle.[6] The electrical motor unit recorded by the EMG needle is called the motor unit action potential (MUAP) and represents only a portion of the anatomic motor unit, because the electrical uptake area of the electrode is less than 1 to 2 mm in diameter. Thus, the MUAP includes only about 7 to 15 fibers of an anatomic motor unit, for both concentric and monopolar electrodes. The MUAP waveform varies with slight needle movement based on the intimate proximity of the needle tip to 1 to 3 muscle fibers of the anatomic motor unit that contribute most to the waveform amplitude and shape.

The EMG study is performed in 2 stages. The first stage is assessment for the presence of abnormal spontaneous muscle fiber activity when the muscle is at rest, and the second is assessment of MUAPs during voluntary activation of the muscle. The presence of abnormal spontaneous activity is assessed at high EMG screen display sensitivity or gain, 20 to 50 μV per division. The presence of positive waves and fibrillation potentials indicates denervation and, in the context of a peripheral neuropathy, denervation from axonal loss (neurogenic denervation). Note that the waveform differences between positive waves and fibrillation potentials depend on the relationship between the electrode tip and the spontaneously active muscle fiber and thus are of equal clinical significance.[7] The presence of very low amplitude abnormal spontaneous activity, less than approximately 50 μV, suggests very long-standing and slowly progressive denervation.

There are about overlapping 20 motor units in the electrode's uptake area, and during voluntary muscle activation the number of active motor units increases from zero at rest toward the 20 with increasing effort. Of note, most routine EMG studies are performed at low levels of activation so that individual MUAPs can be observed. Accordingly, during low levels of activation, the electrode records from 3 to 5 MUAPs close to the needle. At low levels of muscle activation, the recruitment pattern of MUAPs can be assessed for MUAP discharge frequencies.[8] The EMG screen display sensitivity or gain is set at 200 μV per division and sweep speed at 10 milliseconds per division. If the screen has 10 horizontal divisions, the beam sweep time will be 10/s: thus, it is rare for a single MUAP to consistently discharge at 20 Hz (twice/sweep), and observation of several MUAPs discharging at rates greater than 20 Hz support motor unit loss. MUAP waveforms can be inspected for increased amplitude by determining if they exceed 2000 to 3000 μV, an approximate upper limit of normal for distal muscles. MUAP complexity in terms of polyphasia (>4 phases) or polyturn (>5 turns) can be assessed by a trigger and delay line, which permits individual MUAPs to be electronically captured and spread out.[8] It is to be noted that up to 10% of motor units can be polyphasic and excessive emphasis should not be placed on occasional complex motor units.

The goal of these observations is to estimate pathophysiologic changes. In the context of a neuropathy, abnormal spontaneous activity supports denervation of muscles. The remaining motor nerve fibers sprout collateral branches to reinnervate orphaned muscle fibers and the anatomic motor increases in muscle fiber density but not in area. Reinnervated muscle fibers no longer discharge spontaneously, but abnormal spontaneous activity usually persists for 2 reasons. There is subsequent ongoing denervation from the neuropathy and the degree of collateral reinnervation is limited, all of which leads to permanently orphaned (denervated) muscle fibers. With reinnervation, the increased density of the anatomic motor unit is reflected in larger and more complex MUAPs. In neuropathies that are progressing relatively rapidly, there will be ongoing denervation, marked by abnormal spontaneous activity, mildly decreased recruitment, and complex MUAPs. In very slowly progressive neuropathies, there is sufficient time for maximal reinnervation; positive waves and fibrillation potentials from permanently orphaned muscle fibers will be of very low amplitude; and the motor units will be few in number and of very high amplitude, but not complex, because there has been sufficient time for polyphasia and polyturns to simplify. Thus, when MUAPs are observed whose amplitudes are 5 to 10 times normal (10,000–20,000 mV), consideration should be given for a hereditary neuropathy, the most slowly developing form of neuropathy. The extent of denervation (distal-proximal gradient) can be assessed by identifying the most proximal muscle with abnormal needle EMG findings.

LIMITS OF NORMAL

As with most biologic data, "normal limits" are derived from distributions of values from subjects who have no apparent disease. The pool of subjects should include a wide spectrum of ages and body sizes (height). How limits of normal are set is controversial, but most laboratories use upper and lower limits (ULN of distal latency and F-wave latency, LLN for amplitude and conduction velocity) set at 2 to 3 SDs, but data for the different nerve conduction metrics may not be normally distributed and other limits such as confidence intervals may be more appropriate.[9] Although it is preferable for each laboratory to gather its own normal data, this is rarely done, and most limits are handed down. An obscure origin of a laboratory's normal values seems unscientific, but values are generally similar. Some metrics are influenced by body habitus and, although difficult to take into account precisely, should be part of the general considerations. Thin fingers in women can result in very high amplitude digital SNAP amplitudes, and vice versa for thick fingers. Conduction velocities can be reduced and F-wave latencies in particular can be long in very tall individuals, and vice versa in very short patients. Thus, ULN and LLN should be viewed as references and not absolute values and should be interpreted in the overall clinical context. Nerve conduction metrics in the elderly are especially challenging, and although good sural responses can be obtained in the very elderly, absent responses may not be abnormal.[10]

ELECTRODIAGNOSTIC MANIFESTATIONS OF NEUROPATHY

Nerve conduction tests help in distinguishing 3 basic conditions of peripheral nerves. The first state is normal conduction, seen when most nerve fibers and axons are intact. The second situation is axonal injury, seen when the primary injury occurs to axons. The third case is loss of myelin, seen with demyelination, which generally occurs at multiple focal sites along a nerve. This causes variation in nerve action potential propagation resulting in slowing of conduction velocities or slowing to zero (conduction block). Slowed conduction velocity causes abnormal dispersion of arrival times of nerve action potentials at the recording electrode (abnormal temporal dispersion). Of note, there can be mixed patterns with primary demyelination and secondary axonal loss. Finally, there may be slowed conduction from reversible metabolic causes with no obvious damage to myelin.

Normal Conduction

SNAP and CMAP waveforms are influenced by normal temporal dispersion: SNAP amplitude decreases markedly over greater distances, whereas CMAP amplitude decreases minimally and the CMAP negative peak duration increases only minimally (see **Fig. 1**; **Fig. 3**). Normal conduction is defined as values within the laboratory limits of normal. Distal latency, F-wave latency and conduction velocity are influenced by limb length and limb temperature.

Axonal Injury

Loss of axons disconnects fibers from their receptors (sensory nerves) or muscles (motor nerves). Not all fibers may be affected, and the remaining unaffected fibers conduct normally, or all fibers may be affected in severe neuropathies. Generally, axonal loss occurs at the distal ends of fibers, a process called "axonal dying-back." This results in reductions in both SNAP and CMAP amplitudes. The SNAP amplitude is especially sensitive to axon loss because of the lack of compensatory collateral reinnervation. Essentially, there is a linear relationship between the number of axons lost and the amplitude of the SNAP, and with loss of greater than 50% of axons, the amplitude may be unrecordable. The CMAP amplitude, in contrast, is less sensitive to early axonal injury because of the supportive effects of collateral rein-nervation. With mild denervation, collateral reinnervation preserves the number of innervated muscle fibers and the CMAP amplitude remains high, but with either further axonal loss or a very rapid rate of loss, greater numbers of muscle fibers remain dener-vated and the CMAP amplitude decreases. The effects of collateral sprouting can, in some cases, maintain CMAP amplitude at greater than the LLN until greater than 80%

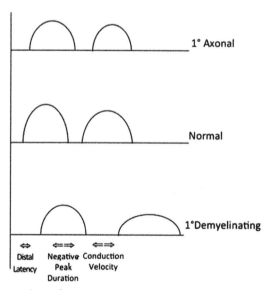

Fig. 3. Stylized comparisons between motor nerve conduction findings in normal and primarily axon and primarily demyelinating neuropathies. Differences in CMAP between waveforms are noted when stimulating at distal and proximal sites (P:D amplitude ratio). Normal: a short distal latency and short latency from proximal stimulation site yield a normal conduction velocity. Normal temporal dispersion results in a very small reduction in CMAP amplitude to proximal stimulation (normal ratio). Primary axonal loss: the distal latency and latency from a proximal stimulation site are only slightly longer than normal because of the loss of rapidly conducting fibers with a normal P:D amplitude ratio. Primary demye-lination: the distal latency is prolonged and the conduction velocity is slowed. The P:D amplitude ratio is low because of phase cancellation.

of axons are lost. When the CMAP is within normal limits, the needle EMG can detect the effects of motor unit enlargement and verify that axonal loss has occurred.

With axonal loss, each remaining nerve fiber conducts at its innate speed. Thus, measures of timing (distal latency, F-wave latency, and conduction velocity) are reduced only to the extent of loss of large axons (see **Fig. 3**). The limits of slowing in axonal neuropathy can be empirically assessed by reviewing data from patients with amyotrophic lateral sclerosis (ALS), a disorder characterized by reduced numbers of axons with no predilection to axon size: distal latency and F-wave latency are rarely longer than 125% of the ULN, and conduction velocity is rarely slower than 75% of the LLN.[11] Temporal dispersion, as measured by negative CMAP peak duration, is largely unaffected in axonal neuropathies. Overall, with moderate to major axonal loss, the SNAP response will be absent and thus provide no information about conduction velocity.

Demyelination

Damage to myelin affects nerve conduction at multiple sites along nerve fibers and nerve roots, resulting in varying degrees of slowed conduction in affected fibers. Thus, distal latency and F-wave latency are prolonged, and conduction velocity is slowed. The increased variability of nerve fiber conduction velocities results in greater degrees of phase cancellation within the SNAP and CMAP waveforms, causing low-amplitude responses (see **Fig. 3**). The sites of demyelination are generally not uniformly distributed along the length of a nerve, and thus the effects of multifocal demyelination can best be demonstrated by measurements over longer nerve conduction distances. Abnormal temporal dispersion (and secondary axonal loss) can markedly reduce SNAP amplitude, frequently to zero, and thus motor responses are more robust and more commonly used to assess conduction velocity and abnormal temporal dispersion. Conduction of individual nerve fibers may be infinitely slowed (conduction block), which can contribute to the reduction in the response amplitude. The degree of temporal dispersion can be measured in the CMAP wave-form by the ratio of the amplitude or area of the proximal to the distal response (P:D ratio); however, the P:D ratio can also be affected by conduction block of axons between the 2 stimulation sites (**Fig. 4**). A more direct measure of temporal dispersion is the CMAP negative peak duration value, comparing values from the proximal to the

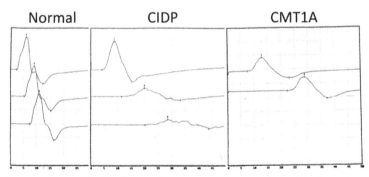

Fig. 4. Changes in actual CMAP waveforms comparing normal with slowed conduction velocities (20 m/s), highlighting differences between acquired primary demyelinating neuropathy (eg, CIDP) and hereditary neuropathy (eg, Charcot-Marie-Tooth type 1). Wave-forms in CIDP show effects of abnormal temporal dispersion, whereas in Charcot-Marie-Tooth, the waveforms show effects of uniform slowing and normal temporal dispersion.

distal response; normally, the negative peak duration increases by less than 10% even over long distances (CMAP from Erb point stimulation compared with wrist stimulation; see **Figs. 1** and **4**).

There is one neuropathy that is an exception with slowed conduction velocity without abnormal temporal dispersion. In Charcot-Marie-Tooth type 1, the CMAP amplitude does not markedly decrease between distal and proximal stimulation sites (see **Fig. 4**). This is because of uniform changes to myelin along nerve fibers. Conduction can also be mildly slowed by metabolic causes that do not affect myelin structurally, and diabetic neuropathies frequently show this pattern.

There have been many efforts to design sets of nerve conduction criteria that can distinguish between primary axonal and primary demyelination in terms of the degree of slowing. The degree of demyelination in such neuropathies is variable: when mild, there will be only small prolongations in distal and F-wave latency and slowing of conduction velocity that may be within (or just beyond) normal limits. When demyelination is more marked, there will be slowing greater than expected for the degree of axonal loss, and the amount of slowing can be referred back to timing values from patients with ALS.[11] The published criteria are complex to apply, and a more simple set of guidelines, based on the degree of slowing in ALS, is given in **Table 1**.[12] These guidelines are not intended to be strict or exclusive but to assist deciding whether there is a demyelinating component in a neuropathy.

Focal Conduction Block

Conduction block refers to blockage of a large number of axons over a short segment of nerve. Focal conduction block occurs most frequently at sites of entrapment (median nerve at the wrist, carpal tunnel syndrome; ulnar nerve at the elbow, tardy ulnar palsy; peroneal nerve at the knee) resulting in mononeuropathies. In the context of peripheral neuropathies, focal conduction block is sought at sites unaffected by entrapment. The pathologic condition may represent focal demyelination (or alteration to myelin at the node of Ranvier) or block by other mechanisms such as alteration or block of membrane ion channels.[13,14] Focal conduction block can be demonstrated by showing loss of CMAP amplitude across the site of block and normal amplitudes along nerve segments above and below the site. The blocking mechanism can be very specific with block only of motor axons with sensory axons

Table 1
Electrodiagnostic guidelines that can be applied to help identify primary demyelination show greater slowing than expected for the degree of axonal loss for motor nerves

Distal latency	>125% of ULN
Conduction velocity	<70% of LLN
F-wave latency	>125% of ULN
CMAP negative peak duration (measured at return to baseline of last negative peak)	Median >6.6 ms Ulnar >6.7 ms Peroneal >7.6 ms Tibial >8.8 ms
P:D CMAP negative peak duration ratio	>0.3

Recording 2 or more values beyond limits raises the question of a primary demyelinating neuropathy. Limits of slowing based on data from patients with pure axonal neuropathy (ALS).

Modified from Bromberg MB. Review of the evolution of electrodiagnostic criteria for chronic inflammatory demyelinating polyradicoloneuropathy. Muscle Nerve 2011;43(6):780–94.

unaffected (multifocal motor neuropathy with conduction block)[15] or with block of both motor and sensory fibers (Lewis-Sumner syndrome).[16] Although the electrodiagnostic hallmark of conduction block is reduction in the CMAP amplitude or area across the site of block, the effects of abnormal temporal dispersion can also produce CMAP amplitude reductions as a result of increased phase cancellation that may be misinterpreted as conduction block. Pure focal conduction block has been defined as a greater than 50% reduction of CMAP area (area is less affected by abnormal temporal dispersion than is amplitude) across the site of block without an increase in negative peak CMAP duration (<20%).[17]

DESIGNING AN ELECTRODIAGNOSTIC STUDY

Patients may be initially seen in a clinic, where a detailed history is obtained and a neurologic examination is performed. However, patients are frequently referred to the EMG laboratory for electrodiagnostic tests only. Under these circumstances, a brief and focused history and examination are required to properly design and interpret the studies.[3]

Patient History

A pertinent history and examination allow for a rational selection of electrodiagnostic tests.[18] Referrals may be for complaints that do not accurately represent the true clinical issue. Important topics to review and specific points to clarify include (1) time course: acute, chronic, or insidious; (2) symptoms: sensory (including numbness or pain) or motor (including cramps, fasciculations, or weakness); (3) distribution: distal legs, distal and proximal limbs, or single nerve; (4) medical history: such as diabetes or collagen vascular diseases; (5) family history: family members with neuropathy, high arches, or hammertoes; and (6) medications: neurotoxic chemotherapeutic drugs or others. A focused neurologic examination should confirm the clinical suspicion for the presence and distribution of sensory loss and weakness. Tendon reflexes are helpful because they are usually absent, at least distally (Achilles reflex), in axonal neuropathies and more diffusely absent or reduced in demyelinating neuropathies.

Study Design

At the conclusion of the clinical evaluation, there should be a good notion of the nature of the neuropathy. The electrodiagnostic study should be designed to confirm what is expected from the history and answer questions that may not be evident from the history and examination. Specific issues include (1) type of nerves involved (motor, sensory, or both); (2) degree of involvement (mild, moderate, or severe); (3) anatomy (which nerves are involved); (4) underlying pathologic conditions (axonal, demyelinating, or both); and (5) time course (acute, ongoing, or slowly progressive).

It is argued here that there is benefit to designing an electrodiagnostic study test by test for each patient, as opposed to applying a predetermined study protocol. With the former approach, data from each nerve or muscle should be predicted. If the predicted result is confirmed, the process of confirming the clinical diagnosis is proceeding on course. If there is an unexpected result, a technical error is sought or the clinical diagnosis is questioned and reviewed. With the latter approach, data are reviewed at the end of the study. As such, it may be hard to make clinical sense of disparate findings, and technical errors may escape detection at a time when they could be corrected.

Study Strategies

Sensory nerve conduction

Assess the most distal sensory nerve first, usually the sural or superficial peroneal nerve. Most peripheral neuropathies have a greater effect on sensory than motor nerves and distal than proximal nerves. If the response is absent, to exclude a technical cause, study the contralateral nerve. This will document symmetry, although the history and examination will support symmetry clinically without the need to document symmetry electrodiagnostically for every nerve. If sensory responses are absent in the legs, a sensory nerve in the arm should be assessed for the overall extent (distribution) of axonal loss, and it is reasonable to chose the ulnar instead of the median sensory nerve, because it will not be affected by common focal conduction abnormalities at the wrist.

Motor nerve conduction

Assess the longest motor nerve next, usually the peroneal motor recording from the extensor digitorum brevis, before the tibial nerve; the tibial nerve is less informative because the amplitude is normally relatively large and small reductions resulting from axonal loss will not be detected. If motor responses are absent in the legs, motor nerves in the arms should be studied, and when a primary demyelinating neuropathy is suspected, the ulnar nerves should be tested with stimulation up to the axilla. Motor nerves will provide information about primary axonal versus primary demyelinating neuropathies by inspection of the distal latencies, F-wave latencies, and conduction velocities and the presence of abnormal temporal dispersion. The amplitude of the tibial response stimulating at the knee usually shows a marked loss of amplitude, and the P:D amplitude ratio from this nerve is not a reliable measure of abnormal temporal dispersion or conduction block. The F-wave response should be assessed after 10 maximal stimuli for minimum latency. Response amplitudes and timing values should be compared for fulfillment of guidelines for primary demyelination (see **Table 1**) when suggested by the history and examination.

Needle EMG

The needle EMG study will provide information on the presence of subtle denervation, proximal extent, and chronicity. Assessing the anterior tibialis muscle is useful because it is usually affected to a mild degree and hence provides full information, whereas the extensor digitorum brevis muscle represents a very distal muscle that may be very atrophic. Assessment for abnormal spontaneous activity is to determine whether there is mild motor nerve axonal loss, especially when the CMAP is mildly reduced. Assessment of recruitment and MUAP amplitude and complexity is helpful to determine the time course: moderately reduced recruitment and moderately increased MUAP amplitude and complexity support ongoing denervation, whereas markedly reduced recruitment, markedly increased MUAP amplitude, but simple waveforms support a very longstanding neuropathy.

Electrodiagnostic Report Summary and Interpretation

The electrodiagnostic report should contain sufficient historical and examination features to provide a context for the interpretation.[3] A summary should not repeat in prose nerve conduction and EMG data tables but should present the salient points that will be used in the overall interpretation, in particular technical or physical issues that influence the data. The overall interpretation can include information from the history and examination and must make sense internally (data internally consistent with the conclusions) and clinically (consistent with examination findings, past medical and family histories, and laboratory findings). Overall, the interpretation can be most informative if the study is designed to answer questions formulated from the history and examination with assessment of each metric to determine consistency.

REVIEWING OUTSIDE ELECTRODIAGNOSTIC STUDIES

When reviewing an outside electrodiagnostic study, one should not rely on the interpretation but instead review the data and make your own conclusions and then compare the 2 interpretations. It must be kept in mind that there may be technical issues not recognized and inappropriate interpretations and numbers, and waveforms should be reviewed when provided. In reading the nerve conduction and EMG data tables, it is most efficient and informative if one reads the study as if one were performing the study; that is, look at the data in the order suggested earlier (steps 1–3).

CLINICAL AND ELECTRODIAGNOSTIC FEATURES OF PROTOTYPIC NEUROPATHIES
Primary Axonal Neuropathies

This represents the most common group of polyneuropathies (**Fig. 5**). Axonal neuropathies are typically slowly progressive but also may have an insidious onset that suggests a hereditary neuropathy. The distribution of axonal loss is length dependent with longest nerves affected first and progression to shorter nerves over time.[19] Clinically, patients describe either a loss of function with reduced or loss of sensory perception and poor balance or positive symptoms with discomfort in the feet. Over time, these symptoms progress proximally as a stocking unrolls, and in the extreme can involve upper extremity sensation as a long glove unrolls, and occasionally in a shieldlike distribution across the abdomen. Foot muscle atrophy is evident in the thinness of the feet, and in hereditary forms, with elevation of the arch and hammering of the toes. Weakness of toe movements and ankle dorsiflexion may not be

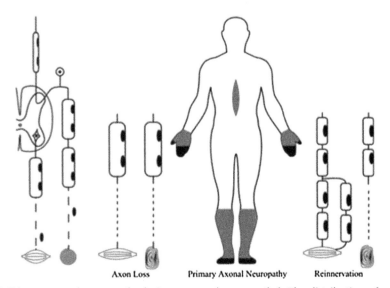

Axon Loss   Primary Axonal Neuropathy   Reinnervation

Fig. 5. Primary axonal neuropathy (primary axonal neuropathy). The distribution of sensory loss is demonstrated, with mild involvement in legs in stocking distribution loss, more severe involvement in legs and arms in stocking-glove distribution loss, and very severe involvement with shield distribution loss.

appreciated by the patient but can be confirmed on examination. Tendon reflexes are usually absent, at least at the ankle.

Electrodiagnostic findings are greatest in distal leg nerves and may not be evident early on in distal arm nerves.[20] SNAP amplitude is decreased earlier and to a greater degree than CMAP amplitude. Distal latency, F-wave latency and conduction velocity are mildly affected (see **Figs. 3** and **5**) and values are within 75% of the LLN or 125% of the ULN. Needle EMG will be more sensitive to mild degrees of denervation when the CMAP amplitude is within the LLN, and the greatest EMG changes will be in most distal muscles. In very chronic forms, such as hereditary neuropathies, there will be expected absent SNAP responses and absent or low amplitude CMAP responses indistinguishable from other causes, but the clue to chronicity will be in the EMG result, which will show markedly reduced motor unit recruitment with very large amplitudes but simple waveforms in distal muscles. Clinical and electrodiagnostic findings are usually symmetric in axonal neuropathies of any cause.

Primary Demyelinating Neuropathies

This group is less common but potentially treatable.[21] The distribution of demyelination is diffuse with multiple foci along nerves and nerve roots, and thus both distal and proximal nerves are affected clinically and electrically (**Fig. 6**). Clinically, patients describe numbness and tingling with a distal emphasis but also along the proximal portion of the limbs. Weakness also has a distal emphasis but can be demonstrated in proximal muscles. The time course can be rapid (within days), as in acute inflammatory demyelinating polyradiculoneuropathy (AIDP), or slow (over months), as in chronic inflammatory demyelinating polyradicoloneuropathy (CIDP). Tendon reflexes are usually uniformly absent, but at least absent in the legs.

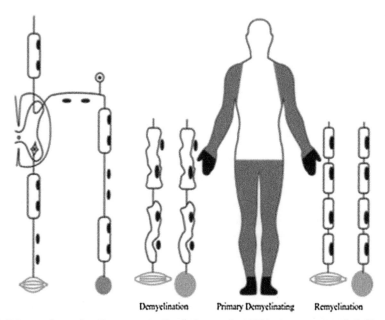

Demyelination   Primary Demyelinating   Remyelination

Fig. 6. Primary demyelinating neuropathy (primary demyelinating neuropathy). The distribution of sensory loss resulting from multifocal demyelination involving nerve and spinal root fibers is shown. Sensory loss involves both legs and arms, both distally and proximally, with distal predominance.

Electrodiagnostic findings are greatest when longer lengths of nerve are studied, and abnormalities are found in leg and arm nerves but more severely in leg nerves. SNAP amplitudes may be markedly reduced and frequently absent because of distal abnormal temporal dispersion and conduction block. CMAP amplitude is usually reduced to distal stimulation and may be markedly reduced to more proximal stimulation caused by multifocal demyelination and conduction block (see **Figs. 3** and **4**). Distal and F-wave latencies are prolonged and conduction velocities slowed. With relatively severe primary demyelinating neuropathies, these values will be markedly slowed, greater than seen in axonal neuropathies, but with more mild degrees of severity, values may overlap with the limits of primary axonal neuropathies.[12] This represents a challenge if electrodiagnostic criteria are not met. A practical approach is to consider the possibility of a demyelinating neuropathy when one or more nerves has values supporting slowing greater than expected for primary axonal neuropathy (see **Table 1**). This may result in false positive demyelinating neuropathies with erring on the side of a possibly treatable neuropathy.

Mixed Primary Axonal and Primary Demyelinating Neuropathies

Several neuropathies may contain a mixture of demyelination and axonal loss. When demyelination is the primary process, axonal loss occurs frequently as a secondary pathologic process. Thus, absent responses in more severe demyelinating neuropathies may be in part the result of secondary axonal loss. Most examples of primary demyelinating neuropathies, AIDP and CIDP, include varying degrees of secondary axonal loss, and responses can be absent in leg nerves. The needle EMG will help determine the degree of axonal loss with the presence of abnormal spontaneous activity and the degree of reduced MUAP recruitment and complexity. Diabetes and uremia are the most common causes of mixed axonal and demyelinating neuropathy, and findings are reduced SNAP and CMAP amplitudes, similar to findings in primary axonal neuropathies, but the slowing of conduction velocities is not as substantial as expected in a primarily demyelinating neuropathy.

Focal Conduction Bock Neuropathies

Multifocal motor neuropathy with conduction block is characterized by focal conduction block over short nerve segments away from entrapment sites and in a mononeuropathy multiplex pattern. There is a potential technical issue in identify this neuropathy in that there may be inadequate activation of axons at the proximal stimulation site leading to a falsely low CMAP response. There is a physiologic issue in that mild reductions in amplitude to proximal stimulation can occur from abnormal temporal dispersion leading to greater phase cancellation, mimicking conduction block. This can be assessed by considering the negative peak duration values: in conduction block, there will be a greater than 50% loss of CMAP amplitude with a less than 15% increase in negative peak duration.[17] In classic multifocal motor neuropathy, sensory conduction across the site is normal, but in the Lewis-Sumner syndrome, there is involvement of sensory nerves at sites of motor block.

SUMMARY

Electrodiagnostic testing follows from the history and is an extension of the neurologic examination. When clinical assessment implicates a peripheral neuropathy, the goal of electrodiagnostic testing is to more fully characterize the neuropathy in terms of the distribution (motor, sensory, symmetric, or asymmetric), extent of a neuropathy (symmetric, legs, or arms), and time course (very chronic or ongoing). Of greatest importance is that electrodiagnostic testing should help identify the type of underlying pathologic condition (primary axonal, primary demyelinating, or conduction block). Once this is accomplished, the differential diagnosis narrows and rational laboratory testing can be ordered or treatment trials initiated.[1]

REFERENCES

1. Donofrio P, Albers J. AAEM minimonograph #34: polyneuropathy: classification by nerve conduction studies and electromyography. Muscle Nerve 1990;13: 889–903.
2. Kimura J. Principles and pitfalls of nerve conduction studies. Ann Neurol 1984;16: 415–29.
3. Jablecki CK, Busis NA, Brandstater MA, et al. Reporting the results of needle EMG and nerve conduction studies: an educational report [Guideline]. Muscle Nerve 2005;32(5):682–5.
4. Kimura J, Machida M, Ishida T, et al. Relation between size of compound sensory or motor action potentials and length of nerve segment. Neurology 1986;36: 647–52.
5. Rutkove SB. Effects of temperature on neuromuscular electrophysiology [Review]. Muscle Nerve 2001;24(7):867–82.
6. Daube JR, Rubin DI. Needle electromyography. Muscle Nerve 2009;39(2): 244–70.
7. Dumitru D. Single muscle fiber discharges (insertional activity, end-plate potentials, positive sharp waves, and fibrillation potentials): a unifying proposal. Muscle Nerve 1996;19:221–6.
8. Bromberg M. Electromyographic (EMG) findings in denervation. Crit Rev Phys Rehabil Med 1993;5:83–127.
9. Robinson L, Temkin N, Fujimoto W, et al. Effects of statistical methodology on normal limits in nerve conduction studies. Muscle Nerve 1991;14:1084–90.
10. Benatar M, Wuu J, Peng L. Reference data for commonly used sensory and motor nerve conduction studies. Muscle Nerve 2009;40(5):772–94.
11. Cornblath D, Kuncl R, Mellits E, et al. Nerve conduction studies in amyotrophic lateral sclerosis. Muscle Nerve 1992;15:1111–5.
12. Bromberg MB. Review of the evolution of electrodiagnostic criteria for chronic inflammatory demyelinating polyradicoloneuropathy [Historical Article]. Muscle Nerve 2011;43(6):780–94.
13. Feasby TE, Brown WF, Gilbert JJ, et al. The pathological basis of conduction block in human neuropathies. J Neurol Neurosurg Psychiatry 1985;48(3):239–44.
14. Arasaki K, Kusunoki S, Kudo N, et al. Acute conduction block in vitro following exposure to antiganglioside sera. Muscle Nerve 1993;16(6):587–93.
15. Lange D, Trojaborg W, Latov N, et al. Multifocal motor neuropathy with conduction block: is it a distinct clinical entity? Neurology 1992;42:497–505.
16. Lewis R, Sumner A, Brown M, et al. Multifocal demyelinating neuropathy with persistent conduction block. Neurology 1982;32:958–64.
17. EFNS/PNSR1. European Federation of Neurological Societies/Peripheral Nerve Society Guideline on management of chronic inflammatory demyelinating polyradiculoneuropathy: report of a joint task force of the European Federation of Neurological Societies and the Peripheral Nerve Society–First Revision. J Peripher Nerv Syst 2010;15(1):1–9.
18. Bromberg MB. An approach to the evaluation of peripheral neuropathies. Semin Neurol 2005;25(2):153–9.

19. Sabin T. Classification of peripheral neuropathy: the long and the short of it. Muscle Nerve 1986;9:711–9.

20. Raynor EM, Ross MH, Shefner JM, et al. Differentiation between axonal and demyelinating neuropathies: identical segments recorded from proximal and distal muscles. Muscle Nerve 1995;18(4):402–8.

21. Albers J, Kelly J. Acquired inflammatory demyelinating polyneuropathies: clinical and electrodiagnostic features. Muscle Nerve 1989;12:435–51.

Electrodiagnosis of Disorders of Neuromuscular Transmission

James F. Howard Jr, MD

KEYWORDS

- Neuromuscular transmission • Myasthenia gravis • Lambert-Eaton syndrome
- MuSK • Repetitive nerve stimulation • Single fiber EMG • EMG • RNS

KEY POINTS

- Conventional needle electrode electromyographic (EMG) examinations are necessary in patients suspected of having myasthenia gravis (MG) to exclude diseases that may mimic or coexist with MG such as peripheral neuropathy and inflammatory or ocular myopathies.
- The lack of attention to temperature requirements in repetitive nerve stimulation testing is the most common error made, rendering the study unhelpful. This is most important when considering presynaptic disorders of neuromuscular transmission.
- There is no one muscle that will be more abnormal in every patient with MG in single-fiber EMG. The muscle(s) to be tested must be selected based on the distribution of weakness in the individual patient.
- Single-fiber EMG provides the most useful information particularly when repetitive nerve stimulation studies are normal and is most always abnormal when there is careful selection of involved muscles including those of the paraspinal region.
- Normal jitter in a clinically weak muscle indicates the weakness is not caused by an abnormality of neuromuscular transmission.

INTRODUCTION

The roles of electrodiagnosis in disorders of neuromuscular transmission are to confirm or reject one's clinical impression regarding the presence or absence of a disorder of neuromuscular transmission (NMT), to determine whether the disorder is either presynaptic or postsynaptic, to exclude other coexisting neuromuscular disorders, and to monitor the disease course in response to its natural history or to treatment.

Funding Sources: National Institutes of Health (National Institute of Neurological Disorders and Stroke, National Institute of Arthritis and Musculoskeletal and Skin Diseases), Cytokinetics Inc, Alexion Pharmaceuticals Inc.
Conflicts of Interest: Consultant to Alexion Pharmaceuticals Inc. Member, Board of Directors of American Board of Electrodiagnostic Medicine. Member, Medical/Scientific Advisory Board of the Myasthenia Gravis Foundation of America.

Neuromuscular Disorders Section, Department of Neurology, The University of North Carolina at Chapel Hill, CB #7025, 2200 Physician Office Building, 170 Manning Drive, Chapel Hill, NC 27599-7025, USA
E-mail address: howardj@neurology.unc.edu

Phys Med Rehabil Clin N Am 24 (2013) 169–192
http://dx.doi.org/10.1016/j.pmr.2012.08.013
1047-9651/13/$ – see front matter © 2013 Elsevier Inc. All rights reserved.

Careful clinical and electrodiagnostic evaluation and sometimes genetic, morphologic, and in vitro microphysiologic studies are necessary to achieve an accurate diagnosis. The electrodiagnostic approach is similar to that of any neuromuscular disorder.

The basis of the clinical electrodiagnostic abnormalities in patients with disorders of NMT (eg, myasthenia gravis [MG], Lambert-Eaton syndrome [LES]) is the failure of the muscle fiber to depolarize sufficiently for the end-plate potential (EPP) to reach action potential (AP) threshold (**Fig. 1**). The resulting impulse blocking accounts for the decremental responses seen on repetitive nerve stimulation (RNS) studies and the impulse blocking seen with single-fiber electromyography (SFEMG). In addition, the time variability of when the EPP reaches AP threshold accounts for the neuromuscular jitter seen in the latter technique. This article will review those electrodiagnostic techniques that are commonly used today and will highlight their specificity, sensitivity, and pitfalls.

NERVE CONDUCTION STUDIES

Standard neurographic studies should be performed on all patients suspected of having disease of the neuromuscular junction (NMJ). Conduction velocities, distal latencies, and late responses are typically normal in these patients. Compound muscle AP (CMAP) amplitude or negative peak area to a single stimulus will be

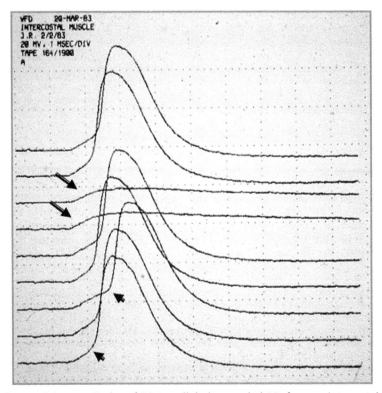

Fig. 1. Sequential raster display of 9 intracellularly recorded APs from an intercostal muscle biopsy specimen from a patient with MG demonstrating neuromuscular jitter and impulse blocking. Note the variation in rise-to-peak of the EPP and the relationship to neuromuscular jitter (*short arrows*). Impulse blocking occurs (traces 3 and 4, *long arrow*) when the EPP fails to reach critical threshold to generate an AP. (*Copyright* JF Howard Jr.)

preserved in postsynaptic disorders (unless the disease is very severe) and typically will be reduced in presynaptic disorders (eg, LES and botulism).

In some congenital myasthenic syndromes, such as the slow channel syndrome and congenital end-plate cholinesterase deficiency, and after exposure to drugs or toxins that inhibit acetylcholinesterase, a single nerve stimulation will evoke more than 1 CMAP response.[1] In this situation, the EPP is abnormally prolonged and remains higher than the AP threshold through the refractory period of the AP. In this situation, each consecutive response is smaller than the previous one and disappears once the EPP amplitude decreases to less than the AP threshold.

NEEDLE EMG

Conventional needle electrode EMG examinations are performed in patients suspected of having MG and other disorders of synaptic transmission to exclude diseases that may mimic or coexist with MG (and LES), such as peripheral neuropathy and inflammatory or ocular myopathies. In the absence of other neuromuscular disorders, the EMG examination will demonstrate, in both presynaptic and postsynaptic disorders of NMT, motor unit action potentials (MUAPs) that vary in configuration with consecutive discharges (**Fig. 2**). This pattern results from intermittent failure of synaptic transmission (impulse blocking) of some of the muscle fibers that comprise the MUAP and is most easily recognized as a variation in amplitude of an isolated MUAP if a slow oscilloscope sweep speed is used. This abnormality may be partially or completely reversed in patients with MG by the administration of edrophonium. This finding may be confused with the abnormality seen in reinnervation in which motor unit instability occurs as a result of immature NMJs. However, patients with reinnervation will have large, prolonged MUAPs. In LES and, to a lesser extent, in botulism, one may see a progressive increase in the EMG envelope amplitude during sustained contraction, as a result of the facilitated release of acetylcholine (ACh) from the nerve terminal.

In rare situations, usually in patients with acute and severe MG, one may find fibrillation potentials, especially in the paraspinal muscles.[2] They may also be seen in patients with severe LES, botulism, and congenital myasthenic syndromes caused by plectin deficiency.[3–5] Their presence, however, should suggest to the electromyographer that there may be an associated disfigurative process. The interference pattern in patients with MG is typically full, although with sustained contraction one may see a reduction in the envelope amplitude as the muscle fatigues and impulse blocking occurs.

Needle EMG is most important in suspected cases of MG associated with antibodies to muscle-specific protein kinase (MuSK), in which MUAP changes (both myopathic and neuropathic) will be recorded in clinically affected muscles, particularly

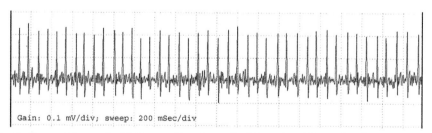

Gain: 0.1 mV/div; sweep: 200 mSec/div

Fig. 2. Concentric needle EMG recordings from the biceps brachii muscle of a patient with MG. Note the marked variation in MUAP amplitude with consecutive discharges caused by intermittent failure of NMT at end-plates within the motor unit. Calibration, 0.1 mV and 200 microseconds per division. (*Copyright* JF Howard Jr.)

those with atrophy.[6,7] Importantly, patients presenting with isolated neck extensor disease or respiratory failure may have normal electrodiagnostic studies in the limbs. It is therefore important that clinically affected muscles be examined to avoid missing the pertinent abnormalities of this disease.

RNS STUDIES

Repetitive motor nerve stimulation has application to a wide variety of clinical disorders that affect the NMJ and is the most frequently used electrodiagnostic test of NMT. Abnormal results from RNS studies are not diagnostic of specific clinical disorders, and abnormalities may be detected in patients with multiple sclerosis, motor neuron disease, peripheral neuropathy, radiculopathy, or primary muscle membrane disease, in addition to patients with primary disorders of the NMJ such as MG, LES, arthropod envenomation, botulism, congenital myasthenic syndromes, and impaired NMT caused by certain commonly used medications (eg, antibiotics) and toxins (eg, organophosphates).[8–20]

General Principles

The technique of RNS is similar to that used in conventional neurographic studies, differing only in the application of stimuli trains or paired stimuli, the use of conditioning exercise, and the careful immobilization of the limb to reduce movement artifact (**Table 1**). The methodology of RNS studies consists of stimulating the peripheral nerve with a supramaximal stimulus (25%–50% greater than the maximum stimulation intensity necessary to activate all the nerve fibers) and recording the CMAP response with an active surface electrode (E1) over the belly of the muscle and a referential electrode (E2) over the tendon of the same muscle. The negative peak amplitude and area of the CMAP response are reflections of the numbers of muscle fibers activated by the nerve stimulus; hence, it is a marker of synaptic efficacy. It is important that measurements of amplitude and area are concordant; a discrepancy implies a technical

Table 1
Comparative features with RNS in presynaptic and postsynaptic disorders

Defect Location	Stimulation Train	Stimulation Frequency	Findings	Exercise Duration	Expected Findings
Presynaptic	5–10 stimuli	2–5 Hz	>10% decrement, reduced CMAP amplitude	10 sec	PAF >100% immediately after exercise
	Stimulation for 5–10 sec	20–50 Hz	>100% increase in intratrain CMAP amplitude	...	...
Postsynaptic	5–10 stimuli	2–5 Hz	>10% decrement, normal CMAP amplitude	30–60 sec / 10 sec	PAE at 3–4 min after exercise / Repair of decrement immediately after exercise

Abbreviations: PAE, postactivation exhaustion; PAF, postactivation facilitation.

problem. Negative peak area should not be used to assess facilitation as some authors have suggested, because there are many technical factors (eg, variable phase cancellation, repolarization, muscle fiber fatigue, and filter settings) that will impede quality recordings.[21]

Supramaximal stimulation must be used because failure to do so will result in a false-positive study because of pseudodecrement. Decrement is defined as the percent change comparing the negative peak amplitude or area between the fifth (or fourth or lowest potential) and the first potential. It can be calculated from the formula[22–24]:

$$\% \; Decrement_n \; = \; [1 \; - \; (Potential_n/Potential_1)] \; \times \; 100\%$$

Facilitatory responses are calculated by the formula:

$$\% \; Facilitation_n \; = \; [(Potential_n/Potential_1)] \; - 1 \; \times \; 100\%$$

where n is the potential number to which the first potential is compared.

The criteria for abnormality will vary to some degree among laboratories.[23] Most electromyographers will accept a decrement greater than 10% or a facilitatory response greater than 100% of the initial CMAP response, although the latter is now being reconsidered.[25]

Muscle Selection

Ideally, one would like to test muscles that are involved clinically, although this is sometimes difficult. Larger muscles are, as a group, more difficult to immobilize and therefore are subject to movement artifact from displacement of either the stimulating or recording electrodes. Smaller muscles, such as those in the hand, are easy to immobilize but often are not involved clinically and most often will not show an abnormality unless the muscle is quite weak. The heterogeneous literature of RNS testing precludes drawing specific estimates of sensitivity and specificity and the literature must be interpreted with caution. However, generalizations can be made that will assist the electromyographer in developing a diagnostic strategy.

The abductor digiti quinti muscle is easily examined and is easily immobilized. Studies in this muscle are well tolerated by patients. The abductor pollicis brevis muscle is more difficult to immobilize because of the large moment of movement caused by thenar contraction. Stimulation of deep nerves requires high stimulus intensity, which may be uncomfortable to the patient and not tolerated well. One can reduce the stimulus-induced discomfort by using monopolar needle stimulation electrodes (eg, musculocutaneous nerve stimulation with biceps brachii recording). These techniques often produce movement artifact when large muscles are examined. Stimulation of the brachial plexus will often elicit contraction of several muscles, inducing movement artifact into the recording. Selective stimulation of the accessory nerve with recording over the upper trapezius muscle is often well tolerated and easy to perform, requires low stimulus intensity, and is an excellent choice for a proximal muscle.[14,26] This study may be performed with the patient either sitting or lying. Facial muscles (nasalis, orbicularis oculi) studies may tend to be uncomfortable for the patient but offer the advantage of a higher diagnostic yield for bulbar and perhaps ocular disease.[27–30] Most investigators begin their evaluation using a distal hand muscle, even though a greater proportion of patients with MG will have abnormalities in proximal muscles, because it allows the patient to experience the procedure with relative comfort. It would be quite unusual to have an abnormality in a distal limb muscle with a normal study in a more proximal location.[29]

There is a paucity of evidence-based literature regarding the sensitivity and specificity of RNS testing in the diagnosis of MG. There are insufficient data to correlate abnormalities of specific nerve–muscle combinations with the clinical severity of disease or the number of nerve–muscle combinations necessary to examine to achieve the highest diagnostic accuracy.[27] In general, the specificity of RNS is very high (~95%) in both ocular MG and generalized MG, whereas the sensitivity of RNS in ocular MG is less than 30% and approaches 80% in generalized MG when clinically affected muscles are examined.[27]

Immobilization

It is critically important to immobilize not only the muscle being examined but also the electrodes used to stimulate the nerve. Muscle and electrode movement artifacts are most often distinguishable by the abrupt change in waveform configuration during a train of stimuli. Failure to immobilize the tested muscle may also result in a pseudo-decremental response as a result of submaximal stimulation of the nerve.[31] Slower rates of stimulation are less likely to cause movement artifact because the muscle will return to its relaxation state before the next contraction. Faster rates of stimulation are more likely to produce movement artifact, primarily because the discomfort causes the patient to contract the muscle. Tetanic stimulation, in addition to the induced discomfort, may alter waveform configuration because of a change in the volume conduction through the muscle produced by change in its shape. Commercially made jigs to restrain movement may be quite useful, but in most instance proper attention to limb position and fixation of the limb by the examiner will suffice for the stimulation rates used in most laboratories. Often, the electromyographer only needs to gently hold the hand in place when recording from hand muscles or, when recording from the trapezius muscle, have the patient place their fingers under their hip when supine or to touch the bottom of the chair when sitting.

Temperature

Increased temperature is known to aggravate the strength of patients with MG, and control of intramuscular temperature is important in performing electrodiagnostic tests of NMT.[26,32] All patients undergoing RNS studies should have their extremities warmed to at least 32°C in the leg and to 34°C in the arm. Shoulder and facial muscles do not need warming in most situations. This may be accomplished by bathing the limb to be studied in a warm bath or using a heating lamp or a thermostatically controlled radiant warmer. Failure to warm the limb properly may result in a masking of the decremental response in patients with disorders of NMT because temperature changes of only a few degrees Celsius can reverse mild decrements (**Fig. 3**).[33,34] Presynaptic disorders may be misdiagnosed because the CMAP amplitude will be large and a facilitatory response masked if the muscle is cool (**Fig. 4**). The mechanism by which this occurs is not completely understood. Some authors postulate that it results from an increase in EPP amplitude and prolongation of EPP duration presumably as a result of alteration of the ionic channel conductance.[34] Others suggest that cooling potentiates NMT by enhancing transmitter packaging and presentation of neurotransmitter to the release site of the nerve terminal, by reducing the hydrolysis of ACh and by increasing ACh receptor sensitivity to ACh.[35–37]

Stimulation Rates

Typically, stimulation rates of 1, 2, 3, or 5 Hz are used. Desmedt found that stimulation rates between 3 Hz and 5 Hz are most likely to produce a decremental response in MG because of the depression in quantal release of ACh with a train of stimuli.[22] We and others have not found a difference between 2-Hz and 3-Hz stimulation.[38] Others think that decremental responses may be missed with stimulation rates less than 7 Hz.[39]

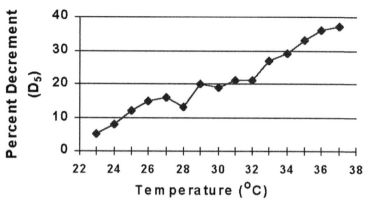

Fig. 3. Effects of temperature on percent decrement in MG. The change in percent decrement in a patient with generalized MG as the intramuscular temperature is changed from 23°C to 27°C. The percent decrement increases with increasing temperature. (*Copyright* JF Howard Jr.)

Stimulation rates in excess of 10 Hz frequently produce artifact and should be avoided except when high-frequency, short-duration stimulation is used to demonstrate the presence of a presynaptic disorder of NMT, such as LES. Excessively fast rates of stimulation or coexisting voluntary muscle contraction may produce an increase in CMAP amplitude with a reduction in the duration of the potential duration but no change in the negative peak area, a phenomenon termed pseudofacilitation. This results from an increase in the synchronization of the propagation velocity of the muscle fibers.[40] In normal individuals, there is no change in the CMAP amplitude with slow rates of stimulation and one may see a minimal increase (pseudofacilitation) of the CMAP amplitude at stimulus rates of 5 Hz or greater. At faster stimulus rates (40–50/sec), there is a mild facilitation of the CMAP amplitude within the first 10 stimuli and then a constant response (**Fig. 5**). Paired supramaximal stimulations with varying interstimulus intervals have been used in the past to assess NMT.[41] This technique is laborious and does not offer any advantages over RNS.

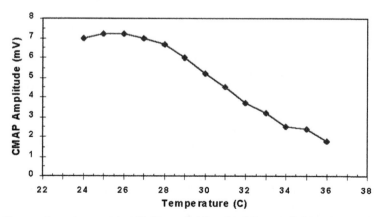

Fig. 4. Temperature response in LES. The reduction in abductor digiti quinti CMAP amplitude (7–2 mV) in a patient with LES as the intramuscular temperature is increased from 24°C to 26°C. Normal amplitude is greater than 4.5 mV. An abnormal response is not seen until the intramuscular temperature is 32°C. (*Copyright* JF Howard Jr.)

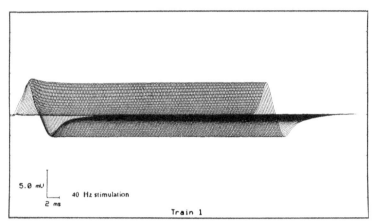

5.0 mV
40 Hz stimulation
2 ms
Train 1

Fig. 5. A train of 189 stimulations at 40 Hz in the abductor digiti quinti muscle in a normal subject. Note the normal initial CMAP amplitude (7.5 mV), the slight increase in amplitude within the first 10 stimuli (pseudofacilitation), and then a constant response. (*From* Howard JF, Sanders DB, Massey JM. The electrodiagnosis of myasthenia gravis and the lambert-eaton myasthenic syndrome. Neurol Clin 1994;12:305–30; with permission.)

Activation Techniques and Provocative Measures

The diagnostic yield of RNS may be increased through several activation techniques or other provocative measures. This is necessary because not all muscles will show the same degree of abnormality. However, these techniques are liable to artifact because many of them require limb movement, rapid rates of stimulation, or noxious procedures.

The most commonly used muscle activation procedure involves having the patient contract the muscle maximally for 10 to 60 seconds or by delivering a high-frequency train of stimuli. Such efforts produce an accumulation of calcium in the nerve terminal, which mobilizes the release of ACh. In a presynaptic disorder, this produces a marked increase in the CMAP amplitude. This phenomenon is termed postactivation facilitation or postexercise facilitation. Following maximum voluntary contraction or tetanic stimulation, there is a depression of end-plate excitability. This response is most often seen 2 to 4 minutes after exercise and is referred to as postactivation exhaustion or postexercise exhaustion. The electrophysiologic accompaniment of this phenomenon is a worsening of the decremental response compared with the preexercise values. In some individuals, particularly those with mild disease, an abnormal decrement may be seen only during the during the exhaustion stage.

Ischemia will enhance the neuromuscular block of presynaptic and postsynaptic disease. Harvey and Masland were the first to describe the effects of ischemia on NMT.[42] The "double-step" RNS test involves prolonged stimulation of a muscle in the hand before and after ischemia of the limb and has been proposed to increase the sensitivity of RNS.[41,43] In patients with MG, this test was found to be only slightly more sensitive than RNS of the trapezius muscle alone and only 60% as sensitive as SFEMG of a hand muscle.[41] The mechanism that accounts for the worsening decrement is not completely understood. Investigators postulate that ischemia depletes acetyl-coenzyme A, resulting in a failure of ACh synthesis, a depression of vesicle packaging, or vesicular recycling.[44] This technique is not in common use today given the increasing use of SFEMG.

Curare and similar neuromuscular blocking agents will impair synaptic transmission at the NMJ by producing a competitive, nondepolarizing neuromuscular block.[45] It is our belief that the use of curare should not be used in the diagnosis of MG given the sensitivity of SFEMG. The reader is cautioned that if curare is to be administered to patients with suspected neuromuscular disease, it should be done in a setting where there is appropriate critical care and respiratory support.

Quality Control in RNS Studies

As with other electrophysiologic techniques, the issue of quality control is paramount. The electromyographer must be able to review the actual waveform obtained in each train of stimuli to ensure that each is similar to the other. Electrode movement, submaximal stimulation, and muscle contraction will produce unique changes in waveform configuration that may be mistaken for either a decremental or incremental response (**Fig. 6**). The review of only a stick diagram will not give clues as to any alteration in the waveform, and the sole use of these diagrams must not be relied on for accurate assessment of the study. Acceptable decrements, or increments, are characterized by similar or gradual changes in CMAP amplitude or area with the greatest change occurring between the first and second potentials (**Fig. 7**). Decrements should be reproducible on repeated testing after appropriate rest periods. The lack of attention to temperature requirements in RNS testing is the most common error made

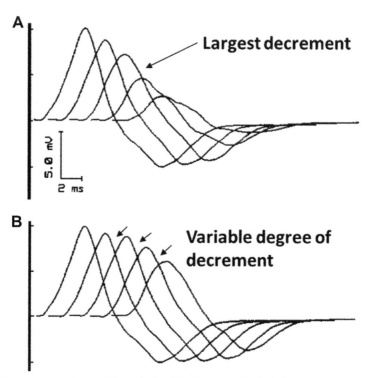

Fig. 6. Common waveform artifacts during RNS that are mistaken for a true abnormality. (*A*) The greatest change occurs between potentials 3 and 4 instead of between 1 and 2. (*B*) There is variable change between successive potentials and the typical envelope pattern is not seen (see **Fig. 7**). (*Copyright* JF Howard Jr.)

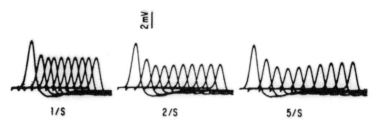

Fig. 7. Rate-dependent decremental responses in a patient with MG. Note that the greatest change always occurs between the first and second potentials, with subsequent intervals being successively less, creating a smooth envelope pattern. (*Copyright* JF Howard Jr.)

rendering the study unhelpful in this author's experience. This is most important when considering presynaptic disorders of NMT.

SFEMG

SFEMG is a highly selective recording technique in which a concentric needle electrode is used to identify and record extracellular APs from individual muscle fibers.[46] The selectivity of the technique results from the small recording surface (25 μm in diameter) that is exposed at a port on the side of the recording electrode, 3 mm from the tip. The amplitude of signals recorded with this surface decreases rapidly as the distance between the electrode and the signal source increases. Thus, APs from distant muscle fibers are much smaller than those from close fibers. The signals are recorded with a high pass (low frequency) filter of 500 Hz, which heightens the selectivity of the recording because the high-frequency components of EMG signals are attenuated by distance to a much greater degree than are low-frequency components. Thus, filtering the low-frequency components excludes predominantly signals from distant fibers and also helps ensure a stable baseline. The concerns for infectious risk have precluded the use of this reusable electrode in some countries. Investigations are under way to determine the validity of jitter measurements using a concentric needle electrode (see later).

When the SFEMG electrode is positioned to record from 2 or more muscle fibers in 1 voluntarily activated motor unit, variations in the time intervals between pairs of APs from these fibers can be seen. This variation is the neuromuscular jitter, most of which is produced by fluctuations in the time it takes for EPPs at the NMJ to reach the threshold for AP generation (see **Fig. 1**).

Jitter is the most sensitive clinical electrophysiologic measure of the safety factor of NMT.[47] It is increased whenever the ratio of the AP threshold and the EPP is greater than normal. When NMT is sufficiently impaired, nerve impulses fail to elicit muscle APs and SFEMG demonstrates intermittent impulse blocking. When blocking occurs in many end-plates in a muscle there is clinical weakness. SFEMG can demonstrate abnormal NMT (as increased jitter) in muscles that are clinically normal and have no decrement to RNS. Jitter varies among different end-plates in a muscle, even among several end-plates within one muscle, and from muscle to muscle. To adequately sample the distribution of jitter within a muscle, at least 20 potential pairs should be measured. With increased age, there is a slight increase in jitter in normal subjects.[48]

Analysis of Neuromuscular Jitter

Neuromuscular jitter may be measured from SFEMG recordings performed during voluntary activation of the tested muscle or during electrical stimulation of the nerve.

Recordings made during voluntary activation require that the electrode be placed so that APs are recorded from 2 or more muscle fibers in the same motor unit. Jitter is then measured as the variation in the length of the intervals between the 2 APs in the pair (interpotential interval [IPI]). This paired jitter represents the combined jitter in 2 end-plates. Jitter recorded during nerve stimulation is calculated as the variation in the intervals between the stimulus and APs from single muscle fibers. This jitter comes from single end-plates. Jitter values calculated from these 2 different techniques will differ and normal ranges have been developed for each technique (see later).

The variation in intervals can be expressed as the SD of a series of intervals. However, the intervals may slowly increase or decrease as a result of electrode movement, cooling of the muscle, or other factors, in which case the SD is not an accurate measure of NMT. To minimize the effects of such slow trends, one can calculate the mean value of consecutive differences of successive IPIs (MCD) from the following formula:

$$MCD = \frac{|IPI_1 - IPI_2| + \ldots + |IPI_{n-1} - IPI_n|}{n - 1}$$

where IPI_i is the IPI (or, when nerve stimulation is used, the stimulus-response interval). In the absence of trends and when the data have a Gaussian distribution, MCD = 1.13 SDs.

In certain situations, the IPI may be influenced by variations in the firing rate. This effect may be minimized by sorting the IPIs in the order of the preceding interdischarge interval and then calculating the mean of consecutive differences in the new sequence. This is called the mean sorted-data difference (MSD). If the ratio MCD/MSD exceeds 1.25, then variations in the firing rate have contributed to the jitter and the MSD should be used to represent the neuromuscular jitter. MCD is used if the ratio is between 0.8 and 1.25. If the MCD/MSD ratio is less than 0.8, there are trends in the data, in which case the MCD is used. The effect of firing rate on jitter is most marked when the IPI is long. If it is not possible to calculate the MSD, this effect can be minimized by having the patient maintain a constant firing rate during voluntary activation, by measuring jitter during nerve stimulation at constant rates, or by excluding from analysis IPIs greater than 4 milliseconds.

Jitter can be calculated most precisely if the IPIs are measured directly with an interval counter or clock. Many commercially available EMG machines now have the capability to measure IPIs and calculate MCD and MSD directly. Most require the electromyographer to set a threshold level to detect the APs of interest and thus to exclude undesired signals. Some systems use a peak-detection algorithm to identify APs for jitter analysis. No system can automatically distinguish spurious triggering potentials from true blocking, however, and the electromyographer should make this distinction and be able to enter this into the record.

The severity of abnormality within a muscle may be quantified by calculating for each muscle tested:

- The mean jitter of all potential pairs tested
- The percentage of potential pairs in which blocking is seen
- The percentage of potential pairs in which jitter is normal

The distribution and severity of jitter and blocking among the potential pairs within a muscle can best be appreciated when the results are displayed graphically (**Fig. 8**).

Quality Control in SFEMG

To ensure that acceptable signals are being acquired, feedback is provided to the electromyographer in different ways during data acquisition. Some systems electronically store and redisplay the waveforms for review. The electromyographer can select

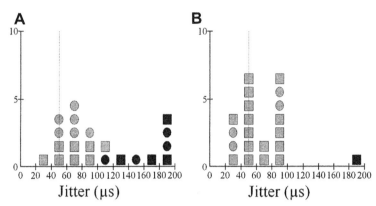

Fig. 8. SFEMG volitional: (left) extensor digitorum. Histogram plots of jitter results in the Extensor digitorum communis muscle of a 54-year-old patient with recent onset of severe generalized MG. Each symbol represents the jitter measured in one pair of potentials. Square symbols represent the MCD; round symbols represent the MSD. Dark symbols represent those potentials with impulse blocking. The vertical dashed lines represent the normal jitter value for age. (*A*) Histogram plot at the time of diagnosis and while untreated. (*B*) Histogram plot following 8-month treatment with mycophenolate mofetil and prednisone. (*Copyright* JF Howard Jr.)

and exclude those that are not acceptable before final calculations are made. The IPI values can also be displayed graphically by some systems, which permits easy visualization of the distribution of data and any trends. Such a display also makes it easier to detect extreme values that do not follow the expected data distribution. The measurement of jitter cannot be completely automated by any system because the electromyographer selects the signal to be analyzed and determines the quality of that signal. To help ensure that the data obtained are valid, quality control should be exerted by the electromyographer throughout the process.

Normal Jitter Values

Normal values for the jitter among potential pairs and the mean jitter of a population of potential pairs within a muscle have been determined for many muscles.[48,49] To determine if a muscle is normal, jitter should be measured in 20 potential pairs. A study is abnormal if either of the following criteria is met:

a. The mean jitter of all potential pairs recorded exceeds the upper limit of mean jitter for that muscle.
b. Ten percent or more of potential pairs have jitter that exceeds the upper limit of normal for paired jitter in that muscle.

In most abnormal studies, both criteria will be met. For example, in 409 SFEMG studies of the EDC in patients with MG, 78% of the 409 were abnormal by both criteria and only 8% of the 409 were abnormal by only 1 criterion.[50]

In some recordings, the jitter is less than 10 microseconds. This is seen rarely in normal muscles and more often in myopathies. These low values probably represent recordings made from split muscle fibers, both branches of which are activated by a single NMJ. These recordings should not be included in the analysis.

SFEMG During Axonal Microstimulation

Single-fiber investigations are most commonly performed during voluntary activation of the muscle. Occasionally it is useful and sometimes it is necessary to use a second technique termed electrical axonal microstimulation.[51] One advantage of electrical stimulation is that these studies can be performed in uncooperative patients (infants, small children, patients with tremor and unconscious patients) or animals. However, the technical pitfalls of this technique are considerable and, therefore, the electromyographer must be rigorous with his or her technique.

For stimulation, an insulated monopolar needle with a bare tip is inserted in the muscle near the motor end-plate zone. Another needle electrode or surface electrode placed close is used as the anode. The stimulus intensity is adjusted to produce a small visible twitch in a part of the muscle. Usually less that 5 mA is necessary. A stimulation frequency of 2 to 10 Hz is often used. The SFEMG electrode is inserted about 2 cm distally to the cathode into the twitching part of the muscle. With increasing stimulus strength, increasing numbers of single-fiber APs (SFAPs) appear, initially with intermittent blocking and high jitter. This increased jitter is caused by subliminal stimulation. Jitter is measured when further increases in the stimulus intensity no longer decrease the jitter of a particular SFAP. The jitter is measured between the stimulus artifact and the AP.

Jitter measured during axonal stimulation will be less than that measured during voluntary activation of the muscle because only the contribution from single endplates is being assessed during axonal stimulation. The theoretical relationship between these 2 values is expressed by the formula[52]:

$$\text{Mean MCD (axonal stim)} = \text{Mean MCD (vol activation)} / \sqrt{2}$$

Normal values for jitter during axonal stimulation determined in the EDC are 40 microseconds (individual muscle fibers) and 25 microseconds (mean of 30 muscle fibers).[51]

Concentric Needle Jitter Recordings

There is increasing interest in the use of disposable concentric or monopolar needle EMG electrodes to perform jitter measurements because of the concern for infectious risk when reusing invasive medical devices. The use of a monopolar needle is not feasible because of its large recording surface and because activity is included in the recording as a result of the referential electrode being outside of the recording area. Small concentric electrodes with an elliptical recording surface of 0.019 μm^2 are currently the most appropriate electrodes to use.[53] The larger recording surface of the concentric electrode predisposes to several technical errors, and much of the literature to date has not taken these into account. The larger recording surface produces a greater shunting effect of the electrical field, and recorded potentials will be smaller than those recorded with the standard SFEMG electrode. Further, the larger recording surface will "see" more SFAPs resulting in a summated signal. This phenomenon is the greatest disadvantage of the technique. The larger recording surface, the recording from multiple SFAPs, and the resulting signal summation produce an underestimation of jitter.[53] Recordings made with concentric electrodes are no different from those made with an SFEMG electrode. However, critical attention must be paid to separation of signals and the absence of shape variation to ensure that SFAPs and not summated signals are being recorded. Details of the technical procedure are described by Stålberg.[53]

Few studies have been published of concentric jitter studies in disease of the NMJ. There are differences in methodology and normative values, and most are fraught with technical errors. There has been no standardization of technique to date. There is limited information available on normative values and that in the literature is for a very limited number of muscles.[54–57] In general. all authors demonstrate that concentric jitter is increased in MG.[58–61] There is only one study in which both techniques were performed on the same muscle; concentric jitter was found to be 5.6 microseconds lower.[53]

Technical Considerations

Most adult patients are able to cooperate well enough to permit adequate SFEMG studies. Patient discomfort rarely limits the use of this test, even when several muscles must be examined. The potential complications of SFEMG are those of needle electromyography in general (ie, hemorrhage and infection). Other than an occasional small hematoma, we have had no complications of the procedure.

If the patient has a tremor, it may be impossible to make adequate recordings from distal arm muscles during voluntary activation. In such cases, recordings can usually be made from facial or more proximal arm muscles, especially the biceps brachii. Alternatively, recordings of jitter can be made during nerve stimulation.

Children older than 8 years old can usually cooperate well enough for adequate studies. In uncooperative children or infants, jitter studies can be performed during nerve stimulation, as described, while the child is sedated or under anesthesia.

EMG FINDINGS IN DISORDERS OF SYNAPTIC TRANSMISSION
Autoimmune MG

Characteristically, in MG the CMAP amplitude is normal, although in severely weak muscles, the amplitude may be slightly reduced. There is a decrementing response to trains of 3- to 7-Hz stimulation. There is partial repair of the decrement after the third or fourth response of the train, producing a "U-shaped" curve (**Fig. 9**). Postactivation facilitation may be seen after periods of 30 to 60 seconds of activation, but this is usually in the range of 10% to 25% and rarely greater than 50%. Postactivation exhaustion is commonly seen 3 to 4 minutes after 30 seconds to 1 minute of maximum voluntary exercise (see **Fig. 9**). One is more likely to demonstrate an abnormality in proximal muscles such as the trapezius or in a facial muscle such as the nasalis or orbicularis oculi than in distal hand or foot muscles.

Standard needle EMG recordings will demonstrate beat-to-beat variability in the amplitude of individual MUAPs, and the fullness of the interference pattern may wane with continued contraction in muscles that are moderate to severely weak.

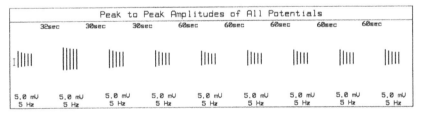

Fig. 9. RNS paradigm in a patient with MG, demonstrating characteristic electrodiagnostic features of this disorder. Trains of 5 stimuli at 5 Hz are administered at variable intervals. The initial train is followed by 30 seconds of activation (maximum voluntary contraction) and subsequent 5-Hz trains of 5 stimuli for 7 minutes. Note the initial decremental response (60%), the minimal postactivation facilitation (13%, comparing the initial response of train 1 to the initial response of train 2), and the postactivation exhaustion that is seen in trains 7 and 8 (68% decrement). Calibration, 5 mV per division. (*From* Howard JF, Sanders DB, Massey JM. The electrodiagnosis of myasthenia gravis and the lambert-eaton myasthenic syndrome. Neurol Clin 1994;12:305–30; with permission.)

The typical SFEMG finding in MG is that within one muscle, there are some end-plates with normal jitter, others with increased jitter, and still others with increased jitter and impulse blocking (**Fig. 10**). This spectrum of findings may even be seen within the end-plates of a single motor unit. SFEMG demonstrates abnormal jitter in virtually all (98%) patients with MG. One muscle, the EDC, is abnormal in most patients with this disease, but to obtain the maximum diagnostic sensitivity it may be necessary to examine other muscles, especially ones that are more involved clinically. There is no one muscle that will be more abnormal in every patient with MG. The muscle or muscles to be tested must be selected based on the distribution of weakness in the individual patient. In patients with symptoms or signs of weakness in any extremity muscles, the EDC is usually tested first. This muscle is easily activated by most patients and is relatively free of age-dependent changes. Abnormal jitter was found in this muscle in 89% of patients with MG who had weakness in any limb muscle and in 63% of those with weakness restricted to the ocular muscles.[50] If the first muscle studied is normal, another muscle should be examined, selected based on the distribution of clinical weakness. If this is done, increased jitter can be demonstrated in 98% of patients with ocular MG and in 99% of patients with weakness in any limb muscle.[50]

In patients whose symptoms are restricted to the ocular muscles, the frontalis, orbicularis oculi, or orbicularis oris muscle may be examined first. Abnormal jitter can be demonstrated in the EDC in more than 60% of patients with ocular MG, confirming that the physiologic abnormality is more widespread than can be determined by clinical examination alone. In those patients whose forearm study is normal, examination of the frontalis or orbicularis oculi muscles will demonstrate abnormalities in 98% of patients.

We would not consider a jitter study to be normal unless we had tested a clinically affected muscle or, in the case of purely ocular weakness, the orbicularis oculi or

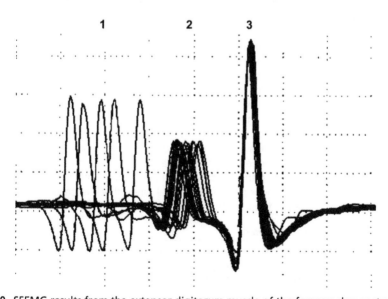

Fig. 10. SFEMG results from the extensor digitorum muscle of the forearm demonstrating 3 muscle fiber APs under the control of the same motor neuron. Potential 1 demonstrates increased jitter and impulse blocking; potential 2 demonstrates increase jitter without impulse blocking; and potential 3 is the triggering potential. The decremental response seen on RNS study is equivalent to potential 1 (impulse blocking). (*Copyright* JF Howard Jr.)

orbicularis oris muscle. Jitter is more often abnormal in any given muscle in patients with more severe disease. However, there is marked variability of the abnormality within each clinical group, so that no conclusions about disease severity can be drawn from the amount of jitter alone. Jitter is usually increased even in muscles with normal strength but is worse in weak muscles in patients with MG. Jitter is usually worse in facial muscles than in limb muscles but the opposite is true in occasional patients.

In most patients with MG, changes in disease severity correlate with changes in jitter measurements. The mean MCD increases by at least 10% in the tested muscle in two-thirds of patients who become worse between SFEMG studies. Conversely, in more than 80% of instances when the mean MCD decreases by at least 10% between 2 studies, there has been definite clinical improvement.[50] Thus, there is a strong correlation between the overall change in clinical status in patients with MG and a change of at least 10% in mean jitter in any muscle. Serial SFEMG studies may be of value in predicting changes in disease severity under certain circumstances.[62] For example, when the jitter values in one muscle have been constant for several months, any subsequent increase in jitter is usually accompanied or followed by clinical deterioration. Although therapeutic decisions should always be based on clinical considerations, jitter measurements may be useful in providing one part of the clinical picture.

It is the opinion of this author that concentric jitter studies must be interpreted with caution and are an underestimation of the severity of the abnormality. Hence, their use in mild or restricted disease is limited.

MG With Antibodies to MuSK

Neurographic studies are typically normal in the limbs of patients with MG with positive MuSK antibodies (MuSK MG) but may demonstrate reduced CMAP amplitudes in axial or facial muscles because of their associated muscle atrophy. Needle EMG is most important in suspected cases of MuSK MG when short-duration, small-amplitude MUAPs will be recorded in clinically affected muscles, particularly those with atrophy.[6,7] Fibrillation potentials may be seen in some patients.[5] Importantly, patients presenting with isolated neck extensor disease or respiratory failure may have normal electrodiagnostic studies in the limbs. It is therefore necessary that clinically affected muscles be examined to avoid missing the pertinent abnormalities of this disease. The RNS findings of MuSK MG will be reflected by the phenotype of the disease.[63] Studies in the limb will often demonstrate no decrement or a decrement that is disproportionately smaller for the degree of muscle weakness. Studies are abnormal in 52% with examination of multiple muscles compared with 69% of Ach receptor antibody–positive patients.[63] Proximal muscles are more often abnormal, similar to that found in Ach receptor antibody–positive patients with MG, and facial muscles are most often abnormal.[64] SFEMG provides the most useful information, particularly when RNS studies are normal, and is most always abnormal when there is careful selection of involved muscles, including those of the paraspinal region.[5,65,66]

Congenital Myasthenic Syndromes

Congenital myasthenic syndromes are a heterogeneous group of genetically determined structural disorders of the presynaptic, synaptic, and postsynaptic elements of the NMJ. Most of these disorders have been elegantly elucidated by Andrew Engel and were recently summarized.[10] The electrophysiologic abnormalities reflect the phenotype of the disorder and, in general, have many of the same characteristics of the prototypical presynaptic and postsynaptic disorders, LES and MG. Specific differentiation of these disorders requires microphysiologic study of synaptic transmission, molecular chemical examination of the membrane proteins, and genetic analysis.

Unique clinical electrodiagnostic features do exist. Prolongation of the EPP, as seen in the slow channel syndrome and congenital acetylcholinesterase deficiency, causes a repetitive CMAP after a single stimulation, because the EPP duration exceeds the refractory period of the AP (**Fig. 11**).[67] They are usually found in the small muscles of the hand and foot. Afterdischarges are abolished by repetitive stimulation in contrast to artifact, which will persist.

Congenital choline acetyltransferase deficiency demonstrates decremental responses to slow rates of stimulation that worsen with prolonged continuous 5- or 10-Hz stimulation for 5 minutes. Although a similar pattern may be seen in severe auto-immune MG or congenital ACh receptor deficiency, the recovery pattern in congenital choline acetyltransferase is very prolonged, lasting up to 30 minutes.[68] SFEMG is similar to other NMJ disorders. Needle EMG will often demonstrate normal or small varying amplitude MUAPs. Neurographic studies are normal.

LES

RNS studies are the most specific test available to confirm the diagnosis of LES. The characteristic electrophysiologic findings on RNS studies in presynaptic disorders of NMT are a reduction in the initial CMAP amplitude, a decremental response to slow stimulation rates (1 Hz through 5 Hz), marked postactivation facilitation following a brief period of maximum voluntary contraction or following a tetanic stimulation, and the absence of significant postactivation exhaustion (**Fig. 12**). These decrements are most often seen at 3/s stimulation and tend to be less at faster rates of stimulation such as 5/s. Postactivation facilitation is in excess of twice the initial CMAP amplitude and is much more pronounced than that seen in postsynaptic disorders. Care must be taken not to exercise the muscle too long because this will deplete neurotransmitter release and mask the facilitatory response. Unlike postsynaptic disorders in which 30 seconds to 1 minute of maximum exercise is best, 10 seconds is all that is necessary in these disorders. Rapid rates of stimulation will produce a marked facilitatory response in excess of 60% and often much greater (**Fig. 13**).

SFEMG demonstrates abnormal jitter in virtually all patients with LES. The degree of jitter and blocking for any degree of muscle weakness tends to be greater in these patients compared with those with MG. In presynaptic neuromuscular abnormalities, such as LES and botulism, jitter typically decreases as the firing rate increases.[69] These effects of firing rate are not always seen in these conditions, however, and we have seen jitter and blocking that decreases at high firing rates in some potential pairs in patients with neuropathy or MG.[70] The effects of different firing rates may be assessed by measuring jitter from one pair of potentials while the patient maintains a low activation rate, and again at a higher rate or by using axonal microstimulation techniques.

Botulism

The electrodiagnostic abnormalities seen in botulism are very similar to those seen in LES. Neurographic studies are normal other than a reduction in CMAP amplitude. The resting CMAP amplitude is reduced in virtually all cases. Needle EMG recordings will demonstrate fibrillation potentials because there is a functional denervation of muscle. A decremental response is seen with slow stimulation rates, but this may be masked if the CMAP amplitude is markedly reduced. A moderate facilitatory response is seen with rapid stimulation rates or following very brief maximum isometric contraction if the patient is able. This is more likely in children and may be initially absent in the adult form of the disease. In the adult, facilitation may require more prolonged rapid-rate stimulation duration (10–20 seconds) and also lasts longer (5–30 minutes) compared with other presynaptic disorders. The degree of postactivation facilitation is usually

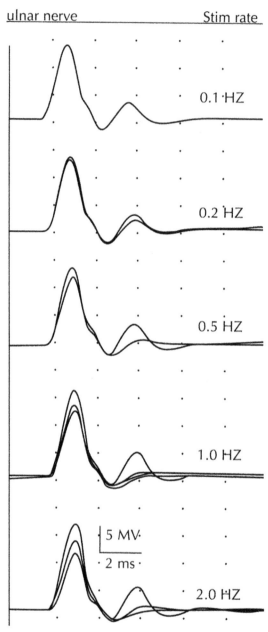

Fig. 11. Repetitive discharges in the abductor digiti quinti muscle in a patient with congenital acetylcholinesterase deficiency. Four consecutive superimposed CMAPs are shown with increasing stimulus rates. Stimulation faster than 0.5 Hz abolishes the repetitive discharge. (*From* Engel AG. Myasthenia gravis and myasthenic disorders. In Harper CM, editor. Electrodiagnosis of myasthenic disorders. New York: Oxford University Press; 2012. p. 37–59, Figs. 2.1 and 2.10; with permission of Oxford University Press, Inc.)

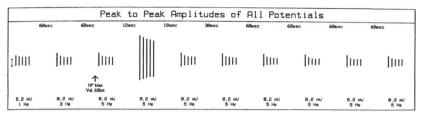

Fig. 12. Peak-to-peak amplitudes of all Potentials. Stimulus paradigm in a patient with LES demonstrating the characteristic electrodiagnostic features of this syndrome. Trains of 5 stimuli are administered at stimulus rates of 1, 3, and 5 Hz followed by 10 seconds of activation (maximum voluntary contraction) and subsequent intermittent 5-Hz trains of 5 stimuli maximum for 4.5 minutes. Note the initial low CMAP amplitude (trains 1–3), the decremental response to slow rates of stimulation (train 1–3, 20%, 40%, and 40%, respectively), and the marked postactivation facilitation after 10 seconds of exercise (167%, comparing the initial response of train 4 to the initial response of train 3). Postactivation exhaustion is not easily seen because of the small CMAP responses. Calibration, 0.2 mV per division. (*From* Howard JF, Sanders DB, Massey JM. The electrodiagnosis of myasthenia gravis and the lambert-eaton myasthenic syndrome. Neurol Clin 1994;12:305–30; with permission.)

less than that seen in LES, ranging from 40% to 200%.[71] Postactivation exhaustion is not seen in botulism.[72] SFEMG recordings show increased jitter and impulse blocking disproportionately more severe than in MG and similar to that seen in LES.

COMPARISON OF DIAGNOSTIC TECHNIQUES IN MG

RNS studies show an abnormal decrement in a hand or shoulder muscle in approximately 75% of patients with generalized MG and in less than 50% of those with ocular myasthenia.[73] The "double-step" RNS test is only slightly more sensitive than RNS of the trapezius muscle alone and only 60% as sensitive as SFEMG of a hand muscle.[43] SFEMG is the most sensitive test of NMT and is abnormal in up to 95% of patients with MG.[27] SFEMG, because of its high sensitivity, may demonstrate abnormal NMT in diseases other than MG or LES, which must be excluded. It is most valuable in demonstrating abnormal NMT in patients with mild MG or those with purely ocular disease. In addition, it can be helpful in excluding a disorder of NMT; the demonstration of normal jitter in the presence of muscle weakness suggests that the weakness is not caused by a disorder of synaptic transmission.[50] About 25% of patients with MG do not have elevated anti–ACh receptor antibody levels, and SFEMG can be of great value in confirming or excluding the diagnosis of MG in patients in whom these antibodies are not found.

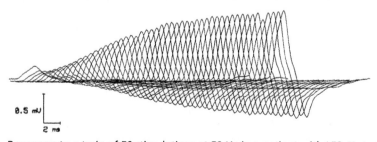

Fig. 13. Responses to a train of 50 stimulations at 50 Hz in a patient with LES. Note the low initial CMAP amplitude (0.3 mV) and the marked facilitation (to 1.5 mV, 400%). Calibration, 0.5 mV and 2 mSec per division. (*From* Howard JF, Sanders DB, Massey JM. The electrodiagnosis of myasthenia gravis and the Lambert-Eaton myasthenic syndrome. Neurol Clin 1994;12:305–30; with permission.)

SUMMARY

The electrophysiologic examination of a patient suspected of having a disorder of synaptic transmission should be an extension of the physical examination and history. Patients should first undergo standard measures of nerve conduction and needle EMG for the reasons mentioned earlier. The amplitude of the CMAP response to a single shock in an appropriately warmed muscle will give clues as to whether the problem is presynaptic or postsynaptic in origin. Cholinesterase inhibitors should be withdrawn for 72 hours to minimize the risk of masking an abnormality of NMT.[74]

RNS studies should be performed on a clinically involved muscle, typically the trapezius or nasalis muscle, in patients suspected of having MG. A distal hand muscle (eg, abductor digiti quinti) may be used if it is necessary to condition the patient to the procedure. Attention to the caveats previously discussed should be adhered to as careful attention to technique is critical for an optimal study. Should these studies be normal, SFEMG recordings performed initially on the forearm will be abnormal in most cases, and if necessary, a second muscle should be chosen based on the distribution of the clinical weakness. One should not consider a study to be completely normal until a clinically affected muscle or, in the case of suspected ocular MG, the orbicularis oculi muscle has been examined.

Abnormal jitter is also seen in diseases of nerve and muscle; these diseases must be excluded by other electrophysiologic and clinical examinations before diagnosing MG. If neuronal or myopathic disease is present, increased jitter does not indicate that MG is also present. Rarely, MG may be present in the presence of a normal SFEMG study. However, if jitter is normal in a muscle with definite weakness, the weakness is not caused by an abnormality of NMT.

When abnormal NMT has been demonstrated by RNS, the finding of abnormal jitter does not add to the diagnosis, although it may be useful in providing baseline values for comparison with the results of subsequent studies. SFEMG is most valuable clinically in the patient with suspected MG in whom other tests of NMT and anti–ACh receptor antibody titers are normal. Serial measurements of jitter can be useful in following the course of disease and in assessing the effect of treatment, but the results from these studies must always be interpreted in light of the overall clinical picture. It may be necessary to perform SFEMG studies on facial or axial muscles to establish a diagnosis of MuSK MG.

An easy screening test in patients suspected of having LES is to rest an appropriately warmed limb, stimulate the nerve once, and, if the CMAP amplitude is low, voluntarily activate the muscle maximally for 10 seconds before stimulating the nerve a second time. In nearly all cases, there will be a marked facilitation of the CMAP amplitude. More formal studies can then be undertaken to demonstrate the decremental response to slow rates of stimulation and the facilitation following postactivation or tetanic stimulation.

REFERENCES

1. Harper CM. Congenital myasthenic syndromes. Semin Neurol 2004;24(1):111–23.
2. Barbieri S, Weiss GM, Daube JR. Fibrillation potentials in myasthenia gravis. Muscle Nerve 1982;5:S50.
3. Banwell BL, Russel J, Fukudome T, et al. Myopathy, myasthenic syndrome, and epidermolysis bullosa simplex due to plectin deficiency. J Neuropathol Exp Neurol 1999;58(8):832–46.
4. Cruz MA, Anciones B, Ferrer MT, et al. Electrophysiologic study in benign human botulism type B. Muscle Nerve 1985;8(7):580–5.

5. Sanders DB, El-Salem K, Massey JM, et al. Clinical aspects of MuSK antibody positive seronegative MG. Neurology 2003;60(12):1978–80.
6. Farrugia ME, Kennett RP, Hilton-Jones D, et al. Quantitative EMG of facial muscles in myasthenia patients with MuSK antibodies. Clin Neurophysiol 2007; 118(2):269–77.
7. Padua L, Tonali P, Aprile I, et al. Seronegative myasthenia gravis: comparison of neurophysiological picture in MuSK+ and MuSK– patients. Eur J Neurol 2006; 13(3):273–6.
8. Bernstein LP, Antel JP. Motor neuron disease: decremental responses to repetitive nerve stimulation. Neurology 1981;31:202–4.
9. Dyken ML, Smith DM. An electromyographic diagnostic screening test in McArdle's disease and a case report. Neurology 1967;17:45–50.
10. Engel AG, Shen XM, Ohno K, et al. Congenital myasthenic syndromes. In: Engel AG, editor. Myasthenia gravis and myasthenic syndromes. 2nd edition. New York: Oxford University Press; 2012. p. 173–230.
11. Gilchrist JM, Sanders DB. Myasthenic U-shaped decrement in multifocal cervical radiculopathy. Muscle Nerve 1989;12:64–6.
12. Gutmann L, Bodensteiner J, Gutierrez A. Electrodiagnosis of botulism. J Pediatr 1992;121:835.
13. Lambert EH. Defects of neuromuscular transmission in syndromes other than myasthenia gravis. Ann N Y Acad Sci 1966;135:367–84.
14. Ma DM, Wasserman EJ, Giebfried J. Repetitive stimulation of the trapezius muscle: its value in myasthenic testing. Muscle Nerve 1980;3:439–40.
15. Maselli RA, Soliven BC. Analysis of the organophosphate-induced electromyographic response to repetitive nerve stimulation: paradoxical response to edrophonium and D-tubocurarine. Muscle Nerve 1991;14:1182–8.
16. Patten BM, Hart A, Lovelace R. Multiple sclerosis associated with defects in neuromuscular transmission. J Neurol Neurosurg Psychiatry 1972;35:385–94.
17. Subramony SH, Mitsumoto H, Mishra SK. Motor neuropathy associated with a facilitating myasthenic syndrome. Muscle Nerve 1986;9:64–8.
18. Swift TR, Greenberg MK. Miscellaneous neuromuscular transmission disorders. In: Brumback RA, Gerst J, editors. The neuromuscular junction. Mount Kisco (NY): Futura; 1984. p. 295–340.
19. Vroom FW, Jarrell MA, Maren TH. Acetazolamide treatment of hypokalemic periodic paralysis. Probable mechanism of action. Arch Neurol 1938;32(6):385–92.
20. Wright EA, McQuillen MP. Antibiotic-induced neuromuscular blockade. Ann N Y Acad Sci 1971;182:358–68.
21. Aiello I, Sau GF, Bissakou M, et al. Standardization of changes in M-wave area to repetitive nerve stimulation. Electromyogr Clin Neurophysiol 1986;26(7):529–32.
22. Desmedt JE. The neuromuscular disorder in myasthenia gravis. 1. Electrical and mechanical response to nerve stimulation in hand muscles. In: Desmedt JE, editor. New developments in electromyography and clinical neurophysiology. Basel (Switzerland): Karger; 1973. p. 241–304.
23. Oh SJ. Electromyography neuromuscular transmission studies. Baltimore (MD): William & Wilkins; 1988. p. 1–304.
24. Stålberg EV, Sanders DB. Electrophysiological tests of neuromuscular transmission. In: Stalberg E, Young RR, editors. Clinical Neurophysiology. Severoaks, Kent (United Kingdom): Butterworth and Co; 1981. p. 88–116.
25. Oh SJ, Hatanaka Y, Claussen GC, et al. Electrophysiological differences in seropositive and seronegative Lambert-Eaton myasthenic syndrome. Muscle Nerve 2007;35(2):178–83.

26. Schumm F, Stohr M. Accessory nerve stimulation in the assessment of myasthenia gravis. Muscle Nerve 1984;7(2):147–51.
27. Benatar M. A systematic review of diagnostic studies in myasthenia gravis. Neuromuscul Disord 2006;16(7):459–67.
28. Niks EH, Badrising UA, Verschuuren JJ, et al. Decremental response of the nasalis and hypothenar muscles in myasthenia gravis. Muscle Nerve 2003;28(2):236–8.
29. Zambelis T, Kokotis P, Karandreas N. Repetitive nerve stimulation of facial and hypothenar muscles: relative sensitivity in different myasthenia gravis subgroups. Eur Neurol 2011;65(4):203–7.
30. Zinman LH, O'Connor PW, Dadson KE, et al. Sensitivity of repetitive facial-nerve stimulation in patients with myasthenia gravis. Muscle Nerve 2006;33(5):694–6.
31. Borenstein S, Desmedt JE. New diagnostic procedures in myasthenia gravis. In: Desmedt JE, editor. New developments in electromyography and clinical neurophysiology, vol.3. Basel (Switzerland): Karger; 1973. p. 50–74.
32. Rutkove SB. Effects of temperature on neuromuscular electrophysiology. Muscle Nerve 2001;24(7):867–82.
33. Howard JF. The diagnosis of myasthenia gravis and other disorders of neuromuscular transmission. In: Engel AG, editor. Myasthenia gravis and myasthenic disorders. 2nd edition. New York: Oxford University Press; 2012. p. 108–29.
34. Ricker K, Hertel G, Stodieck S. Influence of temperature on neuromuscular transmission in myasthenia gravis. J Neurol 1977;216:273–82.
35. Foldes FF, Kuze S, Vizi ES, et al. The influence of temperature on neuromuscular performance. J Neural Transm 1978;43:27–45.
36. Harris JB, Leach GDH. The effect of temperature on end-plate depolarization of the rat diaphragm produced by suxamethonium and acetylcholine. J Pharm Pharmacol 1968;20:194–8.
37. Hubbard JI, Jones SF, Landau EM. The effect of temperature change upon transmitter release, facilitation and post-tetanic potentiation. J Physiol 1971;216:591–608.
38. Phillips LH. Electromyography in myasthenia gravis. Semin Neurol 1982;2:239–49.
39. Sun YT, Lin TS. Is the stimulation frequency of the repetitive nerve stimulation test that you choose appropriate? Acta Neurol Taiwan 2004;13(4):186–91.
40. Trontelj JV. Muscle fiber conduction velocity changes with length. Muscle Nerve 1993;16(5):506–12.
41. Gilchrist JM, Sanders DB. Double-step repetitive stimulation in myasthenia gravis. Muscle Nerve 1987;10:233–7.
42. Harvey AM, Masland RL. A method for the study of neuromuscular transmission in human subjects. Bull Johns Hopkins Hosp 1941;68:81–93.
43. Temucin CM, Arsava EM, Nurlu G, et al. Diagnostic value of double-step nerve stimulation test in patients with myasthenia gravis. Clin Neurophysiol 2010;121(4):556–60.
44. Heuser JE, Reese TS. Evidence for recycling of synaptic vesicle membrane during transmitter release at the frog neuromuscular junction. J Cell Biol 1973;57:315–44.
45. Ricker KW, Hertel G, Reuther P, et al. Repetitive proximal nerve stimulation and systemic curare test in myasthenia gravis. Ann N Y Acad Sci 1981;377:877–8.
46. Stålberg EV, Trontelj JV, Sanders DB. Single fiber EMG. Fiskenbäcksil (Sweden): Edshagen Publishing House; 2010. p. 1–400.
47. Sanders DB. Clinical impact of single-fiber electromyography. Muscle Nerve 2002;(Suppl 11):S15–20.

48. Bromberg MB, Scott DM. Single fiber EMG reference values: reformatted in tabular form. AD HOC Committee of the AAEM Single Fiber Special Interest Group. Muscle Nerve 1994;17(7):820–1.
49. Ad Hoc Committee of the AAEM SFEMG Special Interest Group. Single fiber EMG reference values: a collaborative effort. Muscle Nerve 1992;15:151–61.
50. Sanders DB, Howard JF. AAEE minimonograph #25: single-fiber electromyography in myasthenia gravis. Muscle Nerve 1986;9:809–19.
51. Trontelj JV, Stålberg EV. Jitter measurement by axonal micro-stimulation. Guidelines and technical notes. Electroencephalogr Clin Neurophysiol 1992;85:30–7.
52. Trontelj JV, Stålberg EV, Mihelin M, et al. Jitter of the stimulated motor axon. Muscle Nerve 1992;15:449–54.
53. Stalberg EV, Sanders DB. Jitter recordings with concentric needle electrodes. Muscle Nerve 2009;40(3):331–9.
54. Kouyoumdjian JA, Stalberg EV. Concentric needle single fiber electromyography: comparative jitter on voluntary-activated and stimulated Extensor Digitorum Communis. Clin Neurophysiol 2008;119(7):1614–8.
55. Kouyoumdjian JA, Stalberg EV. Reference jitter values for concentric needle electrodes in voluntarily activated extensor digitorum communis and orbicularis oculi muscles. Muscle Nerve 2008;37(6):694–9.
56. Kouyoumdjian JA, Stalberg EV. Concentric needle jitter on stimulated Orbicularis Oculi in 50 healthy subjects. Clin Neurophysiol 2011;122(3):617–22.
57. Kouyoumdjian JA, Stalberg EV. Concentric needle jitter in stimulated frontalis in 20 healthy subjects. Muscle Nerve 2012;45(2):276–8.
58. Ertas M, Baslo MB, Yildiz N, et al. Concentric needle electrode for neuromuscular jitter analysis. Muscle Nerve 2000;23(5):715–9.
59. Farrugia ME, Weir AI, Cleary M, et al. Concentric and single fiber needle electrodes yield comparable jitter results in myasthenia gravis. Muscle Nerve 2009;39(5):579–85.
60. Kouyoumdjian JA, Fanani AC, Stalberg EV. Concentric needle jitter on stimulated frontalis and extensor digitorum in 20 myasthenia gravis patients. Muscle Nerve 2011;44(6):912–8.
61. Sarrigiannis PG, Kennett RP, Read S, et al. Single-fiber EMG with a concentric needle electrode: validation in myasthenia gravis. Muscle Nerve 2006;33(1):61–5.
62. Howard JF, Sanders DB. Serial single-fiber EMG studies in myasthenic patients treated with corticosteroids and plasma exchange. Muscle Nerve 1981;4:254.
63. Stickler DE, Massey JM, Sanders DB. MuSK-antibody positive myasthenia gravis: clinical and electrodiagnostic patterns. Clin Neurophysiol 2005;116(9):2065–8.
64. Oh SJ, Hatanaka Y, Hemmi S, et al. Repetitive nerve stimulation of facial muscles in MuSK antibody-positive myasthenia gravis. Muscle Nerve 2006;33(4):500–4.
65. Evoli A, Tonali PA, Padua L, et al. Clinical correlates with anti-MuSK antibodies in generalized seronegative myasthenia gravis. Brain 2003;126(Pt 10):2304–11.
66. Nemoto Y, Kuwabara S, Misawa S, et al. Patterns and severity of neuromuscular transmission failure in seronegative myasthenia gravis. J Neurol Neurosurg Psychiatry 2005;76(5):714–8.
67. Van Dijk JG, Lammers GJ, Wintzen AR, et al. Repetitive CMAPs: mechanisms of neural and synaptic genesis. Muscle Nerve 1996;19(9):1127–33.
68. Kraner S, Laufenberg I, Strassburg HM, et al. Congenital myasthenic syndrome with episodic apnea in patients homozygous for a CHAT missense mutation. Arch Neurol 2003;60(5):761–3.
69. Schwartz MS, Stalberg E. Myasthenic syndrome studied with single fiber electromyography. Arch Neurol 1975;32(12):815–7.

70. Sanders DB. The effect of firing rate on neuromuscular jitter in Lambert-Eaton myasthenic syndrome. Muscle Nerve 1992;15:256–8.

71. Cornblath DR, Sladky JT, Sumner AJ. Clinical electrophysiology of infantile botulism. Muscle Nerve 1983;6(6):448–52.

72. Cherington M. Electrophysiologic methods as an aid in diagnosis of botulism: a review. Muscle Nerve 1982;5(9S):S28–9.

73. Howard JF Jr, Sanders DB, Massey JM. The electrodiagnosis of myasthenia gravis and the Lambert-Eaton myasthenic syndrome. Neurol Clin 1994;12(2): 305–30.

74. Massey JM, Sanders DB, Howard JF. The effect of cholinesterase inhibitors on SFEMG in myasthenia gravis. Muscle Nerve 1989;12:154–5.

Electrodiagnostic Evaluation of Myopathies

Sabrina Paganoni, MD, PhD[a],*, Anthony Amato, MD[b]

KEYWORDS

- Electromyography • Muscle biopsy • Muscle membrane irritability
- Motor unit action potential • Recruitment

KEY POINTS

- Electrodiagnostic studies are an extension of the physical examination.
- In the appropriate clinical setting, they are an important tool in the evaluation of patients with suspected myopathies.
- Electrodiagnostic patterns may help recognize the underlying pathophysiologic process and help direct further testing.

INTRODUCTION

The evaluation of patients suspected of having a myopathy begins with a thorough history and clinical examination. This process leads to the elaboration of a clinical impression, based on symptoms, progression, family history, and examination findings. Further diagnostic tests are then ordered using a hypothesis-driven approach to add laboratory evidence in support of or against the clinical suspicion. Electrodiagnostic (EDX) studies, in this respect, are an extension of the physical examination and may help establish the diagnosis of myopathy.

EDX studies, however, are not always needed to diagnose a myopathy. This is particularly true in the pediatric and, occasionally, the adult population. Oftentimes, patients with inherited myopathies present with characteristic phenotypes, and, possibly, a positive family history. In these cases, it is reasonable to proceed directly to genetic testing. In addition, at times, the diagnosis ultimately requires a muscle biopsy, regardless of the EDX study results. Therefore, if clinical suspicion for a myopathy is high, generally corroborated by elevated creatine kinase (CK) levels, it is often

[a] Department of Physical Medicine and Rehabilitation, Spaulding Rehabilitation Hospital, Harvard Medical School, 125 Nashua Street, Suite 753, Boston, MA 02114, USA; [b] Department of Neurology, Brigham and Women's Hospital, Harvard Medical School, 75 Francis Street, Boston, MA 02115, USA
* Corresponding author.
E-mail address: spaganoni@partners.org

Phys Med Rehabil Clin N Am 24 (2013) 193–207
http://dx.doi.org/10.1016/j.pmr.2012.08.017
1047-9651/13/$ – see front matter © 2013 Elsevier Inc. All rights reserved.

pmr.theclinics.com

reasonable to skip or limit the extent of the EDX studies. Finally, EDX studies may be normal in selected muscle diseases (certain endocrine, metabolic, congenital, and mitochondrial myopathies). Thus, in the appropriate clinical context, normal EDX studies do not necessarily rule out the presence of a myopathy.

EDX studies are most useful to diagnose a myopathy when further data are needed to exclude alternative diagnoses, confirm the presence of a muscle disease, and narrow down the differential. The role of EDX studies is summarized in **Box 1**. First of all, the results of nerve conduction studies (NCSs) and electromyography (EMG) are used to exclude neuromuscular conditions that may mimic a myopathy (such as motor neuron disease and neuromuscular junction disorders or, occasionally, motor neuropathies). Second, EMG is often able to confirm the diagnosis of a muscle disorder, when motor units with characteristic morphology and recruitment pattern are identified (**Figs. 1** and **2**). In such cases, EMG may also add diagnostic information relating to the location, type, and severity of the underlying process. For example, the presence of abnormal spontaneous activity may help narrow down the differential among different myopathic processes (**Box 2**). Finally, EMG may be useful in identifying target muscles for biopsy. This is particularly helpful when the only clinically weak muscles are not easily accessible for biopsy (such as the gluteal muscles, the hip flexors, or the paraspinals). The yield of a muscle biopsy increases when a weak (Medical Research Council grade 4 of 5), but not end-stage, muscle is biopsied. EMG analysis allows the evaluation of multiple sites and the identification of affected muscles that are not weak on neurologic examination.

ELECTRODIAGNOSTIC APPROACH

A practical EDX approach for patients with suspected myopathy is outlined in **Box 3** (adapted from other sources).[1,2]

Nerve Conduction Studies

The authors usually perform routine NCSs first, expecting sensory NCSs to be normal in myopathies, unless there is a coexistent neuropathy. Motor NCSs are also generally normal, because routine motor NCSs assess distal muscles that are preserved in most myopathic processes. Exceptions in this respect are distal

---

Box 1
Role of electrodiagnostic studies in the diagnosis of myopathies

1. Exclude neuromuscular conditions that may mimic a myopathy
   a. Motor neuron disease
   b. Motor neuropathies
   c. Neuromuscular junction disorders
2. Provide EMG evidence of the presence of a myopathy (although EMG may be normal in the presence of selected myopathic processes)
3. Characterize the myopathy
   a. Location (proximal, distal, symmetric, or asymmetric)
   b. Presence/absence of abnormal spontaneous activity
   c. Severity
4. Identify target muscles for biopsy

Normal

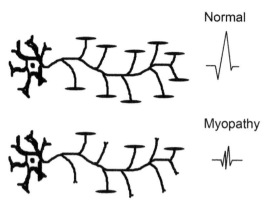

Myopathy

Fig. 1. Physiologic model of motor units in myopathies. The pathologic process in myopathies results in dysfunction and dropout of individual muscle fibers located randomly within the motor unit. Motor neurons and motor axons are not affected. As a result, each MUAP is generated by fewer motor fibers. MUAPs become polyphasic, short in duration, and low in amplitude.

myopathies (which preferentially affect distal muscles), the myopathy of intensive care (which is often generalized and may be associated with a polyneuropathy), or severe cases of myopathies that start proximally but then extend to involve distal muscles in the end-stage. If motor NCSs are affected, CMAP amplitudes are expected to be reduced, with preserved distal latencies and conduction velocities, reflecting muscle damage in the face of normal nerve function. The motor NCSs of a myopathy affecting distal muscles may be similar to the ones seen in motor neuron disorders and presynaptic neuromuscular junction transmission disorders. The former are differentiated from a myopathy based on clinical history and needle EMG findings. The latter are ruled out with additional studies (discussed later).

The authors usually perform at least one motor and one sensory conduction study from one upper extremity and one lower extremity (eg, ulnar motor, ulnar sensory, tibial, and sural NCSs).

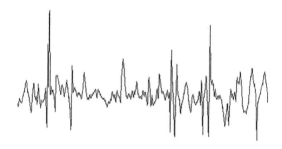

10 ms 200 uV

Fig. 2. Morphology and recruitment pattern of MUAPs in myopathies. Myopathies are characterized by the presence of polyphasic, short-duration, low-amplitude MUAPs. Because each small motor unit is able to generate only a reduced amount of force compared with normal, with little muscle contraction, many MUAPs are recruited.

Box 2
Myopathies associated with muscle membrane irritability/myotonic discharges on EMG

1. Inflammatory myopathies (often)
   a. Polymyositis
   b. Dermatomyositis
   c. Inclusion body myositis (IBM)
   d. Immune-mediated necrotizing myopathy (with or without association with cholesterol-lowering agents)
2. Toxic/necrotic myopathies (often)
   a. Cholesterol-lowering agent myopathies (eg, statin myopathies)
   b. Critical illness myopathy
   c. Chloroquine/hydroxychloroquine
   d. Amiodarone
   e. Colchicine
3. Muscular dystrophies, including the distal muscular dystrophies/myopathies, hereditary inclusion body myopathies, and the myofibrillar myopathies
4. Congenital myopathies (some)
   a. Nemaline rod myopathy
   b. Centronuclear/myotubular myopathy
   c. Central core myopathy
   d. Multicore/minicore myopathy
5. Myopathies associated with selected infectious agents
   a. HIV and human T-lymphotropic virus 1–associated myositis
   b. Trichinosis
   c. Toxoplasmosis
6. Metabolic myopathies (some)
   a. GDS II (acid alpha-glucosidase deficiency or Pompe disease)
   b. GSD III (debrancher enzyme deficiency)
   c. GSD IV (branching enzyme deficiency)
   d. Lipid storage myopathies
7. Myotonic disorders
   a. Myotonic dystrophy type 1 (DM1) and myotonic dystrophy type 2 (DM2)
   b. Myotonia congenita, paramyotonia congenita (PMC), potassium-aggravated myotonias
   c. Hyperkalemic periodic paralysis

Depending on the differential diagnosis and the patient comorbidities, additional studies may be needed. Neuromuscular junction disorders generally present with fatigable proximal more than distal muscle weakness. In these circumstances, repetitive nerve stimulation studies of at least one distal and one proximal muscle should be performed. If the amplitudes of the CMAPs are reduced, it is necessary to rule out a presynaptic neuromuscular junction disorder, such as Lambert-Eaton myasthenic

---

Box 3
Suggested EDX protocol for the assessment of a suspected myopathy

1. Routine NCSs

   a. At least one motor and one sensory conduction study from one upper extremity and one lower extremity (eg, ulnar motor, ulnar sensory, tibial, or sural)

   Comments

   • If there is a clinical history of fatigability, consider repetitive nerve stimulation studies of at least one distal and one proximal muscle to evaluate for neuromuscular junction disorders.

   • If the amplitudes of the compound muscle action potentials (CMAPs) are reduced, exercise the muscle maximally for 10 seconds, then repeat a single supramaximal stimulation. A significant (>100% of baseline) increment in CMAP amplitude is suggestive of a presynaptic neuromuscular junction disorder.

   • If there is clinical suspicion for a myotonic disorder, consider performing short and long exercise tests.

2. EMG

   a. At least one proximal and one distal muscle from one upper extremity (eg, deltoid, biceps, extensor digitorum communis, or first dorsal interosseous)

   b. At least one proximal and one distal muscle from one lower extremity (eg, iliopsoas, vastus lateralis, tibialis anterior, or gastrocnemius)

   c. Thoracic paraspinals

   Comments

   • The number and location of muscles studied depends on the pattern of weakness.

   • It is best to study muscles that are clinically weak.

   • If both sides are affected equally, perform EDX on the dominant side. Muscle biopsy then is performed on the nondominant side.

   • It is best to study muscles that can be easily biopsied on the contralateral side (eg, deltoid, biceps, extensor digitorum communis, or vastus lateralis).

   • If results of routine EMG are indeterminate, consider quantitative MUAP analysis.

---

syndrome. This can be generally accomplished by exercising the muscle maximally for 10 seconds and repeating a single supramaximal stimulation. A significant increment in CMAP amplitude is suggestive of a presynaptic neuromuscular junction disorder (**Fig. 3**). The cutoff for significant CMAP increase has traditionally been considered greater than 100% of baseline, although recent studies suggest that a cutoff of 60% may provide better sensitivity without sacrificing specificity in the appropriate clinical setting.[3] Finally, if there is clinical suspicion for a channelopathy, short and long exercise tests may be considered to help narrow down the differential and direct genetic testing (discussed later and by Fournier and colleagues[4,5]).

Electromyography

Needle EMG examination is the most informative part of the EDX study in myopathic disorders.[6,7] It can confirm the presence of a myopathy, narrow down the differential, and identify an appropriate biopsy site. The number and location of muscles studied depends on the pattern of weakness. At a minimum, the authors recommend studying one proximal and one distal muscle from one upper extremity and from one lower extremity as well as the thoracic paraspinals. This may be sufficient when there is

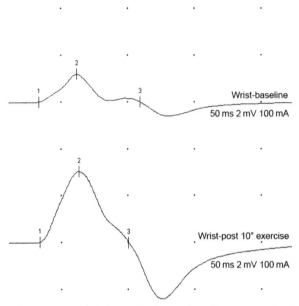

Fig. 3. Incremental response to brief exercise in Lambert-Eaton myasthenic syndrome. The upper trace shows the baseline ulnar-abductor digiti minimi CMAP stimulating at the wrist. Baseline CMAP amplitude was reduced compared with normal (1.2 mV). The lower trace shows the ulnar CMAP stimulating at the wrist immediately after 10 seconds of isometrically resisted finger abduction. The amplitude of the ulnar CMAP post 10 seconds of exercise was 3 mV.

a high clinical suspicion of myopathy and a patient does not have comorbidities that may affect the needle study (such as a radiculopathy or entrapment neuropathy). Commonly assessed muscles include the deltoid, biceps, triceps, pronator teres, extensor digitorum communis, first dorsal interosseous, gluteal muscles, iliopsoas, vasti, tibialis anterior, and gastrocnemius. Additional muscles may be selected depending on a patient's pattern of weakness and the clinical suspicion. For example, finger flexors are often evaluated in suspected IBM because they tend to be preferentially affected in this condition. Because most myopathies generally involve proximal muscles first, the diagnostic yield increases when more proximal muscles are sampled. The paraspinals are the most proximal muscles that can be examined and may be the only ones with abnormalities in selected myopathies, such as Pompe disease. Instead of cervical or lumbosacral thoracic paraspinals are examined because they are less likely to be affected by unrelated processes, such as nerve root impingement secondary to degenerative spine disease.

The yield of needle EMG increases if clinically weak muscles are studied. EMG is more sensitive than clinical examination and may reveal abnormalities in muscles that, clinically, were believed spared. This is particularly helpful when a decision needs to be made with regards to which muscle to biopsy. Commonly biopsied muscles include the deltoid, biceps, and vasti, and, occasionally, the extensor digitorum communis and tibialis anterior. The gastrocnemius is also easily accessible, but muscle biopsy results may be confounded by the presence of unrelated chronic neurogenic changes secondary to preganglionic neuropathy, which are commonly encountered in asymptomatic individuals. In some patients, the only clinically weak muscles are not readily accessible for biopsy, such as the hip girdle muscles. In these circumstances, the value of the EMG is to identify suitable targets for biopsy. It is best not to biopsy a muscle where needle EMG has been recently performed in order not to mistake inflammatory changes secondary to needle insertion for true pathologic findings. If both sides are affected equally, the authors perform needle EMG on the dominant side. Muscle biopsy then is performed on the nondominant side, which is generally more comfortable for the patient, especially if an upper extremity is biopsied.

The analysis of spontaneous activity is helpful in narrowing down the differential diagnosis. Muscle membrane irritability, in the form of increased insertional activity, fibrillation potentials, and positive sharp waves (PSWs), is characteristic of certain myopathies but not others (inflammatory and toxic/necrotic processes, muscular dystrophies, and selected congenital and metabolic disorders [see **Box 2**]). Although fibrillation potentials and PSWs are often colloquially referred to as denervating potentials, the authors do not favor this term. Denervation implies the presence of an underlying neurogenic pathophysiologic mechanism. Fibrillation potentials and PSWs may, however, also be present in myopathic disorders when the muscle membrane is irritable due to the presence of inflammation or necrosis. Thus, these myopathies are reported as myopathy with muscle membrane irritability or membrane instability and include inflammatory and toxic/necrotic processes, muscular dystrophies and selected congenital and metabolic disorders.

Occasionally, in chronic myopathies, complex repetitive discharges (CRDs) may be seen. This type of abnormal spontaneous activity is nonspecific and simply speaks to the chronic nature of the underlying process. Alternatively, myotonic discharges yield additional diagnostic information (see **Box 2**). Myotonic discharges, similarly to fibrillations, PSWs and CRDs, are generated at the muscle fiber level. Although their morphology is similar to fibrillations and PSWs, they characteristically wax and wane in both frequency and amplitude. They are typically seen in myotonic disorders, such as DM1 and DM2, myotonia congenita, PMC, potassium-aggravated myotonias, and potassium-sensitive periodic paralysis. In addition, electrical myotonia may be occasionally encountered in selected myopathies that do not present with clinical myotonia, including inflammatory myopathies, metabolic myopathies (eg, Pompe disease), and toxic myopathies (see **Box 2**).

Finally, there are some circumstances when the normal insertional activity generated by needle insertion is decreased. This may occur in chronic end-stage myopathies, when electrically active muscle fibers are replaced by fat or connective tissue, typically in muscular dystrophies or, occasionally, in long-standing inflammatory myopathies. The electromyographer may also feel increased resistance to needle advancement due to the fibrotic nature of the remaining muscle. Decreased insertional activity may also been seen in patients with certain glycogen storage disorders, such as McArdle disease, experiencing a contracture in that muscle or during an episode of severe weakness from periodic paralysis.

Analysis of motor unit action potential (MUAP) morphology and recruitment pattern is the key element of needle EMG that helps establish the diagnosis of a myopathy. In myopathic processes, there is dropout or dysfunction of individual muscle fibers (see **Fig. 1**). Thus, the size of the motor unit decreases. The number of available motor units does not change because the pathologic process occurs distal to the motor axons. This results in the emergence of short, small, polyphasic MUAPs (see **Figs. 1** and **2**). Sometimes, this combination of findings is referred to as myopathic unit. The authors discourage the use of this term because similar MUAPs may be occasionally found in neurogenic and neuromuscular junction disorders and, therefore, do not always imply a primary muscle disease. Most notably, they may be seen in early reinnervation after severe denervation (nascent motor units) when each motor unit is composed of only few fibers that have successfully reinnervated. More rarely, they may be seen in neuromuscular junction disorders when there is significant block resulting in functional dropout of individual muscle fibers within each motor unit.

When analyzing MUAP morphology, 3 parameters are evaluated: duration, amplitude, and number of phases. In myopathies, MUAP duration and amplitude both decrease, whereas the number of phases increases; hence MUAPs are brief, small, and polyphasic (see **Figs. 1** and **2**). The most important of these parameters is MUAP duration. The decrease in MUAP duration most closely reflects the decrease in the total number of muscle fibers per motor unit, including those that are located at a distance from the recording electrode. Acoustically, this corresponds to a crisp, high-pitch sound. To diagnose a myopathy, however, many MUAPs should be analyzed per muscle and the results compared with what is normally expected for that particular muscle. There is a range of MUAP duration, influenced by age (MUAP duration increases with age) and muscle studied (eg, some small facial muscles normally have much smaller MUAPs than big limb muscles). Mean MUAP duration is reduced in myopathies, although some of the MUAPs may still be normal.

Occasionally, the results of qualitative needle EMG are indeterminate. This may occur when there are only subtle MUAP changes. In such cases, if there is a high clinical suspicion of an underlying myopathy, quantitative MUAP analysis may be performed to increase the diagnostic yield. This is accomplished using standard EMG equipment. Quantitative data regarding the duration of at least 20 MUAPs are collected. Results are then compared with established age-matched, muscle-specific normative values (for a complete description of quantitative EMG and normative data, see Nandedkar and colleagues[8]).

In a myopathy, these short, small, polyphasic, high-pitch MUAPs display a characteristic early recruitment pattern. Because each motor unit is smaller than normal, it can generate only a small amount of force. Therefore, to produce even a small amount of power, individuals need to recruit many MUAPs that fill the screen early on during muscle contraction (see **Fig. 2**). Only the electromyographer performing the study can adequately identify recruitment as early because how much force is being generated to make such an assessment needs to be known. Importantly, in myopathies, a full interference pattern is seen even in very weak muscles, with many units firing at the same time but producing little power. This is in contrast to weakness secondary to neurogenic processes or central processes. In the former, the interference pattern is not full due to the loss of available motor units. The remaining motor units fire rapidly as a compensatory mechanism creating the pattern of reduced recruitment with rapid firing. In the latter, recruitment is actually normal, but the interference pattern is not full due to lack of activation, with resulting slow firing rate.

The only exception to the pattern of short, small, polyphasic MUAPs with early recruitment (described previously) is cases of end-stage muscle that may occasionally be seen in severe chronic myopathies. If all the muscle fibers of an individual motor unit are lost, there is a reduction in the number of available motor units resulting in reduced recruitment. Some reinnervation and motor unit remodeling may also occur overtime and a mixed population of short and long duration MUAPs may occasionally be seen in severe chronic myopathies, such as IBM, long-standing polymyositis and dermatomyositis, and end-stage muscular dystrophies. Finally, as discussed previously, short, small, polyphasic MUAPs may also be seen in nascent motor units. In these cases, recruitment of such units is reduced, reflecting the reduced number of motor units available due to the underlying neurogenic process.

EDX PATTERNS IN SELECTED MYOPATHIES
Muscular Dystrophies

The muscular dystrophies are a group of hereditary, progressive muscle disorders characterized by necrosis of muscle tissue and replacement by connective and fatty tissue.[9] The best-known muscular dystrophies are the dystrophinopathies (Duchenne muscular dystrophy [DMD] and Becker muscular dystrophy [BMD]), which are caused by mutations in the gene encoding the muscle protein dystrophin.[10] EDX testing is of limited utility in the dystrophinopathies, particularly when there is a positive family history. Definitive diagnosis requires genetic testing and, at times, muscle biopsy. EDX testing may be helpful, however, in sporadic cases of DMD and in BMD, which may have a more benign phenotype and a broader differential diagnosis. If needle EMG is performed in a patient with a dystrophinopathy, it typically reveals increased insertional and spontaneous activity in the form of fibrillation potentials and PSWs, along with brief, small, polyphasic MUAPs with early recruitment. In the end stages of the disease, however, when muscle is replaced by connective and fatty tissue, the insertional activity is reduced and a mixed population of short and long duration MUAPs might be appreciated, reflecting the chronicity of the disease process.[11,12]

EDX testing is more helpful in the other muscular dystrophies, in which CK levels may be only mildly elevated and the differential diagnosis is broader. EDX findings again include abnormal spontaneous activity (fibrillation potentials and PSWs) and short, small, polyphasic MUAPs with early recruitment. The pattern of muscle involvement, such as limb girdle versus distal, depends on the specific disease process.

Polymyositis/Dermatomyositis

Polymyositis and dermatomyositis are idiopathic inflammatory myopathies that are characterized on needle EMG by the presence of prominent muscle membrane irritability (fibrillations, PSWs, and even myotonic discharges), especially in proximal muscles.[13,14] MUAPs are small, short, and polyphasic and recruit early. These abnormal features do not distinguish inflammatory myopathies from other myopathies with muscle membrane instability. In long-standing disease, a mixed population of small and long duration MUAPs may be seen (discussed previously).

The degree of abnormal muscle membrane irritability is believed to reflect the ongoing disease activity. Many patients with inflammatory myopathies are treated with high-dose steroids. Some may develop new weakness after a period of symptom improvement on steroids. In these cases, it needs to be determined whether the new weakness is secondary to an increase in disease activity or is attributable to type 2 muscle fiber atrophy, which may occur from disuse or chronic steroid administration. Abnormal spontaneous activity is expected in active myositis, although it is not associated with isolated type 2 muscle fiber atrophy (discussed later).

Inclusion Body Myositis

IBM is an idiopathic inflammatory myopathy that presents generally after the age of 50 years with slowly progressive weakness. The clinical hallmark of IBM is early involvement of the quadriceps, wrist and finger flexors, and ankle dorsiflexors. The clinical diagnosis is often elusive and many patients have been misdiagnosed with other inflammatory myopathies.[15] Unfortunately, patients with IBM do not typically respond to immunosuppressive therapies. EDX studies are nonspecific and may actually provide additional diagnostic confusion. Fibrillations and PSWs are common and, early in the course, are associated with small, short, polyphasic MUAPs. Due to the insidious nature of the myopathic process, however, many patients also exhibit large, long MUAPs, reflecting the chronicity of the disease.[15,16] Although the morphology of these units may resemble those seen in a chronic neurogenic process, the recruitment pattern in IBM is early pointing toward a myogenic basis. In addition, approximately a third of the patients also demonstrate a mild axonal sensory polyneuropathy on nerve conduction studies.

Toxic/Necrotic Myopathies

Toxic/necrotic myopathies may be induced by several drugs, such as the lipid-lowering agents, or by multifactorial mechanisms, such as in the setting of a critical illness. Asymptomatic CK elevation is common in patients taking lipid-lowering agents. In the absence of symptoms, EMG is often normal. More rarely, these same agents may trigger a toxic myopathy and result in clinical weakness. In these circumstances, fibrillations, PSWs, and even myotonic discharges with early recruitment of short-duration MUAPs become apparent in weak muscles.[17,18]

Patients in an ICU may develop generalized weakness due to critical illness polyneuropathy or myopathy.[19,20] It can be difficult to differentiate between these two conditions and patients can present with a combination of the two. Distal and proximal muscles are both affected. Nerve conduction studies demonstrate low CMAP amplitudes without any evidence of demyelination. Sensory nerve action potential may also be reduced in amplitude if there is a concomitant polyneuropathy or from technical reasons if there is third spacing and edema, which are not uncommon in critically ill patients. Needle EMG shows prominent muscle membrane irritability as well as early recruitment of short-duration MUAPs.

Steroid Myopathy

Steroid myopathy manifests as proximal muscle weakness and atrophy, affecting the leg more than the arms. The needle EMG is typically normal.[21] On histopathology, steroid myopathy is characterized by type 2B muscle fiber atrophy, which explains the paucity of findings on EDX testing. The evaluation of MUAP morphology on needle EMG is limited to the analysis of type 1 fibers, which, based on the size principle of recruitment, are the first recruited fibers. Because type 2 fibers are preferentially affected in steroid myopathy, the abnormal MUAPs they generate are not detectable because these are obscured by their initially recruited type I counterparts.

Pompe Disease

Pompe disease (GSD II or acid alpha-glucosidase deficiency) is a metabolic myopathy caused by deficiency of a lysosomal enzyme, which is important in carbohydrate metabolism causing muscle weakness. It may present in a classic severe infantile form or have a later childhood or adult onset. The diagnosis of the adult-onset form may be elusive because CK levels may be normal and the pattern of weakness (generally proximal) may be confused with several other myopathies. There can be a predilection for involvement of the muscles of ventilation, with dyspnea the presenting symptom in some patients. Recognition of this disease is important because infusion of the recombinant enzyme is available. Characteristically, needle EMG in Pompe disease is irritable.[22] Abundant spontaneous activity may be present in proximal muscles and may include not only fibrillations and PSWs but also CRDs and myotonic discharges. These findings, however, in mild cases, may be limited to the paraspinal muscles.

Dystrophic Myotonias and Nondystrophic Myotonias

Myotonic disorders include the myotonic dystrophies and the nondystrophic myotonias. The former, DM1 and DM2 (or proximal myotonic myopathy), are characterized by dystrophy of the muscle tissue, progressive weakness, and clinical myotonia. Most patients with DM1 and DM2 exhibit electrical myotonia, although myotonia may not necessarily be present in every muscle.[23] The distribution of electrical myotonia is predominantly distal in both the arms and legs in DM1. In DM2, electrical myotonia is seen distally in the arms, but it often affects both the proximal and distal leg muscles.[23] Finally, classic waxing-waning discharges (true electrical myotonia) predominate in DM1. Alternatively, in DM2, a less specific waning pattern (ie, spontaneous discharges that only wane in frequency or amplitude, or pseudomyotonia) is more common, making the electrodiagnosis of DM2 more challenging.[23]

The nondystrophic myotonias are caused by mutations in different ion channels (hence, the alternative name, channelopathies) and manifest with various phenotypes (stiffness, myotonia, and episodes of transient weakness in variable combinations) without dystrophic changes in the muscle tissue.[24] Needle EMG may identify myotonic discharges in myotonia congenita, PMC, potassium-aggravated myotonias, and, at times, hyperkalemic periodic paralysis. Clinical and electrical myotonia are absent in hypokalemic periodic paralysis. Nerve conduction studies play an important role in differentiating among these disorders because specific patterns may be recognized on short and long exercise tests helping to direct genetic testing.

The short and long exercise tests are variations of standard motor nerve conduction studies.[5,6] They are typically performed on the ulnar nerve, recording from the abductor digiti minimi. The CMAP amplitude is measured 3 to 5 times before exercise to ensure a stable baseline. For the short exercise test, the patient is instructed to isometrically activate the selected muscle for 10 seconds. This is followed by serial assessment of the CMAP amplitude immediately after exercise and then every 10 seconds for 1 minute. A normal response includes a transient 5% to 10% increase in CMAP amplitude immediately after exercise with normalization within 10 seconds. Typically, 3 subsequent trials are performed. The same protocol may also be repeated after limb cooling, particularly if PMC is suspected (discussed later).

Box 4
Myopathies that may have a normal EMG

1. Type II muscle atrophy

    a. Steroid myopathy

    b. Disuse myopathy

2. Some mitochondrial myopathies

3. Some congenital myopathies

4. Metabolic myopathies with dynamic[a] phenotype if not performed during acute exacerbations

    a. GSD V (McArdle disease or myophosphorylase deficiency)

    b. GDS VII (phosphofructokinase deficiency)

    c. Carnitine palmityltransferase II deficiency

[a] Here, metabolic myopathies are referred to as having a dynamic phenotype when they are associated with exercise-induced symptoms (exertional myalgias, cramps, and myoglobinuria) as the dominant clinical features.

Box 5
Myopathies that may have a normal CK level

A normal or only mildly elevated CK level does not preclude the following diagnoses in the appropriate clinical context:

- Dermatomyositis

- IBM

- Congenital myopathies

- Metabolic myopathies

- Mitochondrial myopathies

More rarely, some of the muscular dystrophies (limb-girdle, facioscapulohumeral, scapuloperoneal, Emery-Dreifuss, and oculopharyngeal and distal) may be present with normal or only mildly elevated CK levels.

The long exercise test involves isometric contraction of the selected muscle for 5 minutes, with periods of brief rest (3 to 4 seconds) every 30 to 45 seconds during the exercise. This is followed by sequential CMAP measurements immediately after exercise, then every minute for the first 5 minutes after exercise, and finally every 5 minutes for approximately 45 minutes. In normal subjects, a transient mild decrease in CMAP amplitude (5%–10%) is observed immediately after exercise, but the CMAP amplitude normalizes within 1 min and remains stable for the remainder of the test.

Box 6
Diagnostic studies used to characterize myopathic processes

Often performed to diagnose a myopathy

1. CK levels

2. Thyrotropin, electrolytes, renal and liver function tests, complete blood count, erythrocyte sedimentation rate, and serum protein electrophoresis/immunofixation

3. Genetic testing (hypothesis-driven, step-wise; avoid panels)

4. NCS/EMG

5. Muscle biopsy (if above are nondiagnostic)

Used only within the appropriate clinical context, to further characterize a myopathy

1. ECG and echocardiogram

2. Pulmonary function tests

3. Videofluoroscopic swallow studies

4. Exercise forearm test with measurement of lactate and ammonia.

5. Malignancy work-up (occult malignancies may be associated with inflammatory and necrotizing myopathies)

6. Antinuclear antibody, rheumatoid factor, and antibodies to extractable nuclear antigens (connective tissue disorders may be associated with inflammatory and necrotizing myopathies)

7. Myositis-specific antibodies (especially Jo-1, which may indicate concurrent interstitial lung disease in patients with inflammatory and necrotizing myopathies)

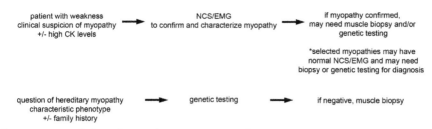

Fig. 4. Suggested algorithm to diagnose a myopathic process.

The short exercise test may identify characteristic response patterns in some patients with PMC and myotonia congenital (MC). In PMC, there may be a decrement in the CMAP amplitude compared with baseline that worsens with successive stimuli and trials.

Typically, performing the short exercise test after limb cooling bring out even more marked reductions in CMAP amplitude. In MC, the short exercise test may be normal (usually in the autosomal dominant form) or abnormal (in the autosomal recessive form). The abnormal pattern seen in autosomal recessive MC includes an initial CMAP reduction immediately after exercise that improves with successive stimuli returning to baseline within 1 minute. Such CMAP amplitude reduction is less marked during subsequent trials. The long exercise test is most useful to identify hereditary periodic paralysis. In periodic paralysis, there is an early increase in CMAP amplitude immediately after exercise that is followed by a gradual delayed decrease over a prolonged period of time. The long exercise test is also abnormal in PMC, with early decrease in CMAP amplitude immediately after exercise that may persist for hours. For a more detailed description of these techniques, readers are referred to the seminal articles by Fournier and colleagues.[5,6]

SUMMARY

In summary, EDX studies may play an important role in the evaluation of patients with suspected myopathies (**Boxes 4** and **5**). Although multiple diagnostic tests are often used to work-up a patient (**Box 6**), they are often expensive and uncomfortable for the patient. Thus, the authors cannot emphasize enough that these tools should be used judiciously in a step-wise, hypothesis-driven fashion. A comprehensive history and physical examination along with pattern recognition are invaluable in directing further testing, so as to avoid unnecessary tests and, most importantly, interpret test results correctly (**Fig. 4**).

REFERENCES

1. Amato AA, Russell J. Testing in neuromuscular disease-electrodiagnosis and other modalities. In: Sydor AM, Naglieri C, editors. Neuromuscular disorders. 1st edition. New York: McGraw-Hill; 2008. p. 17–69.
2. Preston D, Shapiro B. Myopathy. In: Preston D, Shapiro B, editors. Electromyography and neuromuscular disorders. 2nd edition. Philadelphia: Elsevier; 2005. p. 575–89.
3. Oh SJ, Kurokawa K, Claussen GC, et al. Electrophysiological diagnostic criteria of Lambert-Eaton myasthenic syndrome. Muscle Nerve 2005;32(4):515–20.

4. Fournier E, Arzel M, Sternberg, et al. Electromyography guides toward subgroups of mutations in muscle channelopathies. Ann Neurol 2004;56(5): 650–61.

5. Fournier E, Viala K, Gervais H, et al. Cold extends electromyography distinction between ion channel mutations causing myotonia. Ann Neurol 2006;60(3): 356–65.

6. Petajan JH. AAEM minimonograph #3: motor unit recruitment. Muscle Nerve 1991;14(6):489–502.

7. Daube JR. AAEM minimonograph #11: needle examination in clinical electromyography. Muscle Nerve 1991;14(8):685–700.

8. Nandedkar SD, Stalberg EV, Sanders D. Quantitative EMG. In: Dumitru D, Amato AA, Swartz MJ, editors. Electrodiagnostic medicine. 2nd edition. Philadelphia: Hanley & Belfus; 2002. p. 293–356.

9. Cardamone M, Darras BT, Ryan MM. Inherited myopathies and muscular dystrophies. Semin Neurol 2008;28(2):250–9.

10. Hoffman EP, Fischbeck KH, Brown RH, et al. Characterization of dystrophin in muscle-biopsy specimens from patients with Duchenne's or Becker's muscular dystrophy. N Engl J Med 1988;318(21):1363–8.

11. Emeryk-Szajewska B, Kopeć J. Electromyographic pattern in duchenne and becker muscular dystrophy. Part I: electromyographic pattern in subsequent stages of muscle lesion in duchenne muscular dystrophy. Electromyogr Clin Neurophysiol 2008;48(6–7):265–77.

12. Emeryk-Szajewska B, Kopeć J. Electromyographic pattern in duchenne and becker muscular dystrophy. Part II. Electromyographic pattern in becker muscular dystrophy in comparison with duchenne muscular dystrophy. Electromyogr Clin Neurophysiol 2008;48(6–7):279–84.

13. Amato AA, Barohn RJ. Evaluation and treatment of inflammatory myopathies. J Neurol Neurosurg Psychiatry 2009;80(10):1060–8.

14. Buchthal F, Pinelli P. Muscle action potentials in polymyositis. Neurology 1953; 3(6):424–36.

15. Lotz BP, Engel AG, Nishino H, et al. Inclusion body myositis. Observations in 40 patients. Brain 1989;112(Pt 3):727–47.

16. Joy JL, Oh SJ, Baysal AI. Electrophysiological spectrum of inclusion body myositis. Muscle Nerve 1990;13(10):949–51.

17. Grable-Esposito P, Katzberg HD, Greenberg SA, et al. Immune-mediated necrotizing myopathy associated with statins. Muscle Nerve 2010;41(2): 185–90.

18. Meriggioli MN, Barboi AC, Rowin J, et al. HMG-CoA reductase inhibitor myopathy: clinical, electrophysiological, and pathologic data in five patients. J Clin Neuromuscul Dis 2001;2(3):129–34.

19. Lacomis D, Petrella JT, Giuliani MJ. Causes of neuromuscular weakness in the intensive care unit: a study of ninety-two patients. Muscle Nerve 1998;21(5): 610–7.

20. Lacomis D, Giuliani MJ, Van Cott A, et al. Acute myopathy of intensive care: clinical, electromyographic, and pathological aspects. Ann Neurol 1996;40(4): 645–54.

21. Buchthal F. Electrophysiological abnormalities in metabolic myopathies and neuropathies. Acta Neurol Scand 1970;46(Suppl 43):129+.

22. Hobson-Webb LD, Dearmey S, Kishnani PS. The clinical and electrodiagnostic characteristics of Pompe disease with post-enzyme replacement therapy findings. Clin Neurophysiol 2011;122(11):2312–7.

23. Logigian EL, Ciafaloni E, Quinn LC, et al. Severity, type, and distribution of myotonic discharges are different in type 1 and type 2 myotonic dystrophy. Muscle Nerve 2007;35:479–85.
24. Matthews E, Fialho D, Tan SV, et al, CINCH Investigators. The non-dystrophic myotonias: molecular pathogenesis, diagnosis and treatment. Brain 2010; 133(Pt 1):9–22.

Electrodiagnosis of Myotonic Disorders

Michael K. Hehir, MD[a],*, Eric L. Logigian, MD[b]

KEYWORDS

- Myotonia • Myotonic dystrophy • Periodic paralysis • Nondystrophic myotonia
- Muscle channelopathies

KEY POINTS

- Clinical or electrical myotonia is caused by a small group of neuromuscular disorders including the dystrophic and nondystrophic myotonias.
- Chloride or sodium muscle channelopathies are the causes of myotonia in the dystrophic and nondystrophic myotonic disorders.
- Electrodiagnostic techniques, including needle electromyogram examination, short and long exercise testing, can help distinguish among the various myotonic disorders.

INTRODUCTION

Clinical and electrical myotonia is caused by a small group of neuromuscular disorders (**Box 1**). Myotonia is due to increased excitability of the muscle membrane often caused by dysfunction of muscle ion channels. Clinical myotonia is manifest by incomplete relaxation of muscle following either voluntary muscle contraction or direct muscle percussion. At the bedside, myotonia is clinically demonstrable by slowed muscle relaxation during repetitive hand grip and eye closure or by delayed relaxation of a muscle contraction evoked by tapping various muscles such as the thenar eminence or the finger extensors.

Electrical myotonia is an abnormal spontaneous muscle fiber discharge observed on needle electromyogram (EMG) examination. Electrical myotonia appears as repetitive muscle fiber potential discharges (eg, positive waves or fibrillation potentials) with waxing and waning frequency and amplitude with a firing rate between 20 and 80 Hz (**Fig. 1A**).[9] When played over the audio, myotonic discharges have a characteristic sound of a dive bomber, or in the modern day, an accelerating and decelerating motorcycle engine. Electrical myotonia must be distinguished from neuromyotonia (frequency of greater than 150 Hz with a pinging sound) and chronic repetitive

[a] Department of Neurology, University of Vermont, 1 South Prospect Street, Burlington, VT 05401, USA; [b] Department of Neurology, University of Rochester, 601 Elmwood Ave, Box 673, Rochester, NY 14642, USA
* Corresponding author.
E-mail address: Michael.Hehir@vtmednet.org

Phys Med Rehabil Clin N Am 24 (2013) 209–220
http://dx.doi.org/10.1016/j.pmr.2012.08.015
1047-9651/13/$ – see front matter © 2013 Elsevier Inc. All rights reserved.

> **Box 1**
> **Neuromuscular disorders with myotonia**
>
> *Muscular dystrophies:*
> - Myotonic dystrophy type 1 and 2
> - Myofibrillar myopathies[1]
>
> *Muscle channelopathies:*
> - Nondystrophic myotonia (myotonia congenita, paramyotonia congenita, sodium channel myotonia)
> - Hyperkalemic periodic paralysis
>
> *Metabolic myopathy:*
> - Acid maltase deficiency[a,2,3]
> - Debrancher deficiency[a,4]
> - McArdle disease (myophosphorylase deficiency)[a,4]
>
> *Toxic myopathies[a]:*
> - Chloroquine/hydroxychloroquine myopathy[5,6]
> - Statin myopathy[7]
> - Colchicine myopathy[8]
>
> *Endocrine myopathies[a]:*
> - Hypothyroidism[4]
>
> *Inflammatory myopathies[a,4]*
> - Polymyositis
> - Dermatomyositis
>
> [a] Electrical myotonia without clinical myotonia.

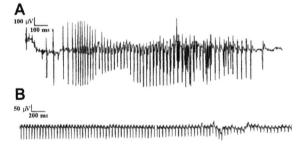

Fig. 1. Electrical myotonia. (*A*) Two-second myotonic discharge in DM1 patient with typical waxing and waning frequency and amplitude. (*B*) Four-second waning only myotonic discharge in a DM2 patient in which frequency and amplitude decline gradually with no waxing component. (*From* Logigian EL, Ciafaloni E, Quinn LC, et al. Severity, type, and distribution of myotonic discharges are different in type 1 and type 2 myotonic dystrophy. Muscle Nerve 2007;35:479–85; with permission. Copyright with Wiley InterScience.)

discharges of constant, or less commonly, waning frequency with a machinelike sound.[9]

This article focuses on electrodiagnosis of the primary myotonic disorders (myotonic dystrophy and the nondystrophic myotonias [NDMs]) as well as the related periodic paralysis (PP) muscle channelopathies.

EVALUATION OF CHANNELOPATHIES

Muscle ion channelopathies alter muscle membrane resting potential, resulting in either muscle hyperexcitability (eg, myotonia) or inexcitability (eg, muscle weakness). In the NDMs, muscle membrane hyperexcitability typically results in muscle "stiffness" during voluntary movement because of delayed skeletal muscle relaxation caused by repetitive muscle fiber action potentials (myotonia) as a result of mutations in the chloride (CLCN1) or sodium (SCN4A) skeletal muscle channel genes.[10] By contrast, in the PPs, skeletal muscle membrane, inexcitability results in prolonged episodic muscle weakness caused by mutations in the sodium (SCN4A), calcium (CACN1A), and potassium (KCNJ2) channels.[11] Of note, patients with both hyperkalemic PP and paramyotonia congenita (PC), due to different SCN4A mutations, have myotonia and episodes of skeletal muscle weakness.

Nondystrophic Myotonia

The NDMs include myotonia congenita (MC), PC, and sodium channel myotonia (SCM). The main clinical symptom of NDM is muscle stiffness from myotonia. Some patients also develop weakness and pain.[10] These conditions must be distinguished from myotonic dystrophy type 1 and 2 (DM1 and DM2), which have significant, extramuscular, systemic manifestations. On clinical grounds alone, there is often an overlap among DM2 and NDM. Electrodiagnostic and genetic testing help differentiate among the NDMs and between NDM and DM. When functionally debilitating, myotonia in NDM is treated with sodium channel blockade.[10,12]

Myotonia congenita

MC presents as either an autosomal recessive form (also known as Becker disease) or a less severe autosomal dominant form (called Thomsen disease.) Both are caused by loss of function mutations in the CLCN-1 chloride channel, resulting in relative depolarization of the muscle membrane.[10,12] Autosomal recessive MC presents between age 4 and 12 years and autosomal dominant MC presents before age 3 years.[10] Myotonia typically develops with vigorous voluntary movement after resting; a warm-up phenomenon, that is, improvement in muscle relaxation with repetitive hand grip or rarely eye closure is often described.[10] Patients with Becker (but not Thomsen) disease may develop transient weakness or "paresis" lasting seconds to minutes that resolves (like the myotonia) with repetitive muscle contractions.[10]

Paramyotonia congenita (Group 1 SCM)

PC is an autosomal dominant disease due to a gain of function mutation in the SCN4A muscle sodium channel, resulting in relative muscle membrane depolarization.[10,12] Patients develop not only muscle stiffness due to myotonia but also flaccid muscle weakness when depolarization progresses to membrane inexcitability. Cold temperature and exercise exacerbate myotonia and weakness in this disease.[10,12] Face and hand muscles are preferentially affected. Most PC patients have paradoxic myotonia of hand grip or eye closure characterized by progressively slower muscle relaxation with repetitive activity, the opposite of the warm-up phenomenon typically seen in the chloride channelopathies.[10,12] Patients present during the first or second decade.[10,12] PC is allelic to hyperkalemic PP and like that condition results in pro-longed episodes of muscle weakness.[10]

Sodium channel myotonias (Group 2 SCM)
This group of autosomal dominant diseases is also caused by gain of function muta-tions of the SCN4A channel similar to PC.[10] However, group 2 SCM patients do not typically develop attacks of weakness (as in PC). In contrast to chloride channelopa-thies, patients with group 2 SCM are often sensitive to potassium, may have eyelid myotonia, lack transient paresis, and more often have pain.[10,13] SCM can also be distinguished from PC and chloride channelopathies based on electrodiagnostic tes-ting(see later discussion).[14–16]

Electrodiagnosis of NDM

Commercial genetic testing is available for some of the causative mutations in NDM, but there is a false-negative rate in these conditions as high as 20%.[17] Electrodiagnos-tic studies are extremely helpful in directing genetic testing and also making the diag-nosis of NDM in patients with negative genetic testing. Evidence of membrane hyperexcitability (eg, myotonic discharges) is sought with needle EMG examination, whereas evidence of membrane inexcitability (eg, drop in motor response amplitude) is investigated with long and short exercise testing.

Needle EMG reveals diffuse myotonic discharges in proximal and distal muscles in NDM[10,12,14,18]; at times the number of myotonic discharges can be so substantial that evaluation of voluntary motor unit potential morphology and recruitment is not possible. In addition to myotonic discharges, low-amplitude (100–600 μV), high-frequency (150–250 Hz) discharges resembling neuromyotonic discharges have recently been observed in some NDM patients.[16] Occasionally, repetitive firing of muscle fibers following a single stimulus termed "postexercise myotonic potentials" can be observed as delayed lower amplitude motor responses following the compound motor action potential (CMAP) during performance of routine nerve conduction studies.[14] Postexer-cise myotonic potentials are described in both SCN4A and CLCN1 mutations.[14]

In general, the pattern and location of electrical myotonia does not distinguish among the NDM disorders,[14] but the long and especially the short exercise test results can be helpful in this regard. Postexercise recording of serial CMAPs evaluates the functional consequences of ion channel mutations. A long-exercise protocol was initially described, which shows 80% sensitivity in PP and 15% to 30% sensitivity in NDM.[19] Subsequently, a short-exercise protocol was developed that has been shown to be more sensitive for the detection of NDMs in general and useful in differentiating among the individual NDM disorders.

Short-exercise protocol
In the short-exercise protocol, serial CMAPs are recorded from the abductor digiti minimi (ADM) after supramaximal stimulation of the ulnar nerve at the wrist. Supra-maximal CMAPs are recorded at baseline and then following 10 seconds of sustained contraction of the ADM. Additional CMAPs are recorded 2 seconds after exercise and then every 10 seconds for a total of 60 seconds; this protocol is repeated 3 times.[14] Postexercise CMAP amplitudes are compared with the patient's preexercise baseline CMAP amplitudes. The short-exercise protocol is easy to perform and causes minimal patient discomfort when compared with other electrodiagnostic tests such as pro-longed repetitive nerve stimulation.

The short-exercise protocol has a high sensitivity of 100% (83%–100%) in PC, 83% (53%–100%) in MC, and 60% in SCM.[12,14,15] Repeating the protocol with limb cooling (to 20–25°C) improves the sensitivity in MC (70%–100%) and exaggerates the abnormality observed in PC.[15,16]

Three patterns are observed in patients with NDM, Fournier I, II, and III.[10,14,15] Patients with PC exhibit Fournier pattern I with a decrement in CMAP amplitude (19%–40% less than preexercise baseline CMAP), which persists for 60 seconds and which increases with subsequent trials and with cooling (**Fig. 2**).[14,15] This decrement reproduces the weakness in PC patients that develops with exercise, especially with muscle cooling.

Patients with MC commonly exhibit Fournier pattern II with an initial postexercise CMAP decrement, which repairs by 60 seconds and is less pronounced on subsequent trials (see **Fig. 2**).[14] The Fournier pattern II is also observed in some patients with DM1 and DM2 whose myotonia, like MC, is due to chloride channel dysfunction.[10] At room temperature, a subset of MC patients (primarily dominant MC) exhibit Fournier pattern III without a postexercise decrement or sometimes an initial increment following exercise with return to baseline (see **Fig. 2**).[14] Fournier III is also observed in normal controls and most patients with SCM.[14,15] However, repeating the short exercise test with cooling reveals the Fournier pattern II in 91% to 100% of patients with recessive MC and in 14% to 71% of patients with dominant MC.[15] Rewarming the limb and repeating the test may identify a small group of additional patients with MC.[16]

Most patients with SCM exhibit the Fournier pattern III at room temperature, similar to normal controls. With cooling, a subset of SCM patients exhibits the Fournier pattern I, similar to PC.[15] In one series, combining the clinical symptom of eye closure myotonia (historical or on clinical examination) with the Fournier pattern III distinguished SCM from MC with a specificity of 94% and sensitivity of 82%.[16] Although helpful in the evaluation of hyperkalemic PP, the long exercise test (LET) adds little to the diagnostic evaluation of NDM. The LET has a sensitivity of 25% in MC and 89% in PC.[12,20]

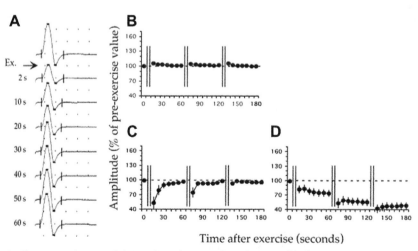

Fig. 2. Short exercise test. (*A*) Transient decrease in CMAP amplitude in myotonia congenita. (*B*) Fournier pattern III: initial increment in CMAP with return to baseline. No change with subsequent tests. (*C*) Fournier pattern II: initial CMAP decrement postexercise with return to baseline on subsequent trials. (*D*) Fournier pattern I: decrement of CMAP amplitude postexercise, which worsens on subsequent trials. (*Modified from* Fournier E, Arzel M, Sternberg D, et al. Electromyography guides toward subgroups of mutations in muscle channelopathies. Ann Neurol 2004;56:650–61; with permission. Copyright with Wiley InterScience.)

Repetitive nerve stimulation

Prolonged repetitive stimulation of the ADM has been studied in NDM. In the typical protocol, the ulnar nerve is stimulated at the wrist at 10 Hz for 10 seconds; the test is repeated after 5 minutes rest with 10 Hz stimulation for 5 seconds.[18] Similar to the short exercise test, repetitive stimulation is repeated with cooling.

At room temperature, patients with autosomal recessive MC and DM exhibit a decrement in CMAP amplitude that is more pronounced with cooling.[18] Patients with PC exhibited a decrement only with cooling.[18] In one series, repetitive nerve stimulation identified two-thirds of patients with recessive MC compared with one-third in the short exercise test.[18] A later trial showed no added diagnostic information with repetitive stimulation when added to the short exercise test.[16] Repetitive stimulation may be useful in identifying patients with recessive MC who exhibit Fournier III pattern on short exercise testing. However, this test causes significant patient discomfort compared with the short exercise test.

Directed genetic testing

Over 100 missense, nonsense, insertion, deletions, and splice site mutations have been identified in the CLCN1 channel gene on chromosome 7q35. More than 40 mutations are described in the SCN4A gene on chromosome 17.[10] Only a portion of these mutations can be evaluated commercially. In addition, genetic testing can be costly and in some cases not covered by the patient's medical insurance policy.

Fournier and colleagues[14,15] propose directed genetic testing based on the results of the short exercise protocol and repetitive nerve stimulation. Patients with the Fournier pattern I should be checked for SCN4A mutations. Patients with the Fournier pattern II should be screened for CLCN1 mutations and if negative SCN4A mutations as a small subset of SCM patients exhibit this pattern. Fournier II patients with negative testing for both CLCN1 and SCN4A should be screened for DM1 and DM2. Patients with the Fournier pattern III who exhibit eyelid myotonia should be screened for SCN4A; those patients without eyelid myotonia should be screened for CLCN1.[16] The 10-Hz repetitive nerve stimulation protocol may help distinguish between SCM and MC in patients with negative genetic testing; this may prove useful if mutation-specific therapies are developed.[18]

Periodic Paralysis

The PPs are autosomal dominant muscle channelopathies that result in muscle inexcitability and recurrent attacks of flaccid paralysis. They include hypokalemic PP, hyperkalemic PP, Andersen-Tawil syndrome (ATS), and thyrotoxic PP. Most weakness episodes are transient and are not life threatening; most affected patients develop persistent mild proximal weakness over time that is not linked to frequency or severity of attacks.[11,12] Patients with ATS may develop life-threatening cardiac arrhythmias.[11] Patients with PP are treated with a combination of lifestyle modification to avoid triggers and medical therapy with carbonic anhydrase inhibition with acetazolamide (125–1000 mg/d) or dichlorphenamide (50–200 mg/d).[11]

Hypokalemic periodic paralysis

Hypokalemic PP is an autosomal dominant muscle channelopathy with incomplete penetrance in women.[11,12,21–23] Prevalence is estimated at 1 per 100,000.[11] Sixty percent of cases are due to mutation in the calcium CACNA1S channel and 20% are due to SCN4A mutations.[11] Patients develop episodes of flaccid focal or generalized weakness that typically spare respiratory and facial muscles. Attacks last for hours or days and usually begin in the first or second decade.[11] Attacks are most common on waking in the morning and may be triggered by prolonged rest after exercise or a carbohydrate rich meal.[11,12] Weakness is typically associated with low serum potassium; attacks can often be aborted with potassium administration.[11]

Thyrotoxic PP is also related to hypokalemia; thyroid-stimulating hormone and free T4 should be evaluated in all cases of suspected hypokalemic PP because patients with this condition often have minimal manifestations of thyrotoxicosis.[11] They do not have a known calcium or sodium channelopathy, but there is genetic data to implicate potassium channel mutations.[24] In addition, patients without channelopathies can develop a subacute proximal myopathy in the setting of severe hypokalemia (serum K <2.5 mEq/L).[25,26]

Hyperkalemic periodic paralysis

Hyperkalemic PP is an autosomal dominant SCN4A channelopathy that is allelic to PC and typically begins in the first decade.[11,12] Attacks of weakness are usually shorter than those in hypokalemic PP (hours) and are associated with elevated levels of potassium in 50% of cases.[11] The remaining 50% have normal potassium levels but are believed to have a relative elevation of potassium level within the normal range, resulting in weakness.[11] Weakness is often triggered by rest after exercise, stress, and fatigue. Unlike hypokalemic PP, electrical myotonia is appreciated in 50% to 75% of cases.[11,12,14] In addition, during attacks of weakness, CMAP amplitude may be decreased or absent as in other causes of PP. Needle EMG examination discloses decreased insertional activity, increased fibrillation potentials/positive waves, and increased polyphasic motor units.[11]

Andersen-Tawil syndrome

ATS is a disorder that combines PP, ventricular arrhythmias, and skeletal anomalies. It is caused by mutations in the inward rectifying muscle potassium channel KCNJ2.[11] Prevalence is estimated to be one-tenth of hypokalemic PP.[11] Episodes of weakness are triggered by rest after exercise and stress.[11] Cardiac abnormalities range from prolongation of the corrected QT interval to ventricular ectopy and runs of ventricular tachycardia.[11] Skeletal anomalies include small mandible, hypertelorism, syndactyly, clinodactyly, broad nose, and short stature.[11,12]

Electrodiagnosis of PP

Similar to NDM, commercial genetic testing for PP is incomplete and in some cases prohibitive because of cost or lack of insurance coverage. Electrodiagnostic testing is helpful in guiding genetic testing and in distinguishing between PP and other forms of weakness. Some patients with hyperkalemic PP show an initial increment during the short exercise protocol.[14] However, the short exercise test does not have significant diagnostic value in PP as most patients show no abnormalities.[14] The LET is more useful in these patients. Some patients with hyperkalemic PP exhibit electrical myotonia; this finding is not described in hypokalemic PP.[11,14]

Long exercise test

LET is also typically performed stimulating the ulnar nerve at the wrist and recording the ADM motor responses. Supramaximal ADM responses are recorded at baseline, throughout 5 minutes of exercise, and then more than 45 to 60 minutes following exercise; investigators vary on the frequency of recordings following exercise.[14,16,19] Patients with PP are expected to show postexercise drop in motor response amplitude or area corresponding to the clinical symptom of flaccid paralysis.

During the LET, baseline supramaximal CMAPs are typically measured every 10 seconds for 1 to 2 minutes to establish a stable baseline. The patient is then exercised for 5 minutes with periodic, short-rest periods every 15 seconds. CMAPs are recorded after each minute of exercise. Some investigators then record postexercise CMAPs every minute for 5 minutes followed by every 5 minute CMAPs for 40 to 45 minutes.[14] Others recommend postexercise CMAPs every 1 to 2 minutes for 30 to 45 minutes.[19] In the initial version of the LET, decrements in amplitude and area were measured from the maximal CMAP obtained during or immediately after exercise.[19,20] Subsequent investigators have measured decrement from the baseline CMAP obtained before exercise.[14] One study shows the methods to be similar, although use of the preexercise baseline may be less sensitive in hyperkalemic PP.[16]

Among the small cohorts studied, the LET has a sensitivity of 80% to 90% in both hypokalemic PP and hyperkalemic PP.[12,14,19,20] In one series of ATS, the LET was demonstrated to have a sensitivity of 80% to 100%, which improved to 100% if CMAP area was examined alone.[16]

Normal controls typically show a small increment in amplitude and area (10%) following exercise and a subsequent decrement of 15% in amplitude and area compared with maximal-exercise CMAP (never more than 30%).[19,20] An abnormal decrease is defined as 40.9% for amplitude and 48% for area (2 SDs).[19,20] When measured from preexercise baseline, an abnormal decrement in CMAP amplitude is defined as greater than 20% of baseline.[14]

Two typical LET patterns are observed in PP, which may help to distinguish between calcium and sodium channel mutations.[14] Patients with a sodium channel mutation often exhibit Fournier pattern IV (**Fig. 3**) manifest by an increment in CMAP amplitude/area with exercise followed by a decrement in amplitude/area 40% to 80% of baseline (dependent on method); maximal decrement is observed between 30 and 45 minutes postexercise.[14,16,20] Fournier pattern V manifest by a maximal decrement in area/amplitude after 20 to 40 minutes is more typical of calcium channel-related PP; this decrement may or may not be preceded by an initial increment in CMAP amplitude/area.[14,16,20] However, there is some cross over between pattern IV and V in hyperkalemic and hypokalemic PP, which may be explained by the proportion of hypokalemic PP patients who have an SCN4A mutation.[14] Pattern V is most typical in ATS.[16]

Directed genetic testing

Genetic testing in PP can be guided by a combination of clinical presentation, serum potassium measurement during an attack, and the LET. Patients with skeletal anomalies and cardiac symptoms should be screened for ATS. In the absence of distinctive clinical or serum K abnormalities, one strategy is to screen patients exhibiting Fournier pattern IV for CACNA1S first and if normal SCN4A. Similarly, patients with Fournier pattern V could be screened for SCN4A first and if normal CACNA1S.

EVALUATION OF MYOTONIC DYSTROPHY

DM1 and DM2 are inherited disorders of skeletal muscle that result in progressive weakness similar to other muscular dystrophies. The presence and pattern of weakness, clinical and electrical myotonia, and extramuscular manifestations distinguish the myotonic dystrophies from NDM and other forms of dystrophy.

Myotonic Dystrophy Type 1

DM1 is an autosomal dominant progressive muscular dystrophy due to an unstable trinucleotide repeat (cytosine-thymine-guanine [CTG]) on chromosome 19q.[27] DM1 exhibits anticipation with more severe disease in subsequent generations who inherit trinucleotide repeats of increasing length.[27,28] Clinically, the age of onset of disease is inversely proportional to the CTG repeat length.[27]

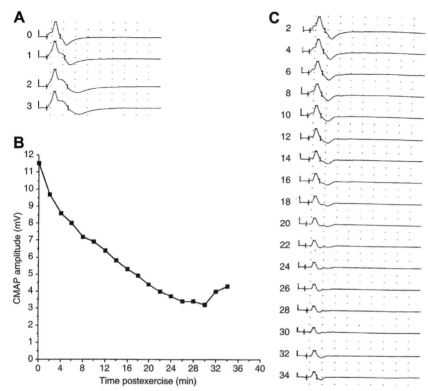

Fig. 3. Long exercise test. Example of long exercise test (Fournier pattern IV) in a patient with hypokalemic PP believed due to SCN4A mutation. (A) CMAPs evoked (5 mV/division) from the ADM during brief pauses (every 1 minute) in a 3-minute exercise with a transient increase in amplitude (17%) and area (81%). (B and C) After exercise, there is a gradual 70% decrease in CMAP amplitude to 70% of postexercise baseline by 30 minutes. (From Logigian EL, Barbano RL. Applied physiology of muscle. In: Disorders of voluntary muscle. 7th Edition. 2001. p. 219–51; with permission. Copyright with Cambridge University Press.)

DM1 patients have a classic pattern of facial weakness, mild ptosis, bulbar weakness, and distal motor (finger flexors/ankle dorsiflexion) weakness with associated clinical and electrical myotonia. Myotonia is typically absent for the first year in infantile onset disease. Myotonia is usually manifest by difficulty relaxing handgrip and with percussion of thenar or finger extensor muscle groups.

DM1 causes significant extramuscular disease, which distinguishes it from NDM. Patients typically develop a combination of early cataracts (before 50 years old), cardiac arrhythmias, psychological dysfunction/cognitive dysfunction, sleep disorders, gastrointestinal irritability, various neoplasms, and glucose intolerance.[27] Disabling myotonia can be treated with sodium channel blockade (eg, mexiletine) and many of the systemic manifestations necessitate referral to other subspecialists.

Myotonic Dystrophy Type 2

DM2, aka proximal myotonic myopathy, is also an autosomal dominant inherited progressive muscular dystrophy due to a CCTG expansion on chromosome 3q.[27] Anticipation is also observed in DM2. In contrast to DM1, patients with DM2 exhibit more prominent proximal hip and shoulder weakness and present later in life (mean age onset fourth/fifth decade).[27] Pain is reported by more than 50% of patients[27] with DM2, and myotonia is less obvious in DM2 than DM1 on clinical and EMG examination.

DM2 is also associated with extramuscular disease. Early development of cataracts, cardiac conduction abnormalities, and endocrine abnormalities are typical. Gastrointestinal and cognitive dysfunctions are atypical in DM2.[27] In contrast to DM1, a congenital form of the disease is not observed in DM2.

Diagnosis of Myotonic Dystrophy

In most patients with DM1 and DM2, the diagnosis is made at the bedside and the EMG laboratory based on the pattern of weakness, presence of myotonia, and extramuscular features. The diagnosis is confirmed with genetic testing that is clinically available and abnormal in 100% of patients with DM1 and 99% of patients with DM2.[29,30]

The role of electrophysiology is to confirm the presence of myotonic discharges that may not be obvious on clinical examination. This is particularly the case for DM2 patients in whom grip and percussion myotonia may be absent or subtle.[31] Differences in muscle histology are described in DM1 and DM2, but muscle biopsy is rarely needed to confirm the diagnosis.

Muscle Biopsy

Similar to other muscular dystrophies, muscle biopsy in DM1 and DM2 typically shows variation in fiber size, rounded atrophic fibers, increased central nuclei, increased connective tissue, and fatty replacement of muscle on H&E and trichrome staining of frozen tissue.[32] Occasional moth-eaten fibers are observed with reduced nicotinamide adenine dinucleotide - tetrazolium reductase (NADH-TR) staining.[32] Nuclear clumps, not typical of other dystrophies, are observed in both types of myotonic dystrophy.[32] DM1 patients generally show preferential atrophy of type 1 fibers, whereas DM2 patients show predominantly type 2 atrophy.[32] The finding of nuclear clumps amidst typical dystrophic histologic changes should prompt workup for DM1 and DM2. The additional presence of selective muscle fiber type atrophy (type 1 fiber atrophy in DM1 and type 2 fiber atrophy in DM2) can potentially help guide the order of genetic testing.

Electrodiagnostic Testing

Widespread electrical myotonia on needle EMG is the electrophysiologic hallmark of myotonic dystrophy, but it is more easily evocable in DM1 than DM2 and tends to be "waxing and waning" in DM1 and "waning" in DM2.[33] Moreover, a subset of patients with DM2 exhibits only subtle "waning" myotonia[31,33]; these waning discharges can easily be misclassified as fibrillation potentials, chronic repetitive discharges, or nonsustained increased insertional activity (see Fig. 3).[31] Electrical myotonia is most prominent in distal limb muscles in both DM1 and DM2. However, myotonia is more prevalent in proximal leg muscles in DM2 than DM1.[33] There is a similar occurrence of thoracic paraspinal myotonia in both conditions.[33] The authors recommend sampling an array of proximal and distal extremity muscles as well as thoracic paraspinal muscles in patients with suspected myotonic dystrophy. The presence of only waning myotonia should prompt genetic testing for DM2 before DM1. Finally, rare patients with DM2 are described without electrical myotonia.[31] Therefore, genetic testing for DM2 may still be indicated in patients with suspicious clinical or histologic features of myotonic dystrophy in the absence of electrical myotonia.

As discussed in the previous section, patients with DM1 and DM2 may show Fournier pattern II on short exercise testing, similar to patients with chloride channel myotonia.[10] Patients exhibiting Fournier pattern II with negative genetic testing for mutations of CLCN1 and SCN4a should have genetic testing for DM1 and DM2.

SUMMARY

Clinical and electrical myotonia is caused by a small group of neuromuscular disorders. Electrodiagnostic testing is used to confirm the presence of myotonia and membership in this group of diseases, to distinguish the specific cause of myotonia, and to guide additional diagnostic testing and treatment.

REFERENCES

1. Selcen D. Myofibrillar myopathies. Neuromuscul Disord 2011;21(3):161–71.
2. Van der Ploeg AT, Reuser AJ. Lysosomal storage disease 2: Pompe's disease. Lancet 2008;372:1342–53.
3. Muller-Felber W, Horvath R, Gempel K, et al. Late onset Pompe disease: clinical and neurophysiological spectrum of 38 patients including long-term follow-up in 18 patients. Neuromuscul Disord 2007;17:698–706.
4. Logigian EL, Barbano RL. Applied physiology of muscle. In: Karpati G, Hilton-Jones D, Griggs RC, editors. Disorders of voluntary muscle. 7th edition. Cambridge (MA): Cambridge University Press; 2001. p. 219–50.
5. Kwon JB, Kleiner A, Ishida K, et al. Hydroxychloroquine-induced myopathy. J Clin Rheumatol 2010;16:28–31.
6. Abdel-Hamid H, Oddis CV, Lacomis D. Severe Hydroxychloroquine myopathy. Muscle Nerve 2008;38:1206–10.
7. Nakahara K, Kuriyama M, Sonoda Y, et al. Myopathy induced by HMG-CoA reductase inhibitors in rabbits: a pathological, electrophysiological, and biochemical study. Toxicol Appl Pharmacol 1998;152:99–106.
8. Rutkove SB, De Girolami U, Preston DC, et al. Myotonia in colchicine myoneuropathy. Muscle Nerve 1996;19:870–5.
9. AANEM. Glossary of terms in electrodiagnostic medicine. Muscle Nerve 2001;(Suppl 10):S1–50.
10. Matthews E, Fialho D, Tan SV, et al. The non-dystrophic myotonias: molecular pathogenesis, diagnosis and treatment. Brain 2010;133:9–22.
11. Venance SL, Cannon SC, Fialho D, et al. The primary periodic paralyses: diagnosis, pathogenesis, and treatment. Brain 2006;129:8–17.
12. Saperstein DS. Muscle channelopathies. Semin Neurol 2008;28(2):260–9.
13. Trip J, Drost G, Giniaar HB, et al. Redefining the clinical phenotypes of non-dystrophic myotonic syndromes. J Neurol Neurosurg Psychiatr 2009;80:647–52.
14. Fournier E, Arzel M, Sternberg D, et al. Electromyography guides toward subgroups of mutations in muscle channelopathies. Ann Neurol 2004;56:650–61.
15. Fournier EM, Viala K, Gervais H, et al. Cold extends electromyography distinction between ion channel mutations causing myotonia. Ann Neurol 2006;60:356–65.
16. Tan SV, Matthews E, Barber M, et al. Refined exercise testing can aid DNA-based diagnosis in muscle channelopathies. Ann Neurol 2011;69:328–40.
17. Cleland J, Logigian EL. Clinical evaluation of membrane excitability in muscle channel disorders: potential applications in clinical trials. Neurotherapeutics 2007;4(2):205–15.
18. Michel P, Sternberg D, Jeannet PY, et al. Comparative efficacy of repetitive nerve stimulation, exercise, and cold in differentiating myotonic disorders. Muscle Nerve 2007;36:643–50.

19. McManis PG, Lambert EH, Daube JR. The exercise test in periodic paralysis. Muscle Nerve 1986;9:704–10.
20. Kuntzer T, Flocard F, Vial C, et al. Exercise test in muscle channelopathies and other muscle disorders. Muscle Nerve 2000;23:1089–94.
21. Elbaz A, Vale-Santos J, Jurkat-Rott K, et al. Hypokalemic periodic paralysis and the dihydropyridine receptor (CACNLIA3): genotype/phenotype correlations for two predominant mutations and evidence for the absence of a founder effect in 16 Caucasian families. Am J Hum Genet 1995;56:374–80.
22. Fouad G, Dalakas M, Servidei S, et al. Genotype-phenotype correlations of DHP receptor alpha 1 subunit gene mutations causing hypokalemic periodic paralysis. Neuromuscul Disord 1997;7:33–8.
23. Miller TM, Dias da Silva MR, Miller HA, et al. Correlating phenotype and genotype in the periodic paralyses. Neurology 2004;63:1647–55.
24. Jongjaroenprasert W, Phusantisampan T, Mahasirimongkol S, et al. A genome-wide association study identifies novel susceptibility genetic variation for thyrotoxic hypokalemic periodic paralysis. J Hum Genet 2012;57:301–4.
25. Comi G, Testa D, Cornelio F, et al. Potassium depletion myopathy: a clinical and morphological study of six cases. Muscle Nerve 1985;8:17–21.
26. Knochel JP. Neuromuscular manifestations of electrolyte disorders. Am J Med 1982;72:521–35.
27. Machuca-Tzili L, Brook D, Hilton-Jones D. Clinical and molecular aspects of the myotonic dystrophies: a review. Muscle Nerve 2005;32:1–18.
28. Logigian EL, Moxley RT, Blood CL, et al. Leukocyte CTG repeat length correlates with severity of myotonia in myotonic dystrophy type 1. Neurology 2004;62: 1081–9.
29. Bird TD. Myotonic dystrophy Type 1. 1999 Sep 17 [updated 2011 Feb 8]. In: Pagon RA, Bird TD, Dolan CR, et al, editors. GeneReviews™ [internet]. Seattle (WA): University of Washington, Seattle; 1993.
30. Dalton JC, Ranum LP, Day JW. Myotonic dystrophy Type 2. 2006 [updated 2007 Apr 23]. In: Pagon RA, Bird TD, Dolan CR, et al, editors. GeneReviews™ [internet]. Seattle (WA): University of Washington, Seattle; 1993.
31. Young NP, Daube JR, Sorenson EJ, et al. Absent, unrecognized, and minimal myotonic discharges in myotonic dystrophy type 2. Muscle Nerve 2010;41: 758–62.
32. Vihola A, Bassez G, Meola G, et al. Histopathological differences of myotonic dystrophy type 1 (DM1) and PROMM/DM2. Neurology 2003;60:1854–7.
33. Logigian EL, Ciafaloni E, Quinn LC, et al. Severity, type, and distribution of myotonic discharges are different in type 1 and type 2 myotonic dystrophy. Muscle Nerve 2007;35:479–85.

Index

Note: Page numbers of article titles are in **boldface** type.

A

ALS. See Amyotrophic lateral sclerosis (ALS)

Amyotrophic lateral sclerosis (ALS)
    clinical features of, 139–141
    electrodiagnosis of, 141–148
        described, 141–144
        MUNE in, 147
        needle EMG in, 145–147
        nerve conduction studies in, 144–145
        TMS in, 147–148

Amyotrophy
    neuralgic
        brachial plexopathy related to, 19

Andersen-Tawil syndrome
    evaluation of, 215

Arm
    lesions in
        radial neuropathy due to, 37

Autoimmune myasthenia gravis (MG)
    EMG findings in, 182–184

Axilla
    lesions in
        radial neuropathy due to, 36–37

Axillary nerve injury
    proximal upper extremity neuropathy related to, 20

Axonal injury
    in peripheral neuropathies
        electrodiagnosis of, 159–160

B

Back pain
    differential diagnosis of, 86–87

Botulism
    EMG findings in, 185–187

Brachial plexopathy(ies), **13–32**
    causes of, 17–19
    clinical presentations of, 21–22
    described, 13–14
    electrodiagnosis of, 22–26
        lateral cord plexopathy, 24–25
        lower trunk plexopathy, 24

Phys Med Rehabil Clin N Am 24 (2013) 221–231
http://dx.doi.org/10.1016/S1047-9651(12)00121-0
1047-9651/13/$ – see front matter © 2013 Elsevier Inc. All rights reserved.

Printed and bound by CPI Group (UK) Ltd, Croydon, CR0 4YY
03/05/2024
01040440-0003

Moving?

Make sure your subscription moves with you!

To notify us of your new address, find your **Clinics Account Number** (located on your mailing label above your name), and contact customer service at:

Email: journalscustomerservice-usa@elsevier.com

800-654-2452 (subscribers in the U.S. & Canada)
314-447-8871 (subscribers outside of the U.S. & Canada)

Fax number: 314-447-8029

Elsevier Health Sciences Division
Subscription Customer Service
3251 Riverport Lane
Maryland Heights, MO 63043

*To ensure uninterrupted delivery of your subscription, please notify us at least 4 weeks in advance of move.

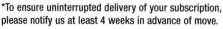